国家卫生和计划生育委员会"十三五"英文版规划教材
全国高等学校教材

供临床医学专业及来华留学生（MBBS）双语教学用

Medical Genetics

U0208286

医学遗传学 改编教学版
Annotated Edition

Lynn B. Jorde　　John C. Carey　　Michael J. Bamshad

主　编　傅松滨
Chief Editor　Songbin Fu

副主编　申本昌　　　　　马长艳
Vice Chief Editor　Benchang Shen　Changyan Ma

编　委（以姓氏笔画为序）

马长艳　　南京医科大学
Changyan Ma　Nanjing Medical University

申本昌　　广州医科大学
Benchang Shen　Guangzhou Medical University

史岸冰　　华中科技大学
Anbing Shi　Huazhong University of Science and Technology

李　枫　　武汉大学
Feng Li　Wuhan University

李　莉　　山西医科大学
Li Li　Shanxi Medical University

吴　丹　　北京大学
Dan Wu　Peking University

何永蜀　　昆明医科大学
Yongshu He　Kunming Medical University

沙　莎　　西藏民族大学
Sha Sha　Xizang Minzu University

张金波　　佳木斯大学
Jinbo Zhang　Jiamusi University

崔晓波　　哈尔滨医科大学
Xiaobo Cui　Harbin Medical University

彭翠英　　南华大学
Cuiying Peng　University of South China

彭鲁英　　同济大学
Luying Peng　Tongji University

傅松滨　　哈尔滨医科大学
Songbin Fu　Harbin Medical University

人民卫生出版社

图书在版编目（CIP）数据

医学遗传学：英文 /（美）林恩·乔德（Lynn B. Jorde）著；傅松滨
主编. —北京：人民卫生出版社，2016
全国高等学校临床医学专业第一轮英文版规划教材
ISBN 978-7-117-23822-9

Ⅰ. ①医…　Ⅱ. ①林…②傅…　Ⅲ. ①医学遗传学－医学院
校－教材－英文　Ⅳ. ①R394

中国版本图书馆 CIP 数据核字（2016）第 293975 号

人卫智网	www.ipmph.com	医学教育、学术、考试、健康，
		购书智慧智能综合服务平台
人卫官网	www.pmph.com	人卫官方资讯发布平台

医学遗传学

主　　编：傅松滨
出版发行：人民卫生出版社（中继线 010-59780011）
地　　址：北京市朝阳区潘家园南里 19 号
邮　　编：100021
E - mail：pmph @ pmph.com
购书热线：010-59787592　010-59787584　010-65264830
印　　刷：北京人卫印刷厂
经　　销：新华书店
开　　本：850×1168　1/16　印张：22
字　　数：650 千字
版　　次：2017 年 2 月第 1 版　2017 年 2 月第 1 版第 1 次印刷
标准书号：ISBN 978-7-117-23822-9/R · 23823
定　　价：118.00 元

ELSEVIER

Elsevier (Singapore) Pte Ltd.

3 Killiney Road

#08-01 Winsland House I

Singapore 239519

Tel: (65) 6349-0200

Fax: (65) 6733-1817

MEDICAL GENETICS, 5/E

Lynn B. Jorde, John C. Carey, Michael J. Bamshad

Copyright 2016 by Elsevier, Inc. All rights reserved.

Copyright © 2010, 2006, 2003, 2000, 1995 by Mosby, Inc., an affiliate of Elsevier Inc. All rights reserved.

ISBN-13: 978-0-323-18835-7

Printed in China by People's Medical Publishing House Co., Ltd under special arrangement with Elsevier (Singapore) Pte Ltd. This edition is authorized for sale in the People's Republic of China only, excluding Hong Kong SAR, Macau SAR and Taiwan. Unauthorized export of this edition is a violation of the contract.

图字号：01-2017-0413

1995 年，我国首次招收全英文授课医学留学生，到 2015 年，接收临床医学专业 MBBS（Bachelor of Medicine & Bachelor of Surgery）留学生的院校达到了 40 余家，MBBS 院校数量、规模不断扩张；同时，医学院校在临床医学专业五年制、长学制教学中陆续开展不同规模和范围的双语或全英文授课，使得对一套符合我国教学实际、成体系、高质量英文教材的需求日益增长。

为了满足教学需求，进一步落实教育部《关于加强高等学校本科教学工作提高教学质量的若干意见（教高 [2001]4 号）》和《来华留学生医学本科教育（英文授课）质量控制标准暂行规定（教外来 [2007]39 号）》等相关文件的要求，规范和提高我国高等医学院校临床医学专业五年制、长学制和来华留学生（MBBS）双语教学及全英文教学的质量，推进医学双语教学和留学生教育的健康有序发展，完善和规范临床医学专业英文版教材的体系，人民卫生出版社在充分调研的基础上，于 2015 年召开了全国高等学校临床医学专业英文版规划教材的编写论证会，经过会上及会后的反复论证，最终确定组织编写一套全国规划的、适合我国高等医学院校教学实际的临床医学专业英文版教材，并计划作为 2017 年春季和秋季教材在全国出版发行。

本套英文版教材的编写结合国家卫生和计划生育委员会、教育部的总体要求，坚持"三基、五性、三特定"的原则，组织全国各大医学院校、教学医院的专家编写，主要特点如下：

1. 教材编写应教学之需启动，在全国范围进行了广泛、深入调研和论证，借鉴国内外医学人才培养模式和教材建设经验，对主要读者对象、编写模式、编写科目、编者遴选条件等进行了科学设计。

2. 坚持"三基、五性、三特定"和"多级论证"的教材编写原则，组织全国各大医学院校及教学医院有丰富英语教学经验的专家一起编写，以保证高质量出版。

3. 为保证英语表达的准确性和规范性，大部分教材以国外英文原版教科书为蓝本，根据我国教学大纲和人民卫生出版社临床医学专业第八轮规划教材主要内容进行改编，充分体现科学性、权威性、适用性和实用性。

4. 教材内部各环节合理设置，根据读者对象的特点，在英文原版教材的基础上结合需要，增加本章小结、关键术语（英中对照）、思考题、推荐阅读等模块，促进学生自主学习。

本套临床医学专业英文版规划教材共 38 种，均为国家卫生和计划生育委员会"十三五"规划教材，计划于 2017 年全部出版发行。

In 1995, China recruited overseas medical students of full English teaching for the first time. Up to 2015, more than 40 institutions enrolled overseas MBBS (Bachelor of Medicine & Bachelor of Surgery) students. The number of MBBS institutions and overseas students are continuously increasing. At the meantime, medical colleges' application for bilingual or full English teaching in different size and range in five-year and long-term professional clinical medicine teaching results to increasingly demand for a set of practical, systematic and high-qualified English teaching material.

In order to meet the teaching needs and to implement the regulations of relevant documents issued by Ministry of Education including "Some Suggestions to Strengthen the Undergraduate Teaching and to Improve the Teaching Quality" and "Interim Provisions on Quality Control Standards of International Medical Undergraduate Education (English teaching)", as well as to standardize and improve the quality of the bilingual teaching and English teaching of the five-year, long-term and international students (MBBS) of clinical medicine in China's higher medical colleges so as to promote the healthy and orderly development of medical bilingual teaching and international students education and to improve and standardize the system of English clinical medicine textbooks, after full investigation, People's Medical Publishing House (PMPH) held the writing discussion meeting of English textbook for clinical medicine department of national colleges and universities in 2015. After the repeated demonstration in and after the meeting, PMPH ultimately determined to organize the compilation of a set of national planning English textbooks which are suitable for China's actual clinical medicine teaching of medical colleges and universities. This set will be published as spring and autumn textbooks of 2017.

This set of English textbooks meets the overall requirements of the Ministry of Education and National Health and Family Planning Commission, the editorial committee includes the experts from major medical colleges and universities as well as teaching hospitals, the main features are as follows:

1. Textbooks compilation is started to meet the teaching needs, extensive and deep research and demonstration are conducted across the country, the main target readers, the model and subject of compilation and selection conditions of authors are scientifically designed in accordance with the reference of domestic and foreign medical personnel training model and experience in teaching materials.

2. Adhere to the teaching materials compiling principles of "three foundations, five characteristics, and three specialties" and "multi-level demonstration", the organization of English teaching experts with rich experience from major medical schools and teaching hospitals ensures the high quality of publication.

3. In order to ensure the accuracy and standardization of English expression, most of the textbooks are modeled on original English textbooks, and adapted based on national syllabus and main content of the eighth round of clinical medicine textbooks which were published by PMPH, fully reflecting the scientificity, authority, applicability and practicality.

4. All aspects of teaching materials are arranged reasonably, based on original textbooks, the chapter summary, key terms (English and Chinese), review questions, and recommended readings are added to promote students' independent learning in accordance with teaching needs and the characteristics of the target readers.

This set of English textbooks for clinical medicine includes 38 species which are among "13th Five-Year" planning textbooks of National Health and Family Planning Commission, and will be all published in 2017.

全国高等学校临床医学专业第一轮英文版规划教材 · 教材目录

	教材名称		主 审	主编
1	人体解剖学	Human Anatomy		刘学政
2	生理学	Physiology		闫剑群
3	医学免疫学	Medical Immunology		储以微
4	生物化学	Biochemistry		张晓伟
5	组织学与胚胎学	Histology and Embryology		李 和
6	医学微生物学	Medical Microbiology		郭晓奎
7	病理学	Pathology		陈 杰
8	医学分子生物学	Medical Molecular Biology		吕社民
9	医学遗传学	Medical Genetics		傅松滨
10	医学细胞生物学	Medical Cell Biology		刘 佳
11	病理生理学	Pathophysiology		王建枝
12	药理学	Pharmacology		杨宝峰
13	临床药理学	Clinical Pharmacology		李 俊
14	人体寄生虫学	Human Parasitology		李学荣
15	流行病学	Epidemiology		沈洪兵
16	医学统计学	Medical Statistics		郝元涛
17	核医学	Nuclear Medicine		黄 钢 李 方
18	医学影像学	Medical Imaging		申宝忠 龚启勇
19	临床诊断学	Clinical Diagnostics		万学红
20	实验诊断学	Laboratory Diagnostics		胡翊群 王 琳
21	内科学	Internal Medicine		文富强 汪道文
22	外科学	Surgery		陈孝平 田 伟
23	妇产科学	Obstetrics and Gynaecology	郎景和	狄 文 曹云霞
24	儿科学	Pediatrics		黄国英 罗小平
25	神经病学	Neurology		张黎明
26	精神病学	Psychiatry		赵靖平
27	传染病学	Infectious Diseases		高志良 任 红

PREFACE

I wish to express our sincere gratitude to Professors Lynn B. Jorde, PhD (University of Utah Health Sciences Center), John P. Carey, MD, MPH (University of Utah Health Sciences Center) and Michael J. Bamshad, MD (University of Washington School of Medicine) for their contributions to this book, which reflect the accumulation of their wisdom and knowledge. This textbook has been well accepted by students for its thorough explanation of key principles of medical genetics integrated with clinical practice, as well as its clear visual layout, which aids in the learning process. We appreciate the endowment from the People's Medical Publishing House, which is responsible for the reorganization of this textbook, and the understanding and support of the Elsevier publishing company in publishing a rearranged version of this book in China.

The rapid development of medical genetics calls for new textbooks to update knowledge of the field for graduate students in China. For this purpose, we reorganized *Medical Genetics*, 5th edition, according to the education protocol in China. The contents of the new edition will be arranged in the following order: background and history; basic cell biology: structure and function of genes and chromosomes; genetic variation: its origin and detection; autosomal dominant and recessive inheritance, sex-linked and nontraditional modes of inheritance, and mitochondrial disorders; multifactorial inheritance and common diseases; clinical cytogenetics: the chromosomal basis of human disease; biochemical genetics: disorders of metabolism; cancer genetics; immunogenetics; genetic testing and gene therapy; genetics and personalized medicine; clinical genetics and genetic counseling.

I would like to acknowledge all of my colleagues for their generous contributions of time and work. Their endeavors and professionalism guarantee the success of the rearranged edition.

I anticipate that this rearranged version will help graduate students in China better understand the principles and concepts of medical genetics.

Songbin Fu
Harbin, China

CONTENTS

Chapter 1

Background and History

Genetics is playing an increasingly important role in the practice of clinical medicine. Medical genetics, once largely confined to relatively rare conditions seen by only a few specialists, is now becoming a central component of our understanding of most major diseases. These include not only the pediatric diseases but also common adult diseases such as heart disease, diabetes, many cancers, and many psychiatric disorders. Because all components of the human body are influenced by genes, genetic disease is relevant to all medical specialties. Today's health-care practitioners must understand the science of medical genetics.

WHAT IS MEDICAL GENETICS?

Medical genetics involves any application of genetics to medical practice. It thus includes studies of the inheritance of diseases in families, mapping of disease genes to specific locations on chromosomes, analyses of the molecular mechanisms through which genes cause disease, and the diagnosis and treatment of genetic disease. As a result of rapid progress in molecular genetics, DNA-based diagnosis is available for hundreds of inherited conditions, and gene therapy—the insertion of normal genes into patients in order to correct genetic disease—is showing promise for some conditions. Medical genetics also includes genetic counseling, in which information regarding risks, prognoses, and treatments is communicated to patients and their families.

WHY IS A KNOWLEDGE OF MEDICAL GENETICS IMPORTANT FOR TODAY'S HEALTH-CARE PRACTITIONER?

There are several reasons health-care practitioners must understand medical genetics. Genetic diseases make up a large percentage of the total disease burden in pediatric and adult populations (Table 1-1). This percentage will continue to grow as our understanding of the genetic basis of disease grows. In addition, modern medicine is placing increasing emphasis on prevention. Because genetics provides a basis for understanding the fundamental biological makeup of the organism, it naturally leads to a better understanding of the disease process. In some cases, this knowledge can lead to prevention of the disorder. It also leads to more effective disease treatment. Prevention and effective treatment are among the highest goals of medicine. The chapters that follow provide many examples of the ways genetics contributes to these goals. But first, this chapter reviews the foundations upon which current practice is built.

A BRIEF HISTORY

The inheritance of physical traits has been a subject of curiosity and interest for thousands of years. The ancient Hebrews and Greeks, as well as later medieval scholars, described many genetic phenomena and proposed theories to account for them. Many of these theories were incorrect. Gregor Mendel (Fig. 1-1), an Austrian monk who is usually considered the father of genetics, advanced the field significantly by performing a series of cleverly designed experiments on living organisms (garden peas). He then used this experimental information to formulate a series of fundamental principles of heredity.

Mendel published the results of his experiments in 1865 in a relatively obscure journal. It is one of the ironies of biological science that his discoveries,

TABLE 1-1   A Partial List of Some Important Genetic Diseases

DISEASE	APPROXIMATE PREVALENCE
Chromosome Abnormalities	
Down syndrome	1/700 to 1/1000
Klinefelter syndrome	1/1000 males
Trisomy 13	1/10,000
Trisomy 18	1/6000
Turner syndrome	1/2500 to 1/10,000 females
Single-Gene Disorders	
Adenomatous polyposis coli	1/6000
Adult polycystic kidney disease	1/1000
α_1-Antitrypsin deficiency	1/2500 to 1/10,000 (whites)[*]
Cystic fibrosis	1/2000 to 1/4000 (whites)
Duchenne muscular dystrophy	1/3500 males
Familial hypercholesterolemia	1/500
Fragile X syndrome	1/4000 males; 1/8000 females
Hemochromatosis (hereditary)	1/300 whites are homozygotes; approximately 1/1000 to 1/2000 are affected
Hemophilia A	1/5000 to 1/10,000 males
Hereditary nonpolyposis colorectal cancer	Up to 1/200
Huntington disease	1/20,000 (whites)
Marfan syndrome	1/10,000 to 1/20,000
Myotonic dystrophy	1/7000 to 1/20,000 (whites)
Neurofibromatosis type 1	1/3000 to 1/5000
Osteogenesis imperfecta	1/5000 to 1/10,000
Phenylketonuria	1/10,000 to 1/15,000 (whites)
Retinoblastoma	1/20,000
Sickle cell disease	1/400 to 1/600 blacks[*] in America; up to 1/50 in central Africa
Tay-Sachs disease	1/3000 Ashkenazi Jews
Thalassemia	1/50 to 1/100 (South Asian and circum-Mediterranean populations)
Multifactorial Disorders	
Congenital Malformations	
Cleft lip with or without cleft palate	1/500 to 1/1000
Club foot (talipes equinovarus)	1/1000
Congenital heart defects	1/200 to 1/500
Neural tube defects (spina bifida, anencephaly)	1/200 to 1/1000
Pyloric stenosis	1/300
Adult Diseases	
Alcoholism	1/10 to 1/20
Alzheimer disease	1/10 (Americans older than 65 years)
Bipolar disorder	1/100 to 1/200
Cancer (all types)	1/3
Diabetes (types 1 and 2)	1/10
Heart disease or stroke	1/3 to 1/5
Schizophrenia	1/100
Mitochondrial Diseases	
Kaerns-Sayre syndrome	Rare
Leber hereditary optic neuropathy (LHON)	Rare
Mitochondrial encephalopathy, lactic acidosis, and stroke-like episodes (MELAS)	Rare
Myoclonic epilepsy and ragged red fiber disease (MERRF)	Rare

[*]The term "white" refers to individuals of predominantly European descent; the term "black" refers to individuals of predominantly sub-Saharan African descent. These terms are used for convenience; some of the challenges in accurately describing human populations are discussed in Chapter 11.

which still form the foundation of genetics, received little recognition for 35 years. At about the same time, Charles Darwin formulated his theories of evolution, and Darwin's cousin, Francis Galton, performed an extensive series of family studies (concentrating especially on twins) in an effort to understand the influence of heredity on various human traits. Neither scientist was aware of Mendel's work.

FIG 1-1 Gregor Johann Mendel. (From Raven PH, Johnson GB. *Biology*. 3rd ed. St Louis: Mosby; 1992.)

Genetics as it is known today is largely the result of research performed during the 20th century. Mendel's principles were independently rediscovered in 1900 by three different scientists working in three different countries. This was also the year in which Landsteiner discovered the ABO blood group system. In 1902, Archibald Garrod described alkaptonuria as the first "inborn error of metabolism." In 1909, Johannsen coined the term **gene** to denote the basic unit of heredity.

The next several decades were a period of considerable experimental and theoretical work. Several organisms, including *Drosophila melanogaster* (fruit flies) and *Neurospora crassa* (bread mold) served as useful experimental systems in which to study the actions and interactions of genes. For example, H. J. Muller demonstrated the genetic consequences of ionizing radiation in the fruit fly. During this period, much of the theoretical basis of population genetics was developed by three central figures: Ronald Fisher, J. B. S. Haldane, and Sewall Wright. In addition, the modes of inheritance of several important genetic

diseases, including phenylketonuria, sickle cell disease, Huntington disease, and cystic fibrosis, were established. In 1944, Oswald Avery showed that genes are composed of **deoxyribonucleic acid** (**DNA**).

Probably the most significant achievement of the 1950s was the specification of the physical structure of DNA by James Watson and Francis Crick in 1953. Their seminal paper, which was only one page long, formed the basis for what is now known as **molecular genetics** (the study of the structure and function of genes at the molecular level). Another significant accomplishment in that decade was the correct specification of the number of human chromosomes. Since the early 1920s, it had been thought that humans had 48 chromosomes in each cell. Only in 1956 was the correct number, 46, finally determined. The ability to count and identify chromosomes led to a flurry of new findings in cytogenetics, including the discovery in 1959 that Down syndrome is caused by an extra copy of chromosome 21.

Technological developments since 1960 have brought about significant achievements at an ever-increasing rate. The most spectacular advances have occurred in the field of molecular genetics. Thousands of genes have been mapped to specific chromosome locations. The Human Genome Project, a large collaborative venture begun in 1990, provided the complete human DNA sequence in 2003 (the term **genome** refers to all of the DNA in an organism). Important developments in computer technology have helped to decipher the barrage of data being generated by this and related projects. In addition to mapping genes, molecular geneticists have pinpointed the molecular defects underlying a number of important genetic diseases. This research has contributed greatly to our understanding of the ways gene defects can cause disease, opening paths to more effective treatment and potential cures.

TYPES OF GENETIC DISEASES

Humans are estimated to have approximately 20,000 to 25,000 genes. Alterations in these genes, or in combinations of them, can produce genetic disorders. These disorders are classified into several major groups:

- **Chromosome disorders**, in which entire chromosomes (or large segments of them) are missing, duplicated, or otherwise altered. These disorders include diseases such as Down syndrome and Turner syndrome.
- Disorders in which single genes are altered; these are often termed *mendelian conditions*, or **single-gene disorders**. Well-known examples include cystic fibrosis, sickle cell disease, and hemophilia.
- **Multifactorial disorders**, which result from a combination of multiple genetic and environmental causes. Many birth defects, such as cleft lip and cleft palate, as well as many adult disorders, including heart disease and diabetes, belong in this category.
- **Mitochondrial disorders**, a relatively small number of diseases caused by alterations in the small cytoplasmic mitochondrial chromosome.

Table 1-1 provides some examples of each of these types of diseases.

Of these major classes of diseases, the single-gene disorders have probably received the greatest amount of attention. These disorders are classified according to the way they are inherited in families: autosomal dominant, autosomal recessive, or X-linked. These modes of inheritance are discussed extensively in Chapters 4 and 5. The first edition of McKusick's *Mendelian Inheritance in Man*, published in 1966, listed only 1368 autosomal traits and 119 X-linked traits. Today, the online version of McKusick's compendium lists nearly 23,000 genes and traits, of which nearly 21,000 are autosomal, more than 1200 are X-linked, 59 are Y-linked, and 65 are in the mitochondrial genome. DNA variants responsible for more than 4000 of these traits, most of which are

inherited diseases, have been identified. With continued advances, these numbers are certain to increase.

Although some genetic disorders, particularly the single-gene conditions, are strongly determined by genes, many others are the result of multiple genetic and nongenetic factors. One can therefore think of genetic diseases as lying along a continuum (Fig. 1-2), with disorders such as cystic fibrosis and Duchenne muscular dystrophy situated at one end (strongly determined by genes) and conditions such as measles situated at the other end (strongly determined by environment). Many of the most prevalent disorders, including many birth defects and many common diseases such as diabetes, hypertension, heart disease, and cancer, lie somewhere in the middle of the continuum. These diseases are the products of varying degrees of genetic and environmental influences.

THE CLINICAL IMPACT OF GENETIC DISEASE

Less than a century ago, diseases of largely nongenetic causation (i.e., those caused by malnutrition, unsanitary conditions, and pathogens) accounted for the great majority of deaths in children. During the 20th century, however, public health vastly improved. As a result, genetic diseases have come to account for an ever- increasing percentage of deaths among children in developed countries. For example, the percentage of pediatric deaths due to genetic causes in various hospitals in the United Kingdom increased from 16.5% in 1914 to 50% in 1976 (Table 1-2).

In addition to contributing to a large fraction of childhood deaths, genetic diseases also account for a large share of admissions to pediatric hospitals. For example, a survey of Seattle hospitals showed that 27% of all pediatric inpatients presented with

FIG 1-2 Continuum of disease causation. Some disease (e.g., cystic fibrosis) are strongly determined by genes, whereas others (e.g., infectious diseases) are strongly determined by environment.

TABLE 1-2 Percentages of Childhood Deaths in United Kingdom Hospitals Attributable to Nongenetic and Genetic Causes

CAUSE	LONDON 1914	LONDON 1954	NEWCASTLE 1966	EDINBURGH 1976
Nongenetic*				
All causes	83.5	62.5	58.0	50.0
Genetic				
Single gene	2.0	12.0	8.5	8.9
Chromosomal	—	—	2.5	2.9
Multifactorial	14.5	25.5	31.0	38.2

Data from Rimoin DL, Connor JM, Pyeritz RE, Korf BR. *Emery and Rimoin's Principles and Practice of Medical Genetics.* London: Churchill Livingstone; 2007.
*Infections, for example.

a genetic disorder, and a survey of admissions to a major pediatric hospital in Mexico showed that 37.8% involved a disease that was either genetic or "partly genetic." It is estimated that mendelian diseases alone account for ≈20% of infant mortality and ≈10% of pediatric hospitalizations.

Another way to assess the importance of genetic diseases is to ask, "What fraction of persons in the population will be found to have a genetic disorder?" This is not as simple a question as it might seem. A variety of factors can influence the answer. For example, some diseases are found more frequently in certain ethnic groups. Cystic fibrosis is especially common among whites, whereas sickle cell disease is especially common among Africans. Some diseases are more common in older persons. For example, colon cancer, breast cancer, and Alzheimer disease are caused by dominant genes in a small fraction (5%-10%) of cases but are not usually manifested until later in life. The prevalence estimates for these genetic diseases would be higher in an older population. Variations in diagnostic and recording practices can also cause prevalence estimates to vary. Accord-

ingly, the prevalence figures shown in Table 1-3 are given as rather broad ranges. Keeping these sources of variation in mind, it is notable that a recognizable genetic disease will be diagnosed in 3% to 7% of the population at some point. This tabulation does not include most cases of the more common adult diseases, such as heart disease, diabetes, and cancer, although it is known that these diseases also have genetic components. If such diseases are included, the clinical impact of genetic disease is considerable indeed.

TABLE 1-3 Approximate Prevalence of Genetic Disease in the General Population

TYPE OF GENETIC DISEASE	LIFETIME PREVALENCE PER 1000 PERSONS
Autosomal dominant	3-9.5
Autosomal recessive	2-2.5
X-linked	0.5-2
Chromosome disorder	6-9
Congenital malformation*	20-50
Total	31.5-73

*Congenital means "present at birth." Most congenital malformations are thought to be multifactorial and therefore probably have both genetic and environmental components.

SUGGESTED READINGS AND WEBSITES

1. Baird PA, Anderson TW, Newcombe HB, Lowry RB. Genetic disorders in children and young adults: a population study. *Am J Hum Genet.* 1988; 42: 677-693.

2. Bell CJ, Dinwiddie DL, Miller NA, et al. Carrier testing for severe childhood recessive diseases by next-generation sequencing. *Sci Transl Med.* 2011; 3(65): 65ra4.

3. Dunn LC. *A Short History of Genetics.* New York: McGraw-Hill; 1965.

4. McKusick VA. History of medical genetics. In: Rimoin DL, Connor JM, Pyeritz RE, Korf BR, eds. *Emery and Rimoin's Principles and Practice of Medical Genetics.* vol. 1. 5th ed. London: Churchill Livingstone; 2007: 3-32.

5. Passarge E. *Color Atlas of Genetics*. 3rd ed. Stuttgart: Georg Thieme Verlag; 2007.

6. Rimoin DL, Connor JM, Pyeritz RE, Korf BR. *Emery and Rimoin's Principles and Practice of Medical Genetics*. 5th ed. London: Churchill Livingstone; 2007.

7. Scriver CR, Sly WS, Childs G, et al. *The Metabolic and Molecular Bases of Inherited Disease*. 8th ed. New York: McGraw-Hill; 2001.

8. Seashore MS, Wappner RS. *Genetics in Primary Care and Clinical Medicine*. Stamford, CT: Appleton & Lange, 1996.

9. Watson JD, Crick FHC. Molecular structure of nucleic acids: A structure for deoxyribose nucleic acid. *Nature*. 1953; 171: 737.

10. Dolan DNA Learning Center, Cold Spring Harbor Laboratory (a useful online resource for learning and reviewing basic principles): http://www.dnalc.org/

11. Genetic Science Learning Center (another useful resource for learning and reviewing basic genetic principles): http://gslc.genetics.utah.edu/

12. Landmarks in the History of Genetics: http://cogweb.ucla.edu/EP/DNA_history.html

13. National Human Genome Research Institute Educational Resources: http://www.genome.gov/Education

14. Online Mendelian Inheritance in Man (OMIM) (a comprehensive catalog and description of single-gene conditions): http://www.ncbi.nlm.nih.gov/Omim/

15. University of Kansas Medical Center Genetics Education Center (a large number of links to useful genetics education sites): http://www.kumc.edu/gec/

(Songbin Fu)

Chapter 2

Basic Cell Biology: Structure and Function of Genes and Chromosomes

All genetic diseases involve defects at the level of the cell. For this reason, one must understand basic cell biology to understand genetic disease. Errors can occur in the replication of genetic material or in the translation of genes into proteins. Such errors commonly produce single-gene disorders. In addition, errors that occur during cell division can lead to disorders involving entire chromosomes. To provide the basis for understanding these errors and their consequences, this chapter focuses on the processes through which genes are replicated and translated into proteins, as well as the process of cell division.

In the 19th century, microscopic studies of cells led scientists to suspect that the nucleus of the cell (Fig. 2-1) contains the important mechanisms of inheritance. They found that **chromatin**, the substance that gives the nucleus a granular appearance, is observable in the nuclei of nondividing cells. Just before a cell undergoes division, the chromatin condenses to form microscopically observable, thread-like structures called **chromosomes** (from the Greek words for "colored bodies"). With the rediscovery of Mendel's breeding experiments at the beginning of the 20th century, it soon became apparent that chromosomes contain **genes**. Genes are transmitted from parent to offspring and are considered the basic

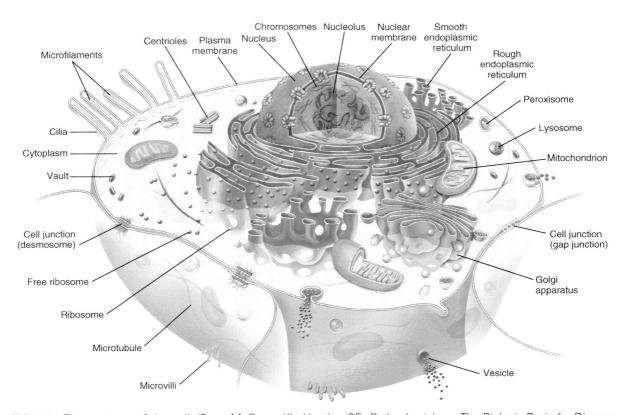

FIG 2-1   The anatomy of the cell. (From McCance KL, Huether SE. *Pathophysiology: The Biologic Basis for Disease in Adults and Children.* 7th ed. St. Louis: Elsevier Mosby; 2014.)

unit of inheritance. It is through the transmission of genes that physical traits such as eye color are inherited in families. Diseases can also be transmitted through genetic inheritance.

Physically, genes are composed of **deoxyribonucleic acid** (**DNA**). DNA provides the genetic blueprint for all proteins in the body. Thus, genes ultimately influence all aspects of body structure and function. Humans are estimated to have 20,000 to 25,000 genes (sequences of DNA that code for ribonucleic acid [RNA] or proteins). An error (or **mutation**) in one of these genes often leads to a recognizable genetic disease.

> Genes, the basic unit of inheritance, are contained in chromosomes and consist of DNA.

Each human **somatic cell** (cells other than the **gametes**, or sperm and egg cells) contains 23 pairs of different chromosomes, for a total of 46. One member of each pair is derived from the individual's father, and the other member is derived from the mother. One of the chromosome pairs consists of the **sex chromosomes**. In normal males, the sex chromosomes are a Y chromosome inherited from the father and an X chromosome inherited from the mother. Two X chromosomes are found in normal females, one inherited from each parent. The other 22 pairs of chromosomes are **autosomes**. The members of each pair of autosomes are said to be **homologs**, or **homologous**, because their DNA is very similar. The X and Y chromosomes are not homologs of each other.

Somatic cells, having two of each chromosome, are **diploid** cells. Human gametes have the **haploid** number of chromosomes, 23. The diploid number of chromosomes is maintained in successive generations of somatic cells by the process of **mitosis**, whereas the haploid number is obtained through the process of **meiosis**. Both of these processes are discussed in detail later in this chapter.

> Somatic cells are diploid, having 23 pairs of chromosomes (22 pairs of autosomes and one pair of sex chromosomes). Gametes are haploid and have a total of 23 chromosomes.

DNA, RNA, AND PROTEINS: HEREDITY AT THE MOLECULAR LEVEL

DNA

Composition and Structure of DNA

The DNA molecule has three basic components: the pentose sugar, deoxyribose; a phosphate group; and four types of nitrogenous **bases** (so named because they can combine with hydrogen ions in acidic solutions). Two of the bases, **cytosine** and **thymine**, are single carbon-nitrogen rings called **pyrimidines**. The other two bases, **adenine** and **guanine**, are double carbon-nitrogen rings called **purines** (Fig. 2-2). The four bases are commonly represented by their first letters: C, T, A, and G.

FIG 2-2   Chemical structure of the four bases, which shows hydrogen bonds between base pairs. Three hydrogen bonds are formed between cytosine-guanine pairs, and two bonds are formed between adenine-thymine pairs.

One of the contributions of Watson and Crick in the mid-20th century was to demonstrate how these three components are physically assembled to form DNA. They proposed the now-famous **double helix** model, in which DNA can be envisioned as a twisted ladder with chemical bonds as its rungs (Fig. 2-3). The two sides of the ladder are composed of the sugar and phosphate components, held together by strong phosphodiester bonds. Projecting from each side of the ladder, at regular intervals, are the nitrogenous bases. The base projecting from one side is bound to the base projecting from the other side by relatively weak hydrogen bonds. The paired nitrogenous bases therefore form the rungs of the ladder.

FIG 2-3 The DNA double helix, with sugar-phosphate backbone and nitrogenous bases.

Figure 2-2 illustrates the chemical bonds between bases and shows that the ends of the ladder terminate in either 3′ or 5′. These labels are derived from the order in which the five carbon atoms composing deoxyribose are numbered. Each DNA subunit, con-

sisting of one deoxyribose, one phosphate group, and one base, is called a **nucleotide**.

Different sequences of nucleotide bases (e.g., ACCAAGTGC) specify different proteins. Specification of the body's many proteins must require a great deal of genetic information. Indeed, each haploid human cell contains approximately 3 billion nucleotide pairs, more than enough information to specify the composition of all human proteins.

> The most important constituents of DNA are the four nucleotide bases: adenine, thymine, cytosine, and guanine. DNA has a double helix structure.

DNA Coiling

Textbook illustrations usually depict DNA as a double helix molecule that continues in a long, straight line. However, if the DNA in a cell were actually stretched out in this way, it would be about 2 meters long. To package all of this DNA into a tiny cell nucleus, it is coiled at several levels. First, the DNA is wound around a **histone** protein core to form a **nucleosome** (Fig. 2-4). About 140 to 150 DNA bases are wound around each histone core, and then 20 to 60 bases form a spacer element before the next nucleosome complex. The nucleosomes in turn form a helical **solenoid**; each turn of the solenoid includes about six nucleosomes. The solenoids themselves are organized into **chromatin loops**, which are attached to a protein scaffold. Each of these loops contains approximately 100,000 base pairs (bp), or 100 **kilobases (kb)**, of DNA. The end result of this coiling and looping is that the DNA, at its maximum stage of condensation, is only about 1/10,000 as long as it would be if it were fully stretched out.

> DNA is a tightly coiled structure. This coiling occurs at several levels: the nucleosome, the solenoid, and 100-kb loops.

Replication of DNA

As cells divide to make copies of themselves, identical copies of DNA must be made and incorporated into the new cells. This is essential if DNA is to serve as the fundamental genetic material. DNA **replica-**

DNA double helix

Histone

DNA

Nucleosomes

200 bp of DNA

Solenoid

Chromatin

Chromatin loop contains approximately 100,000 bp of DNA

Chromatid

FIG 2-4 Patterns of DNA coiling. DNA is wound around histones to form nucleosomes. These are organized into solenoids, which in turn make up the chromatin loops.

tion begins as the weak hydrogen bonds between bases break, producing single DNA strands with unpaired bases. The consistent pairing of adenine with thymine and guanine with cytosine, known as **complementary base pairing**, is the key to accurate replication. The principle of complementary base pairing dictates that the unpaired base will attract a free nucleotide only if that nucleotide has the proper complementary base. For example, a portion of a single strand with the base sequence ATTGCT will bond with a series of free nucleotides with the bases TAACGA. The single strand is said to be a **template** upon which the complementary strand is built. When replication is complete, a new double-stranded molecule identical to the original is formed (Fig. 2-5).

Several different enzymes are involved in DNA replication. One enzyme unwinds the double helix, and another holds the strands apart. Still another

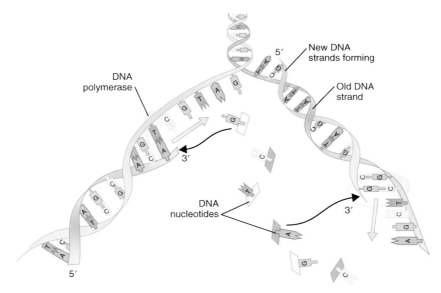

FIG 2-5   DNA replication. The hydrogen bonds between the two original strands are broken, allowing the bases in each strand to undergo complementary base pairing with free bases. This process, which proceeds in the 5′ to 3′ direction on each strand, forms two new double strands of DNA.

enzyme, **DNA polymerase**, travels along the single DNA strand, adding free nucleotides to the 3′ end of the new strand. Nucleotides can be added only to the 3′ end of the strand, so replication always proceeds from the 5′ to the 3′ end. When referring to the orientation of sequences along a gene, the 5′ direction is termed **upstream**, and the 3′ direction is termed **downstream**.

In addition to adding new nucleotides, DNA polymerase performs part of a **proofreading** procedure, in which a newly added nucleotide is checked to make certain that it is in fact complementary to the template base. If it is not, the nucleotide is excised and replaced with a correct complementary nucleotide base. This process substantially enhances the accuracy of DNA replication. When a DNA replication error is not successfully repaired, a mutation has occurred. As will be seen in Chapter 3, many such mutations cause genetic diseases.

 DNA replication is critically dependent on the principle of complementary base pairing (A with T; C with G). This allows a single strand of the double-stranded DNA molecule to form a template for the synthesis of a new, complementary strand.

The rate of DNA replication in humans, about 40 to 50 nucleotides per second, is comparatively slow. In bacteria the rate is much higher, reaching 500 to 1000 nucleotides per second. Given that some human chromosomes have as many as 250 million nucleotides, replication would be an extraordinarily time-consuming process if it proceeded linearly from one end of the chromosome to the other: For a chromosome of this size, a single round of replication would take almost 2 months. Instead, replication begins at many different points along the chromosome, termed **replication origins**. The resulting multiple separations of the DNA strands are called **replication bubbles** (Fig. 2-6). By occurring simultaneously at many different sites along the chromosome, the replication process can proceed much more quickly.

Replication bubbles allow DNA replication to take place at multiple locations on the chromosome, greatly speeding the replication process.

From Genes to Proteins

While DNA is formed and replicated in the cell nucleus, protein synthesis takes place in the cytoplasm. The

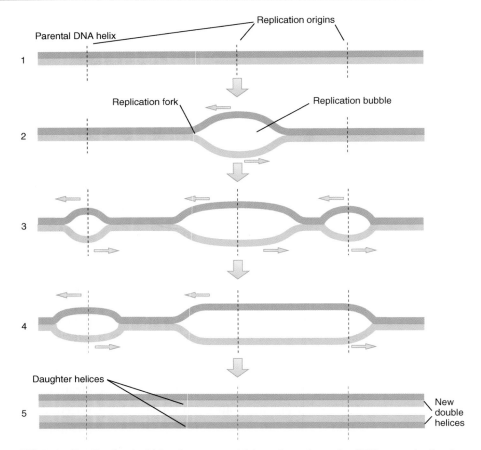

FIG 2-6   Replication bubbles form at multiple points along the DNA strand, allowing replication to proceed more rapidly.

information contained in DNA must be transported to the cytoplasm and then used to dictate the composition of proteins. This involves two processes, transcription and translation. Briefly, the DNA code is **transcribed** into messenger RNA, which then leaves the nucleus to be **translated** into proteins. These processes, summarized in Figure 2-7, are discussed at length later in this chapter. Transcription and translation are both mediated by **ribonucleic acid (RNA)**, a type of nucleic acid that is chemically similar to DNA. Like DNA, RNA is composed of sugars, phosphate groups, and nitrogenous bases. It differs from DNA in that the sugar is ribose instead of deoxyribose, and uracil rather than thymine is one of the four bases. Uracil is structurally similar to thymine, so, like thymine, it can pair with adenine. Another difference between RNA and DNA is that whereas DNA usually occurs as a double strand, RNA usually occurs as a single strand.

 DNA sequences encode proteins through the processes of transcription and translation. These processes both involve RNA, a single-stranded molecule that is similar to DNA except that it has a ribose sugar rather than deoxyribose and a uracil base rather than thymine.

Transcription

Transcription is the process by which an RNA sequence is formed from a DNA template (Fig. 2-8). The type of RNA produced by the transcription process is **messenger RNA (mRNA)**. To initiate mRNA transcription, one of the **RNA polymerase** enzymes (RNA polymerase II) binds to a **promoter** site on the DNA (a promoter is a nucleotide sequence that lies just upstream of a gene). The RNA polymerase then pulls a portion of the DNA strands apart from each other, exposing unattached DNA bases. One

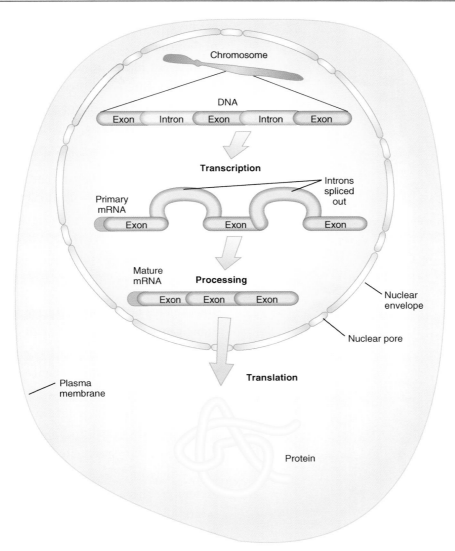

FIG 2-7   A summary of the steps leading from DNA to proteins. Replication and transcription occur in the cell nucleus. The mRNA is then transported to the cytoplasm, where translation of the mRNA into amino acid sequences composing a protein occurs.

of the two DNA strands provides the template for the sequence of mRNA nucleotides. Although either DNA strand could in principle serve as the template for mRNA synthesis, only one is chosen to do so in a given region of the chromosome. This choice is determined by the promoter sequence, which orients the RNA polymerase in a specific direction along the DNA sequence. Because the mRNA molecule can be synthesized only in the 5′ to 3′ direction, the promoter, by specifying directionality, determines which DNA strand serves as the template. This template DNA strand is also known as the **antisense strand**. RNA polymerase moves in the 3′ to 5′ direction along the DNA template strand, assembling the complementary

mRNA strand from 5′ to 3′ (see Fig. 2-8). Because of complementary base pairing, the mRNA nucleotide sequence is identical to that of the DNA strand that does not serve as the template—the **sense strand**—except for the substitution of uracil for thymine.

Soon after RNA synthesis begins, the 5′ end of the growing RNA molecule is capped by the addition of a chemically modified guanine nucleotide. This **5′ cap** appears to help prevent the RNA molecule from being degraded during synthesis, and later it helps to indicate the starting position for translation of the mRNA molecule into protein. Transcription continues until a group of bases called a **termination sequence** is reached. Near this point, a series of 100 to

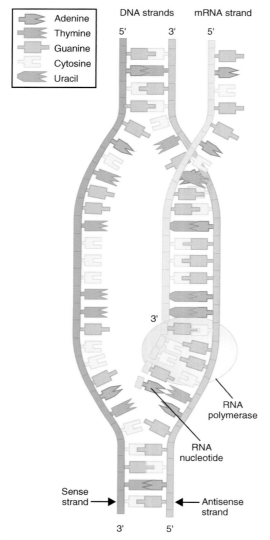

Adenine
Thymine
Guanine
Cytosine
Uracil

DNA strands   mRNA strand

FIG 2-8 Transcription of DNA to mRNA. RNA polymerase II proceeds along the DNA strand in the 3' to 5' direction, assembling a strand of mRNA nucleotides that is complementary to the DNA template strand.

200 adenine bases are added to the 3' end of the RNA molecule. This structure, known as the **poly-A tail**, may be involved in stabilizing the mRNA molecule so that it is not degraded when it reaches the cytoplasm. RNA polymerase usually continues to transcribe DNA for several thousand additional bases, but the mRNA bases that are attached after the poly-A tail are eventually lost. Finally, the DNA strands and the RNA polymerase separate from the RNA strand, leaving a transcribed single mRNA strand. This mRNA molecule is termed the **primary transcript**.

In some human genes, such as the one that can cause Duchenne muscular dystrophy, several differ-

ent promoters exist and are located in different parts of the gene. Thus, transcription of the gene can start in different places, resulting in the production of somewhat different proteins. This allows the same gene sequence to code for variations of a protein in different tissues (e.g., muscle tissue versus brain tissue).

▶ In the process of transcription, RNA polymerase II recognizes a promoter site near the 5' end of a gene on the sense strand and, through complementary base pairing, helps to produce an mRNA strand from the antisense DNA strand.

Transcription and the Regulation of Gene Expression
Some genes are transcribed in all cells of the body. These **housekeeping genes** encode products that are required for a cell's maintenance and metabolism. Most genes, however, are transcribed only in specific tissues at specific points in time. Therefore, in most cells, only a small fraction of genes are actively transcribed. This specificity explains why there is a large variety of different cell types making different protein products, even though almost all cells have exactly the same DNA sequence. For example, the globin genes are transcribed in the progenitors of red blood cells (where they help to form hemoglobin), and the low-density lipoprotein receptor genes are transcribed in liver cells.

Many different proteins participate in the process of transcription. Some of these are required for the transcription of all genes, and these are termed **general transcription factors**. Others, labeled **specific transcription factors**, have more specialized roles, activating only certain genes at certain stages of development. A key transcriptional element is RNA polymerase II, which was described previously. Although this enzyme plays a vital role in initiating transcription by binding to the promoter region, it cannot locate the promoter region on its own. Furthermore, it is incapable of producing significant quantities of mRNA by itself. Effective transcription requires the interaction of a large complex of approximately 50 different proteins. These include general (basal) transcription factors, which bind to RNA polymerase and to specific DNA sequences in the promoter region (sequences such as TATA and others needed for initiating transcription). The general transcription factors allow RNA polymerase to bind to the promoter region so that it can function effectively in transcription (Fig. 2-9).

The transcriptional activity of specific genes can be greatly increased by interaction with sequences called **enhancers**, which may be located thousands of bases upstream or downstream of the gene. Enhancers do not interact directly with genes. Instead, they are bound by a class of specific transcription factors that are termed **activators**. Activators bind to a second class of specific transcription factors called **co-activators**, which in turn bind to the general transcription factor complex described previously (see Fig. 2-9). This chain of interactions, from enhancer to activator to co-activator to the general transcription complex and finally to the gene itself, increases the transcription of specific genes at specific points in time. Whereas enhancers help to increase the tran-

scriptional activity of genes, other DNA sequences, known as **silencers**, help to repress the transcription of genes through a similar series of interactions.

Mutations in enhancer, silencer, or promoter sequences, as well as mutations in the genes that encode transcription factors, can lead to faulty expression of vital genes and consequently to genetic disease. Many examples of such diseases are discussed in the following chapters.

▶ Transcription factors are required for the transcription of DNA to mRNA. General transcription factors are used by all genes, and specific transcription factors help to initiate the transcription of genes in specific cell types at specific points in time. Transcription is also regulated by enhancer and silencer sequences, which may be located thousands of bases away from the transcribed gene.

The large number and complexity of transcription factors allow fine-tuned regulation of gene

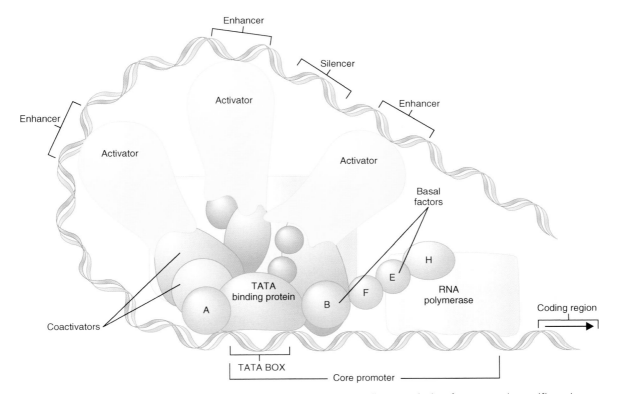

FIG 2-9 Key elements of transcription control include general (basal) transcription factors and specific enhancers and silencers. The activity of enhancers is mediated by activators and coactivators, which are specific transcription factors. (Data from Tjian R. Molecular machines that control genes. *Sci Am.* 1995; 272[2]: 54-61.)

expression. But how do the transcription factors locate specific DNA sequences? This is achieved by **DNA-binding motifs**: configurations in the transcription-factor protein that allow it to fit snugly and stably into a unique portion of the DNA double helix. Several examples of these binding motifs are listed in Table 2-1, and Figure 2-10 illustrates the binding of one such motif to DNA. Each major motif contains many variations that allow specificity in DNA binding.

An intriguing type of DNA-binding motif is contained in the high-mobility group (HMG) class of proteins. These proteins are capable of bending DNA and can facilitate interactions between distantly located enhancers and the appropriate basal factors and promoters (see Fig. 2-9).

> Transcription factors contain DNA-binding motifs that allow them to interact with specific DNA sequences. In some cases, they bend DNA so that distant enhancer sequences can interact with target genes.

Gene activity can also be related to patterns of chromatin coiling or condensation (**chromatin** is the combination of DNA and the histone proteins around which the DNA is wound). Decondensed, or open, chromatin regions, termed **euchromatin**, are typically characterized by histone **acetylation**, the attachment of acetyl groups to lysine residues in the histones. Acetylation of histones reduces their binding to DNA, helping to decondense the chromatin so that it is more accessible to transcription factors. Euchromatin is thus transcriptionally active. In contrast, **heterochromatin** is usually less acetylated, more condensed, and transcriptionally inactive.

Gene expression can also be influenced by **microRNAs** (**miRNA**), which are small RNA molecules (17-27 nucleotides) that are not translated into proteins. Instead, because they are complementary to specific mRNA sequences, they can bind to and down-regulate these mRNAs, thus lowering their expression levels. MicroRNA variation has been found to play important roles in a number of types of cancer (see Chapter 8).

FIG 2-10 A helix-loop-helix motif binds tightly to a specific DNA sequence.

TABLE 2-1	The Major Classes of DNA-Binding Motifs Found in Transcription Factors	
MOTIF	**DESCRIPTION**	**HUMAN DISEASE EXAMPLES**
Helix-turn-helix	Two α helices are connected by a short chain of amino acids, which constitute the turn. The carboxyl-terminal helix is a recognition helix that binds to the DNA major groove.	Homeodomain proteins (HOX): mutations in human *HOXD13* and *HOXA13* cause synpolydactyly and hand-foot-genital syndrome, respectively.
Helix-loop-helix	Two α helices (one short and one long) are connected by a flexible loop. The loop allows the two helices to fold back and interact with one another. The helices can bind to DNA or to other helix-loop-helix structures.	Mutations in the *TWIST* gene cause Saethre-Chotzen syndrome (acrocephalosyndactyly type III)
Zinc finger	Zinc molecules are used to stabilize amino acid structures (e.g., α helices, β sheets), with binding of the α helix to the DNA major groove.	*BRCA1* (breast cancer gene); *WT1* (Wilms tumor gene); *GL13* (Greig syndrome gene); vitamin D receptor gene (mutations cause rickets)
Leucine zipper	Two leucine-rich α helices are held together by amino acid side chains. The α helices form a Y-shaped structure whose side chains bind to the DNA major groove.	*RB1* (retinoblastoma gene); *JUN* and *FOS* oncogenes
β Sheets	Side chains extend from the two-stranded β sheet to form contacts with the DNA helix.	TBX family of genes: *TBX5* (Holt-Oram syndrome); *TBX3* (ulnar-mammary syndrome)

▶ Heterochromatin, which is highly condensed and hypoacetylated, tends to be transcriptionally inactive, whereas euchromatin, which is acetylated and less condensed, tends to be transcriptionally active.

Gene Splicing

The primary mRNA transcript is exactly complementary to the base sequence of the DNA template. In **eukaryotes** (Eukaryotes are organisms that have a defined cell nucleus, as opposed to **prokaryotes**, which lack a defined nucleus), an important step takes place before this RNA transcript leaves the nucleus. Sections of the RNA are removed by nuclear enzymes, and the remaining sections are spliced together to form the functional mRNA that will migrate to the cytoplasm. The excised sequences are called **introns**, and the sequences that are left to code for proteins are called **exons** (Fig. 2-11).Only after gene splicing is completed does the **mature transcript** move out of the nucleus into the cytoplasm. Some genes contain **alternative splice sites**, which allow the same primary transcript to be spliced in different ways, ultimately producing different protein products from the same gene. Errors

in gene splicing, like replication errors, are a form of mutation that can lead to genetic disease.

▶ Introns are spliced out of the primary mRNA transcript before the mature transcript leaves the nucleus. Exons contain the mRNA that specifies proteins.

The Genetic Code

Proteins are composed of one or more **polypeptides**, which are in turn composed of sequences of **amino acids**. The body contains 20 different types of amino acids, and the amino acid sequences that make up polypeptides must in some way be designated by the DNA after transcription into mRNA.

Because there are 20 different amino acids and only four different RNA bases, a single base could not be specific for a single amino acid. Similarly, specific amino acids could not be defined by couplets of bases (e.g., adenine followed by guanine, or uracil followed by adenine) because only 16 (4×4) different couplets are possible. If triplet sets of bases are translated into amino acids, however, 64 ($4 \times 4 \times 4$) combinations can be achieved—more than enough to specify each amino acid. Conclusive proof that amino acids are specified by these triplets of bases, or **codons**, was obtained by manufacturing synthetic nucleotide sequences and allowing them to direct the formation of polypeptides in the laboratory. The correspondence between specific codons and amino acids, known as the **genetic code**, is shown in Table 2-2.

Of the 64 possible codons, three signal the end of a gene and are known as **stop codons**. These are UAA, UGA, and UAG. The remaining 61 codons all specify amino acids. This means that most amino acids can be specified by more than one codon, as Table 2-2 shows. The genetic code is thus said to be **degenerate**. Although a given amino acid may be specified by more than one codon, each codon can designate only one amino acid.

▶ Individual amino acids, which compose proteins, are encoded by units of three mRNA bases, termed codons. There are 64 possible codons and only 20 amino acids, so the genetic code is degenerate.

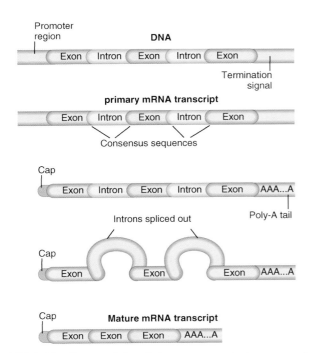

FIG 2-11   Gene splicing. Introns are precisely removed from the primary mRNA transcript to produce a mature mRNA transcript. Consensus sequences mark the sites at which splicing occurs.

TABLE 2-2   The Genetic Code*

FIRST POSITION (5' END) ↓	SECOND POSITION				THIRD POSITION (3' END) ↓
	U	**C**	**A**	**G**	
U	Phe	Ser	Tyr	Cys	U
U	Phe	Ser	Tyr	Cys	C
U	Leu	Ser	STOP	STOP	A
U	Leu	Ser	STOP	Trp	G
C	Leu	Pro	His	Arg	U
C	Leu	Pro	His	Arg	C
C	Leu	Pro	Gln	Arg	A
C	Leu	Pro	Gln	Arg	G
A	Ile	Thr	Asn	Ser	U
A	Ile	Thr	Asn	Ser	C
A	Ile	Thr	Lys	Arg	A
A	Met	Thr	Lys	Arg	G
G	Val	Ala	Asp	Gly	U
G	Val	Ala	Asp	Gly	C
G	Val	Ala	Glu	Gly	A
G	Val	Ala	Glu	Gly	G

Ala, alanine; Arg, arginine; Asn, asparagine; Asp, aspartic acid; Cys, cysteine; Gln, glutamine; Glu, glutamic acid; Gly, glycine; His, histidine; Ile, isoleucine; Leu, leucine; Lys, lysine; Met, methionine; Phe, phenylalanine; Pro, proline; Ser, serine; Thr, threonine; Trp, tryptophan; Tyr, tyrosine; Val, valine.
*Examples: UUG is translated into leucine; UAA is a stop codon; GGG is translated into glycine. Under some circumstances the UGA codon can specify an amino acid called selenocysteine, which is often called the 21st amino acid.

A significant feature of the genetic code is that it is universal: the great majority of organisms use the same DNA codes to specify amino acids. An important exception to this rule occurs in **mitochondria**, cytoplasmic organelles that are the sites of cellular respiration (see Fig. 2-1). The mitochondria have their own extranuclear DNA molecules, and several codons of mitochondrial DNA encode different amino acids than do the same nuclear DNA codons.

Translation

Translation is the process in which mRNA provides a template for the synthesis of a polypeptide. mRNA cannot, however, bind directly to amino acids. Instead, it interacts with molecules of **transfer RNA (tRNA)**, which are cloverleaf-shaped RNA strands of about 80 nucleotides. As Figure 2-12 illustrates, each tRNA molecule has a site at the 3' end for the attachment of a specific amino acid by a covalent bond. At the opposite end of the cloverleaf is a sequence of three nucleotides called the **anticodon**, which undergoes complementary base pairing with an appropri-

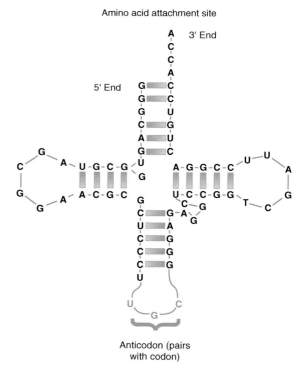

FIG 2-12   The structure of a tRNA molecule. In two dimensions, the tRNA has a cloverleaf shape. Note the 3' site of attachment for an amino acid. The anticodon pairs with a complementary mRNA codon.

ate codon in the mRNA. The attached amino acid is then transferred to the polypeptide chain being synthesized. In this way, mRNA specifies the sequence of amino acids by acting through tRNA.

The cytoplasmic site of protein synthesis is the **ribosome**, which consists of roughly equal parts of enzymatic proteins and **ribosomal RNA (rRNA)**. The function of rRNA is to help bind mRNA and tRNA to the ribosome. During translation, depicted in Figure 2-13, the ribosome first binds to an initiation site on the mRNA sequence. This site consists of a specific codon, AUG, which specifies the amino

FIG 2-13 Translation of mRNA to amino acids. The ribosome moves along the mRNA strand in the 5′ to 3′ direction, assembling a growing polypeptide chain. In this example, the mRNA sequence GUG AGC AAG GGU UCA has assembled five amino acids (Val, Ser, Lys, Gly, and Ser, respectively) into a polypeptide.

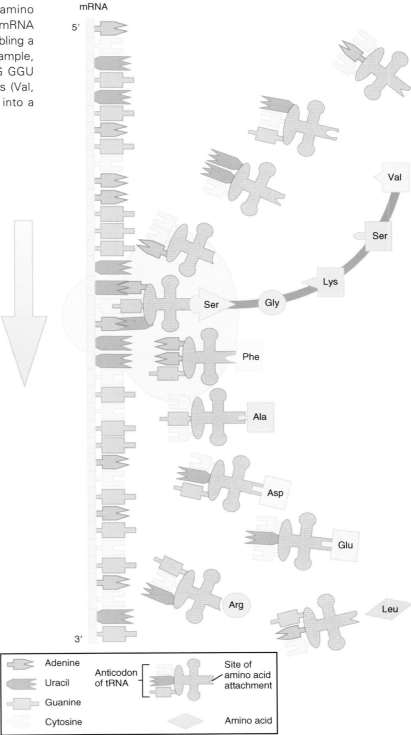

acid methionine (this amino acid is usually removed from the polypeptide before the completion of polypeptide synthesis). The ribosome then binds the tRNA to its surface so that base pairing can occur between tRNA and mRNA. The ribosome moves along the mRNA sequence, codon by codon, in the 5′ to 3′ direction. As each codon is processed, an amino acid is translated by the interaction of mRNA and tRNA.

In this process, the ribosome provides an enzyme that catalyzes the formation of covalent peptide bonds between the adjacent amino acids, resulting in a growing polypeptide. When the ribosome arrives at a stop codon on the mRNA sequence, translation and polypeptide formation cease. The amino (NH_2) terminus of the polypeptide corresponds to the 5′ end of the mRNA strand, and the carboxyl (COOH) terminus corresponds to the 3′ end. After synthesis is completed, the mRNA, the ribosome, and the polypeptide separate from one another. The polypeptide is then released into the cytoplasm.

 In the process of translation, the mRNA sequence serves as a template to specify sequences of amino acids. These sequences, which form polypeptides, are assembled by ribosomes. The tRNA and rRNA molecules interact with mRNA in the translation process.

Before a newly synthesized polypeptide can begin its existence as a functional protein, it often undergoes further processing, termed **posttranslational modification**. These modifications can take a variety of forms, including cleavage into smaller polypeptide units or combination with other polypeptides to form a larger protein. Other possible modifications include the addition of carbohydrate side chains to the polypeptide. Such modifications may be needed, for example, to produce proper folding of the mature protein or to stabilize its structure. An example of a clinically important protein that undergoes considerable posttranslational modification is type I collagen (Clinical Commentary 2-1).

 Posttranslational modification consists of various chemical changes that occur in proteins shortly after they are translated.

CLINICAL COMMENTARY 2-1

Osteogenesis Imperfecta, an Inherited Collagen Disorder

As its name implies, osteogenesis imperfecta is a disease caused by defects in the formation of bone. This disorder, sometimes known as brittle bone disease, affects approximately 1 in 15,000 to 1 in 25,000 births in all ethnic groups.

Approximately 90% of osteogenesis imperfecta cases are caused by defects in type I collagen, a major component of bone that provides much of its structural stability. The function of collagen in bone is analogous to that of the steel bars incorporated in reinforced concrete.

When type I collagen is improperly formed, the bone loses much of its strength and fractures easily. Patients with osteogenesis imperfecta can suffer hundreds of bone fractures (Fig. 2-14), or they might experience only a few, making this disease highly variable in its expression (the reasons for this variability are discussed in Chapter 4). In addition to bone fractures, patients can have short stature, hearing loss, abnormal tooth development (dentinogenesis imperfecta), bluish sclerae, and various bone deformities, including scoliosis. Osteogenesis imperfecta was traditionally classified into four major types, all of which are caused by mutations in either of the two genes that encode type I collagen. Several additional types, caused by mutations in other genes, have subsequently been added (Table 2-3). There is currently no cure for this dis-

ease, and management consists primarily of the repair of fractures and, in some cases, the use of external or internal bone support (e.g., surgically implanted rods). Additional therapies include the administration of bisphosphonates to decrease bone resorption and human growth hormone to facilitate growth. Physical rehabilitation also plays an important role in clinical management.

Type I collagen is a trimeric protein (i.e., having three subunits) with a triple helix structure. It is formed from a precursor protein, type I procollagen. Two of the three subunits of type I procollagen, labeled pro-α1(I) chains, are encoded by an 18-kb (kb = 1000 base pairs) gene on chromosome 17, and the third subunit, the pro-α2(I) chain, is encoded by a 38-kb gene on chromosome 7. Each of these genes contains more than 50 exons. After transcription and splicing, the mature mRNA formed from each gene is only 5 to 7 kb long. The mature mRNAs proceed to the cytoplasm, where they are translated into polypeptide chains by the ribosomal machinery of the cell.

At this point, the polypeptide chains undergo a series of posttranslational modifications. Many of the proline and lysine residues (A residue is an amino acid that has been incorporated into a polypeptide chain.) are hydroxylated (i.e., hydroxyl groups are added) to form hydroxyproline

CLINICAL COMMENTARY 2-1
Osteogenesis Imperfecta, an Inherited Collagen Disorder (Continued)

and hydroxylysine, respectively. (Several rare forms of osteogenesis imperfect, including type VII, are caused by mutations in genes involved in the hydroxylation process.) The three polypeptides, two pro-α1(I) chains, and one pro-α2(I) chain, begin to associate with one another at their COOH termini. This association is stabilized by sulfide bonds that form between the chains near the COOH termini. The triple helix then forms, in zipper-like fashion, beginning at the COOH terminus and proceeding toward the NH₂ terminus. Some of the hydroxylysines are glyco-

TABLE 2-3   Subtypes of Osteogenesis Imperfecta

TYPE	DISEASE FEATURES
I	Mild bone fragility, blue sclerae, hearing loss in 60% of patients, normal or near-normal stature, few bone deformities, dentinogenesis imperfecta in some cases
II	Most severe form, with extreme bone fragility, long bone deformities, compressed femurs, gray-blue sclerae; lethal in the prenatal or perinatal periods (most die of respiratory failure during the first week of life, and survival beyond one year is highly unusual)
III	Severe bone fragility, very short stature, variably blue sclerae, progressive bone deformities, hearing loss in 80% of patients; dentinogenesis imperfecta is common
IV	Short stature, normal-to-gray sclerae, mild to moderate bone deformity, hearing loss in some patients, dentinogenesis imperfecta is common; bone fragility is variable
V	Similar to type IV but also includes calcification of interosseous membrane of forearm, radial head dislocation, and hyperplastic callus formation
VI	Similar to type IV but not caused by type I collagen mutations; calcification in interosseous membranes is not seen; no dentinogenesis imperfecta
VII	White sclerae, early lower limb deformities, shortening of all limbs, congenital fractures, osteopenia
VIII	Severe, often lethal phenotype similar to type II but not caused by type I collagen mutations; severe osteoporosis, shortened long bones, white sclerae

Types I-IV are caused by mutations in the two genes that encode type I collagen protein; types V-VIII have been identified on the basis of distinct bone histology and are caused by mutations in genes involved in posttranslational processing of the gene product. Types VII and VIII have an autosomal recessive mode of inheritance, and several additional rare autosomal recessive forms of osteogenesis imperfect have been identified. There is substantial phenotypic overlap among many of these categories of osteogenesis imperfecta.

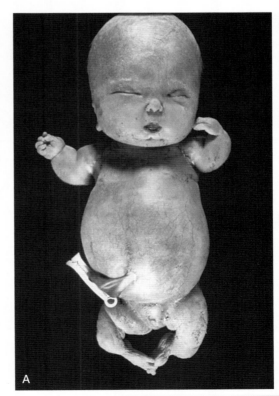

FIG 2-14   A, A stillborn infant with type II osteogenesis imperfecta (the perinatal lethal form). The infant had a type I procollagen mutation and short, slightly twisted limbs. **B,** Radiograph of an infant with type II osteogenesis imperfecta. Note calluses from rib fractures, which are observable as "beads" on the ribs (*arrows*).

CLINICAL COMMENTARY 2-1
Osteogenesis Imperfecta, an Inherited Collagen Disorder (Continued)

sylated (i.e., sugars are added), a modification that commonly occurs in the rough endoplasmic reticulum (see Fig. 2-1). The hydroxyl groups in the hydroxyprolines help to connect the three chains by forming hydrogen bonds, which stabilize the triple helix. Critical to proper folding of the helix is the presence of a glycine in every third position of each polypeptide.

Once the protein has folded into a triple helix, it moves from the endoplasmic reticulum to the Golgi apparatus (see Fig. 2-1) and is secreted from the cell. Yet another modification then takes place: the procollagen is cleaved by proteases near both the NH_2 and the COOH termini of the triple helix, removing some amino acids at each end. These amino acids performed essential functions earlier in the life of the protein (e.g., helping to form the triple helix structure, helping to thread the protein through the endoplasmic reticulum) but are no longer needed. This cleavage results in the mature protein, type I collagen. The collagen then assembles itself into fibrils, which react with adjacent molecules outside the cell to form the covalent cross-links that impart tensile strength to the fibrils.

The path from the DNA sequence to the mature collagen protein involves many steps (Fig. 2-15). The complexity of this path provides many opportunities for mistakes (in replication, transcription, translation, or posttranslational modification) that can cause disease. Of the more than 1500 type I collagen mutations now known to cause osteogenesis imperfecta, the most common type produces a replacement of glycine with another amino acid. Because only glycine is small enough to be accommodated in the center of the triple helix structure, substitution of a different amino acid causes instability of the structure and thus poorly formed fibrils. This type of mutation is often seen in severe forms of osteogenesis imperfecta. Other mutations can cause excess posttranslational modification of the polypeptide chains, again producing abnormal fibrils. Other examples of disease-causing mutations are provided in the suggested readings at the end of this chapter.

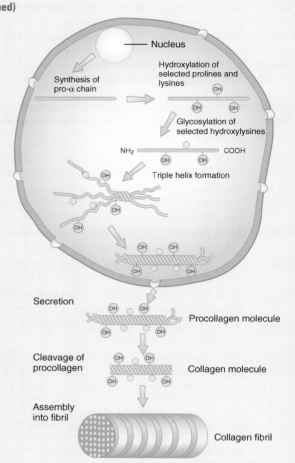

FIG 2-15   The process of collagen fibril formation. After the pro-α polypeptide chain is formed, a series of posttranslational modifications take place, including hydroxylation and glycosylation. Three polypeptide chains assemble into a triple helix, which is secreted outside the cell. Portions of each end of the procollagen molecule are cleaved, resulting in the mature collagen molecule. These molecules then assemble into collagen fibrils.

THE STRUCTURE OF GENES AND THE GENOME

Some aspects of gene structure, such as the existence of introns and exons, have already been touched on. Alterations of different parts of genes can have quite distinct consequences in terms of genetic disease. It is therefore necessary to describe more fully the details of gene structure. A schematic diagram of gene structure is given in Figure 2-16.

Introns and Exons

The intron-exon structure of genes, discovered in 1977, is one of the attributes that distinguishes eukaryotes from prokaryotes. Introns form the major portion of most eukaryotic genes. As noted previously, introns are spliced out of the mRNA before it leaves the nucleus, and this splicing must be under very precise control. Enzymes that carry out splicing are directed to the appropriate locations by DNA sequences known as **consensus sequences** (so named

FIG 2-16   Details of gene structure, showing promoter and upstream regulation (enhancer) sequences and a poly-A addition site.

because they are common in all eukaryotic organisms), which are situated adjacent to each exon.

Because most eukaryotic genes are composed primarily of introns, it is natural to ask whether introns might have some function. One interesting hypothesis is that introns, by lengthening genes, encourage the shuffling of genes when homologous chromosomes exchange material during meiosis (see later discussion). It has also been suggested that introns evolved to modify the amount of time required for DNA replication and transcription.

Surprisingly, some introns contain transcribed genes that are apparently unrelated to the gene in which the introns are contained. For example, introns of the human neurofibromatosis type 1 (*NF1*) gene contain three genes that are transcribed in the direction opposite that of the NF1 gene itself. These genes appear to have no functional relationship to the *NF1* gene. Similar gene inserts have been found within the factor VIII gene (*F8*) on the human X chromosome.

Types of DNA

Although most of the emphasis in genetics is given to the DNA that encodes proteins, only 1% to 2% of the 3 billion nucleotide pairs in the human genome actually perform this role. It has been estimated recently that about 75% of human DNA is transcribed into mRNA at some time in some cells, but the function of most of this mRNA (if any) is unknown. To better understand the nature of all types of DNA, we briefly review the several categories into which it is classified (Fig. 2-17).

The first and most important class of DNA is termed **single-copy DNA**. As the name implies, single-copy DNA sequences are seen only once (or possibly a few times) in the genome. Single-copy DNA accounts for about half of the genome and includes the protein-coding genes. However, protein-coding DNA (exons) represents only a small fraction of all single-copy DNA, most of which is found in introns or in DNA sequences that lie between genes.

The other half of the genome consists of **repetitive DNA**, sequences that are repeated over and over again in the genome, often thousands of times. There are two major classes of repetitive DNA: **dispersed repetitive DNA** and **satellite DNA**. Satellite repeats are clustered together in certain chromosome locations, where they occur as tandem repeats (i.e., the beginning of one repeat occurs immediately adjacent

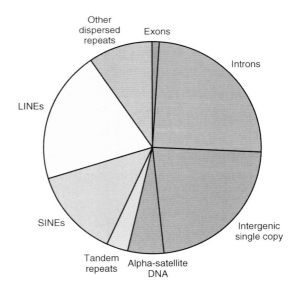

FIG 2-17   Structural composition of the human genome. Because of limitations in mapping repetitive sequences, these figures are approximate. In addition, there is some overlap among categories (e.g., repeat sequences are sometimes found in introns). The category "other dispersed repeats" includes DNA transposons, LTR (long terminal repeat) retrotransposons, and low-copy number duplications.

to the end of another). Dispersed repeats, as the name implies, tend to be scattered singly throughout the genome; they do not occur in tandem.

The term *satellite* is used because these sequences, owing to their composition, can easily be separated by centrifugation in a cesium chloride density gradient. The DNA appears as a satellite, separate from the other DNA in the gradient. This term is not to be confused with the satellites that can be observed microscopically on certain chromosomes (see Chapter 6). Satellite DNA accounts for approximately 8% to 10% of the genome and can be further subdivided into several categories. α-Satellite DNA occurs as tandem repeats of a 171-bp sequence that can extend to several million base pairs or longer. This type of satellite DNA is found near the centromeres of chromosomes. **Minisatellites** are blocks of tandem repeats (each 14 to 500 bp long) whose total length is much smaller, usually a few thousand base pairs. A final category, **microsatellites**, are smaller still: the repeat units are 1 to 13 bp long, and the total length of the array is usually less than a few hundred base pairs. Minisatellites and microsatellites are of special interest in human genetics because they vary in length among individuals, making them highly useful for gene mapping. A minisatellite or microsatellite is found at an average frequency of one per 2 kb in the human genome; altogether they account for about 3% of the genome.

Dispersed repetitive DNA makes up about 45% of the genome, and these repeats fall into several major categories (Fig. 2-18). The two most common categories are short interspersed elements (**SINEs**) and long interspersed elements (**LINEs**). Individual SINEs range in size from 90 to 500 bp, and individual LINEs can be as large as 7000 bp. One of the most important types of SINEs in humans is the 300-bp *Alu* element, so named because each repeat contains a DNA sequence that can be cut by the *Alu* restriction enzyme (see Chapter 3 for further discussion). The *Alu* repeats are a **family** of DNA elements, meaning that all of them have highly similar DNA sequences. About 1 million *Alu* repeats are scattered throughout the genome; they thus constitute approximately 10% of all human DNA. LINE repeats constitute another 20% of the human genome. A remarkable feature of *Alu* sequences, as well as LINEs, is that some of them can generate copies of themselves, which can then be inserted into other parts of the genome. This is how they have achieved such remarkable numbers. These insertions can sometimes interrupt a protein-coding gene, causing genetic disease (examples are discussed in Chapter 4).

 There are several major types of DNA, including single-copy DNA, satellite DNA, and dispersed repetitive DNA. The latter two categories are both classes of repeated DNA sequences. Only about 1% to 2% of human DNA actually encodes proteins.

THE CELL CYCLE

During the course of development, each human progresses from a single-cell **zygote** (an egg cell fertilized

Single-copy DNA (45%)

Dispersed repetitive DNA (45%)

Satellite DNA (10%)

FIG 2-18 Single-copy DNA sequences are unique and are dispersed throughout the genome. Satellite DNA sequences are repetitive elements that occur together in clusters. Dispersed repeats are similar to one another but do not cluster together.

by a sperm cell) to a marvelously complex organism containing approximately 100 trillion (10^{14}) individual cells. Because few cells last for a person's entire lifetime, new ones must be generated to replace those that die. Both of these processes—development and replacement—require the manufacture of new cells. The cell division processes that are responsible for the creation of new diploid cells from existing ones are **mitosis** (nuclear division) and **cytokinesis** (cytoplasmic division). Before dividing, a cell must duplicate its contents, including its DNA; this occurs during **interphase**. The alternation of mitosis and interphase is referred to as the **cell cycle**.

As Figure 2-19 shows, a typical cell spends most of its life in interphase. This portion of the cell cycle is divided into three phases, **G1**, **S**, and **G2**. During **G1** (gap 1, the interval between mitosis and the onset of DNA replication), synthesis of RNA and proteins takes place. DNA replication occurs during the S (synthesis) phase. During G2 (the interval between the S phase and the next mitosis), some DNA repair takes place, and the cell prepares for mitosis. By the time G2 has been reached, the cell contains two identical copies of each of the 46 chromosomes. These identical chromosomes are referred to as **sister chromatids**. Sister chromatids often exchange material during interphase, a process known as **sister chromatid exchange**.

The cell cycle consists of the alternation of cell division (mitosis and cytokinesis) and interphase. DNA replication and protein synthesis take place during interphase.

The length of the cell cycle varies considerably from one cell type to another. In rapidly dividing cells such as those of epithelial tissue (found, for example, in the lining of the intestines and in the lungs), the cycle may be completed in less than 10 hours. Other cells, such as those of the liver, might divide only once each year or so. Some cell types, such as skeletal muscle cells and neurons, largely lose their ability to divide and replicate in adults. Although all stages of the cell cycle have some variation in length, the great majority of variation is due to differences in the length of the G1 phase. When cells stop dividing for a long period, they are often said to be in the G0 stage.

Cells divide in response to important internal and external cues. Before the cell enters mitosis, for example, DNA replication must be accurate and complete and the cell must have achieved an appropriate size. The cell must respond to extracellular stimuli that require increased or decreased rates of division. Complex molecular interactions mediate this regulation. Among the most important of the molecules involved are the **cyclin-dependent kinases** (**CDKs**), a family of kinases that phosphorylate other regulatory proteins at key stages of the cell cycle. To carry out this function, the CDKs must form complexes with various **cyclins**, proteins that are synthesized at specific cell-cycle stages and are then degraded when CDK action is no longer needed. The **cyclins** and CDKs, as well as the many proteins that interact with them, are subjects of intense study because of their vital role in the cell cycle and because their malfunction can lead to cancer (see Chapter 8).

The length of the cell cycle varies in different cell types. Critical to regulation of the cell cycle are CDKs, which phosphorylate other proteins, and cyclins, which form complexes with CDKs. Faulty regulation of the cell cycle can lead to cancer.

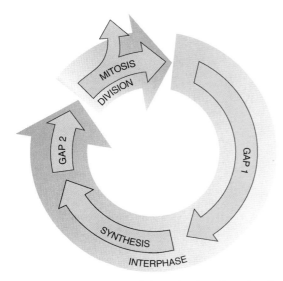

FIG 2-19   Major phases of the mitotic cell cycle, showing the alternation of interphase and mitosis (division).

Mitosis

Although mitosis usually requires only 1 to 2 hours to complete, this portion of the cell cycle involves many critical and complex processes. Mitosis is divided into several phases (Fig. 2-20). During **prophase**, the first mitotic stage, the chromosomes become visible under a light microscope as they condense and coil (chromosomes are not clearly visible during interphase). The two sister chromatids of each chromosome lie together, attached at a point called the **centromere**. The nuclear membrane, which surrounds the nucleus, disappears during this stage. **Spindle**

fibers begin to form, radiating from two **centrioles** located on opposite sides of the cell. The spindle fibers become attached to the centromeres of each chromosome and eventually pull the two sister chromatids in opposite directions.

The chromosomes reach their most highly condensed state during **metaphase**, the next stage of mitosis. Because they are highly condensed, they are easiest to visualize microscopically during this phase. For this reason, clinical diagnosis of chromosome disorders is usually based on metaphase chromosomes. During metaphase, the spindle fibers begin to contract and pull the centromeres of the chromo-

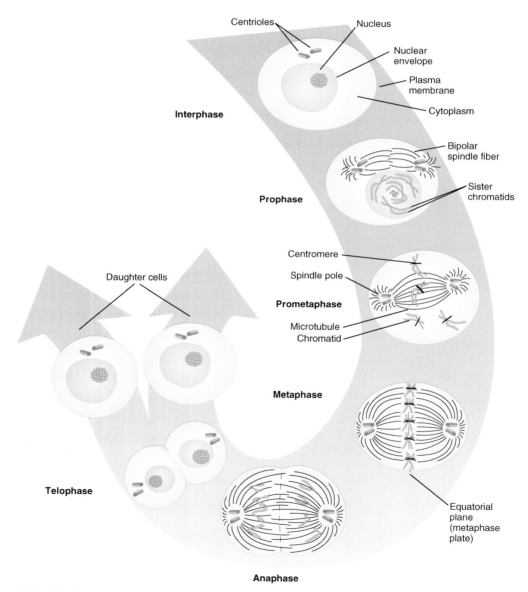

FIG 2-20 The stages of mitosis, during which two identical diploid cells are formed from one original diploid cell.

somes, which are now arranged along the middle of the spindle (the **equatorial plane** of the cell).

During **anaphase**, the next mitotic stage, the centromere of each chromosome splits, allowing the sister chromatids to separate. The chromatids are then pulled by the spindle fibers, centromere first, toward opposite sides of the cell. At the end of anaphase, the cell contains 92 separate chromosomes, half lying near one side of the cell and half near the other side. If all has proceeded correctly, the two sets of chromosomes are identical.

Telophase, the final stage of mitosis, is characterized by the formation of new nuclear membranes around each of the two sets of 46 chromosomes. Also, the spindle fibers disappear, and the chromosomes begin to decondense. Cytokinesis usually occurs after nuclear division and results in a roughly equal division of the cytoplasm into two parts. With the completion of telophase, two diploid **daughter cells**, both identical to the original cell, have been formed.

 Mitosis is the process through which two identical diploid daughter cells are formed from a single diploid cell.

Meiosis

When an egg cell and a sperm cell unite to form a zygote, their chromosomes are combined into a single cell. Because humans are diploid organisms, there must be a mechanism to reduce the number of chromosomes in gametes to the haploid state. Otherwise the zygote would have 92, instead of the normal 46, chromosomes. The primary mechanism by which haploid gametes are formed from diploid precursor cells is **meiosis**.

Two cell divisions occur during meiosis. Each meiotic division has been divided into stages with the same names as those of mitosis, but the processes involved in some of the stages are quite different (Fig. 2-21). During meiosis I, often called the **reduction division stage**, two haploid cells are formed from a diploid cell. These diploid cells are the **oogonia** in females and the **spermatogonia** in males. After

meiosis I, a second meiosis, the **equational division**, takes place, during which each haploid cell is replicated.

The first stage of the meiotic cell cycle is **interphase** I, during which important processes such as replication of chromosomal DNA take place. The second phase of meiosis I, **prophase** I, is quite complex and includes many of the key events that distinguish meiosis from mitosis. Prophase I begins as the chromatin strands coil and condense, causing them to become visible as chromosomes. During the process of **synapsis**, the homologous chromosomes pair up, side by side, lying together in perfect alignment (in males, the X and Y chromosomes, being mostly nonhomologous, line up end to end). This pairing of homologous chromosomes is an important part of the cell cycle that does not occur in mitosis. As prophase I continues, the chromatids of the two chromosomes intertwine. Each pair of intertwined homologous chromosomes is either **bivalent** (indicating two chromosomes in the unit) or **tetrad** (indicating four chromatids in the unit).

A second key feature of prophase I is the formation of **chiasmata** (plural of **chiasma**), cross-shaped structures that mark attachments between the homologous chromosomes (Fig. 2-22). Each chiasma indicates a point at which the homologous chromosomes exchange genetic material. This process, called **crossing over**, produces chromosomes that consist of combinations of parts of the original chromosomes. This chromosomal shuffling is important because it greatly increases the possible combinations of genes in each gamete and thereby increases the number of possible combinations of human traits. Also, this phenomenon is critically important in inferring the order of genes along chromosomes. At the end of prophase I, the bivalents begin to move toward the equatorial plane, a spindle apparatus begins to form in the cytoplasm, and the nuclear membrane dissipates.

Metaphase I is the next phase. As in mitotic metaphase, this stage is characterized by the completion of spindle formation and alignment of the bivalents, which are still attached at the chiasmata, in the equa-

Chiasma

Prophase I

Primary oocyte
Primary spermatocyte

Metaphase I

Anaphase I

Secondary oocyte
Secondary spermatocyte

Telophase I

Metaphase II

Large egg and polar bodies
Spermatids of
equal size

Anaphase II

FIG 2-21 The stages of meiosis, during which haploid gametes are formed from a diploid cell. For brevity, prophase II and telophase II are not shown. Note the relationship between meiosis and spermatogenesis and oogenesis.

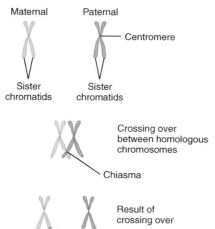

Homologous chromosomes

Maternal   Paternal

Centromere

Sister   Sister
chromatids   chromatids

Crossing over
between homologous
chromosomes

Chiasma

Result of
crossing over

FIG 2-22 The process of chiasma formation and crossing over results in the exchange of genetic material between homologous chromosomes.

torial plane. The two centromeres of each bivalent now lie on opposite sides of the equatorial plane.

During **anaphase I**, the chiasmata disappear and the homologous chromosomes are pulled by the spindle fibers toward opposite poles of the cell. The key feature of this phase is that unlike the corresponding phase of mitosis, the centromeres do not duplicate and divide, so that only half of the original number of chromosomes migrates toward each pole. The chromosomes migrating toward each pole thus consist of one member of each pair of autosomes and one of the sex chromosomes.

The next stage, **telophase I**, begins when the chromosomes reach opposite sides of the cell. The chromosomes uncoil slightly, and a new nuclear membrane begins to form. The two daughter cells each contain the haploid number of chromosomes, and each chromosome has two sister chromatids. In humans, cytokinesis also occurs during this phase. The cytoplasm is divided approximately equally between the two daughter cells in the gametes formed in males. In those formed in females, nearly all of the cytoplasm goes into one daughter cell, which will later form the egg. The other daughter cell becomes a **polar body**, a small, nonfunctional cell that eventually degenerates.

> Meiosis I (reduction division) includes a prophase I stage in which homologous chromosomes line up and exchange material (crossing over). During anaphase I the centromeres do not duplicate and divide. Consequently only one member of each pair of chromosomes migrates to each daughter cell.

The equational division, meiosis II, then begins with **interphase II**. This is a very brief phase. The important feature of interphase II is that, unlike interphase I, no replication of DNA occurs. **Prophase II**, the next stage, is quite similar to mitotic prophase, except that the cell nucleus contains only the haploid number of chromosomes. During prophase II, the chromosomes thicken as they coil, the nuclear membrane disappears, and new spindle fibers are formed. This is followed by **metaphase II**, during which the spindle fibers pull the chromosomes into alignment at the equatorial plane.

Anaphase II then follows. This stage resembles mitotic anaphase in that the centromeres split and each carries a single chromatid toward a pole of the cell. The chromatids have now separated, but, because of chiasma formation and crossing over, the newly separated sister chromatids might not be identical (see Fig. 2-21).

Telophase II, like telophase I, begins when the chromosomes reach opposite poles of the cell. There they begin to uncoil. New nuclear membranes are formed around each group of chromosomes, and cytokinesis occurs. In gametes formed in males, the

cytoplasm is again divided equally between the two daughter cells. The end result of male meiosis is thus four functional daughter cells, each of which has an equal amount of cytoplasm. In female gametes, unequal division of the cytoplasm again occurs, forming the egg cell and another polar body. The polar body formed during meiosis I sometimes undergoes a second division, so three polar bodies may be present when the second stage of meiosis is completed.

> Meiosis is a specialized cell division process in which a diploid cell gives rise to haploid gametes. This is accomplished by combining two rounds of division with only one round of DNA replication.

Most chromosome disorders are caused by errors that occur during meiosis. Gametes can be created that contain missing or additional chromosomes or chromosomes with altered structures. In addition, mitotic errors that occur early in the life of the embryo can affect enough of the body's cells to produce clinically significant disease. Mitotic errors occurring at any point in one's lifetime can, under some circumstances, cause cancer. Cancer genetics is discussed in Chapter 8, and chromosome disorders are the subject of Chapter 6.

The Relationship between Meiosis and Gametogenesis

The stages of meiosis can be related directly to stages in **gametogenesis**, the formation of gametes (see Fig. 2-21). In mature males, the seminiferous tubules of the testes are populated by spermatogonia, which are diploid cells. After going through several mitotic divisions, the spermatogonia produce **primary spermatocytes**. Each primary spermatocyte, which is also diploid, undergoes meiosis I to produce a pair of **secondary spermatocytes**, each of which contains 23 double-stranded chromosomes. These undergo meiosis II, and each produces a pair of **spermatids** that contain 23 single-stranded chromosomes. The spermatids then lose most of their cytoplasm and develop tails for swimming as they become mature

sperm cells. This process, known as **spermatogenesis**, continues throughout the life of the mature male.

 In spermatogenesis, each diploid spermatogonium produces four haploid sperm cells.

Oogenesis, the process by which female gametes are formed, differs in several important ways from spermatogenesis. Whereas the cycle of spermatogenesis is constantly recurring, much of female oogenesis is completed before birth. Diploid oogonia divide mitotically to produce **primary oocytes** by the third month of fetal development. More than 6 million primary oocytes are formed during gestation, and they are suspended in prophase I by the time of birth. Meiosis continues only when a mature primary oocyte is ovulated. In meiosis I, the primary oocyte produces one secondary oocyte (containing the cytoplasm) and one polar body. The **secondary oocyte** then emerges from the follicle and proceeds down the fallopian tube, with the polar body attached to it. Meiosis II begins only if the secondary oocyte is fertilized by a sperm cell. If this occurs, one haploid mature **ovum**, containing the cytoplasm, and another haploid polar body are produced. The polar bodies eventually disintegrate. About 1 hour after fertilization, the nuclei of the sperm cell and ovum fuse, forming a diploid zygote. The zygote then begins its development into an embryo through a series of mitotic divisions.

 In oogenesis, one haploid ovum and three haploid polar bodies are produced meiotically from a diploid oogonium. In contrast to spermatogenesis, which continues throughout the life of the mature male, the first phase of oogenesis is completed before the female is born; oogenesis is then halted until ovulation occurs.

SUMMARY

Human somatic cells contain 23 pairs of chromosomes, whereas gametes contain a total of 23 chromosomes. Genetic information is generally stored in genes, the basic units of inheritance, which are contained in chromosomes as DNA fragments. DNA is composed of 4 nucleotide bases that, along with the pentose sugar deoxyribose and phosphate groups, form a double-helix structure. Based on the principle of complementary base pairing, DNA replication allows a single strand of the double-stranded DNA molecule to form a template for the synthesis of a new complementary strand. Heterochromatin, composed of highly condensed and hypoacetylated DNA, tends to be transcriptionally inactive, whereas euchromatin, which is acetylated and less condensed, is transcriptionally active. During the processes of transcription and translation, mRNA is produced, followed by associated polypeptide synthesized according to codon order. To be functional, most proteins undergo posttranslational modification, in which various chemical changes occur shortly after translation. The cell cycle consists of alternating periods of cell division and interphase. DNA replication and protein synthesis take place during interphase. The length of the cell cycle varies among cell types. Mitosis is the process by which two identical diploid daughter cells are formed from a single diploid cell, whereas meiosis is a specialized cell division process in which a diploid cell gives rise to haploid gametes.

IMPORTANT TERMINOLOGY

chromosome   染色体
gene   基因
deoxyribonucleic acid (DNA)   脱氧核糖核酸
somatic cell   体细胞
gamete   配子
sex chromosome   性染色体
autosome   常染色体
diploid   二倍体
haploid   单倍体
mitosis   有丝分裂
meiosis   减数分裂
nucleotide   核苷酸
histone   组蛋白
nucleosome   核小体

replication   复制

complementary base pairing   互补碱基配对

ribonucleic acid (RNA)   核糖核酸

messenger RNA (mRNA)   信使核糖核酸

promoter   启动子

general transcription factor   通用转录因子

specific transcription factor   特异转录因子

enhancer   增强子

silencer   沉默子

chromatin   染色质

euchromatin   常染色质

acetylation   乙酰化

heterochromatin   异染色质

microRNA   小 RNA

eukaryote   真核生物

prokaryote   原核生物

intron   内含子

exon   外显子

alternative splice site   选择性剪接位点

polypeptide   多肽

codon   密码子

genetic code   遗传密码

degenerate   兼并

translation   翻译

transfer RNA (tRNA)   转运核糖核酸

ribosome   核糖体

ribosomal RNA (rRNA)   核糖体核糖核酸

posttranslational modification   翻译后修饰

single-copy DNA   单拷贝脱氧核糖核酸

repetitive DNA   重复脱氧核糖核酸

cell cycle   细胞周期

zygote   受精卵

interphase   分裂间期

sister chromatid   姐妹染色单体

sister chromatid exchange   姐妹染色单体交换

centromere   着丝粒

crossing over   交换

polar body   极体

gametogenesis   配子发生

oogenesis   卵子发生

REVIEW QUESTIONS

1. Consider the following double-stranded DNA sequence:

   5′-CAG AAG AAA ATT AAC ATG TAA-3′

   3′-GTC TTC TTT TAA TTG TAC ATT-5′

   If the bottom strand serves as the template, what is the mRNA sequence produced by transcription of this DNA sequence? What is the amino acid sequence produced by translation of the mRNA sequence?

2. Arrange the following terms according to their hierarchical relationship to one another: genes, chromosomes, exons, codons, nucleotides, genome.

3. Less than 5% of human DNA encodes proteins. Furthermore, in a given cell type only 10% of the coding DNA actively encodes proteins. Explain these statements.

4. What are the major differences between mitosis and meiosis?

5. The human body contains approximately 10^{14} cells. Starting with a single-cell zygote, how many mitotic cell divisions, on average, would be required to produce this number of cells?

6. How many mature sperm cells will be produced by 100 primary spermatocytes? How many mature egg cells will be produced by 100 primary oocytes?

SUGGESTED READINGS AND WEBSITES

1. Alberts B, Johnson A, Lewis J, et al. *Molecular Biology of the Cell.* 5th ed. New York: Garland Science; 2007.

2. Basel D, Steiner RD. Osteogenesis imperfecta: recent findings shed new light on this once well-understood condition. *Genet Med.* 2009; 11: 375-385.

3. Byers PH, Pyott SM. Recessively inherited forms of osteogenesis imperfecta. *Annu Rev Genet.* 2012; 46: 475-497.

4. Forlino A, Cabral WA, Barnes AM, Marini JC. New perspectives on osteogenesis imperfecta. *Nat Rev Endocrinol.* 2011; 7(9): 540-557.

5. Lewin B, Krebs JE, Goldstein ES, Kilpatrick ST. *Genes XI*. Oxford: Oxford University Press; 2012.

6. Strachan T, Read AP. *Human Molecular Genetics*. 4th ed. London: Garland Science; 2011.

7. Mitosis and meiosis tutorials and animations: http://www.biology.arizona.edu/cell_bio/cell_bio.html

8. Tutorials and animations of DNA replication, transcription, and translation: http://www.hhmi.org/biointeractive/

(Luying Peng)

Chapter 3

Genetic Variation: Its Origin and Detection

Humans display a substantial amount of genetic variation. This is reflected in traits such as height, blood pressure, and skin color. Included in the spectrum of genetic variations are disease states, such as cystic fibrosis or type 1 neurofibromatosis (see Chapter 4). This aspect of genetic variation is the focus of medical genetics.

All genetic variation originates from the process known as **mutation**, which is defined as a change in DNA sequence. Mutations can affect either **germline cells** (cells that produce gametes) or somatic cells (all cells other than germline cells). Mutations in **somatic cells** can lead to cancer and are thus of significant concern. However, this chapter is focused primarily on germline mutations, because they can be transmitted from one generation to the next.

As a result of mutations, a gene can differ among individuals in terms of its DNA sequence. The differing sequences are referred to as **alleles**. A gene's location on a chromosome is termed a **locus** (from the Latin word for "place"). For example, it might be said that a person has a certain allele at the β-globin locus on chromosome 11. If a person has the same allele on both members of a chromosome pair, he or she is said to be a **homozygote**. If the alleles differ in DNA sequence, he or she is a **heterozygote**. The combination of alleles that is present at a given locus is termed the **genotype**.

In human genetics, the term mutation has often been reserved for DNA sequence changes that cause genetic diseases and are consequently relatively rare, with a population frequency less than 1%. DNA sequence variants that are more common in populations are conventionally described as **polymorphisms** ("many forms," describing multiple alleles at a locus). **Loci** (plural of locus) that contain multiple alleles are termed **polymorphic**. Nowadays, however, alleles that have a frequency less than 1% are often called polymorphisms as well. In addition, many common polymorphisms are now known to influence the risks for complex, common diseases such as diabetes and heart disease (see Chapter 5), so the traditional distinction between mutation (rare and disease-causing) and polymorphism (common and benign) has become increasingly blurred.

One of Gregor Mendel's important contributions to genetics was to show that the effects of one allele at a locus can mask those of another allele at the same locus. He performed **crosses** (matings) between pea plants homozygous for a "tall" allele (i.e., having two identical copies of an allele that we will label H) and plants homozygous for a "short" allele (having two copies of an allele labeled h). This cross, which can produce only heterozygous (Hh) offspring, is illustrated in the **Punnett square** shown in Fig. 3-1. Mendel found that the offspring of these crosses, even though they were heterozygotes, were all tall. This is because the H allele is **dominant**, and the h allele is **recessive**. (It is conventional to label the dominant allele in upper case and the recessive allele in lower case.) The term recessive comes from a Latin root meaning "to hide." This describes the behavior of recessive alleles well: in heterozygotes, the consequences of a recessive allele are hidden. A dominant allele exerts its effect in both the homozygote (HH) and the heterozygote (Hh), whereas the presence of the recessive allele is physically observable only when it occurs in homozygous form (hh). Thus, short pea plants can be created only by crossing parent plants that each carry at least one h allele. An example is a heterozygote×heterozygote cross, shown in Figure 3-2.

In this chapter, we examine mutation as the source of genetic variation. We discuss the types of mutation, the causes and consequences of mutation, and the biochemical and molecular techniques that are now used to detect genetic variation in human populations.

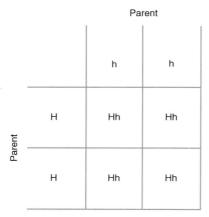

FIG 3-1   Punnett square illustrating a cross between *HH* and *hh* homozygote parents.

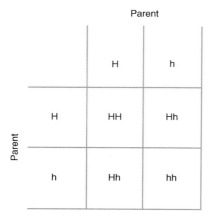

FIG 3-2   Punnett square illustrating a cross between two *Hh* heterozygotes.

MUTATION: THE SOURCE OF GENETIC VARIATION

Types of Mutation

Some mutations consist of an alteration of the number or structure of chromosomes in a cell. These major chromosome abnormalities can be observed microscopically and are the subject of Chapter 6. Here, the focus is on mutations that affect only single genes and are not microscopically observable. Most of our discussion centers on mutations that take place in coding DNA or in regulatory sequences,

because mutations that occur in other parts of the genome usually have no clinical consequences.

One important type of single-gene mutation is the **base-pair substitution**, in which one base pair is replaced by another. In molecular genetics, base-pair substitutions are also termed point mutations. However, "point mutation" was used in classical genetics to denote any mutation small enough to be unobservable under a microscope. Base-pair substitutions can result in a change in the amino acid sequence. However, because of the redundancy of the genetic code, many of these mutations do not change the amino acid sequence and thus typically have no effect. Such mutations are called **silent substitutions**. Base-pair substitutions that alter amino acids consist of two basic types: **missense mutations**, which produce a change in a single amino acid, and **nonsense mutations**, which produce one of the three stop codons (UAA, UAG, or UGA) in the messenger RNA (mRNA) (Fig. 3-3). Because stop codons terminate translation of the mRNA, nonsense mutations result in a premature termination of the polypeptide chain. Conversely, if a stop codon is altered so that it encodes an amino acid, an abnormally elongated polypeptide can be produced. Alterations of amino acid sequences can have profound consequences, and many of the serious genetic diseases discussed later are the result of such alterations.

A second major type of mutation consists of **deletions** or **insertions** of one or more base pairs. These mutations, which can result in extra or missing amino acids in a protein, are often detrimental. An example of such a mutation is the 3-bp deletion that is found in most persons with cystic fibrosis (see Chapter 4). Deletions and insertions tend to be especially harmful when the number of missing or extra base pairs is not a multiple of three. Because codons consist of groups of three base pairs, such insertions or deletions can alter the downstream codons. This is a **frameshift mutation** (Fig. 3-4). For example, the insertion of a single base (an A in the second codon) converts a DNA sequence read as 5′-ACT GAT TGC GTT-3′ to 5′-ACT GAA TTG CGT-3′. This changes the amino acid sequence from Thr-Asp-Cys-Val to

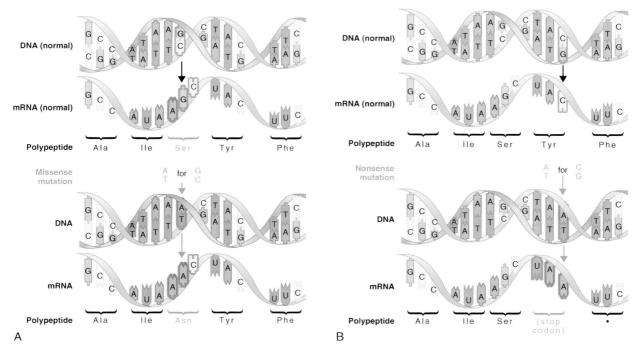

FIG 3-3 Base-pair substitution. Missense mutations (**A**) produce a single amino acid change, whereas nonsense mutations (**B**) produce a stop codon in the mRNA. Stop codons terminate translation of the polypeptide.

Thr-Glu-Leu-Arg. Often, a frameshift mutation produces a stop codon downstream of the insertion or deletion, resulting in a truncated polypeptide.

On a larger scale, **duplications** of whole genes can also lead to genetic disease. A good example is given by Charcot-Marie-Tooth disease. This disorder, named after the three physicians who described it more than a century ago, is a peripheral nervous system condition that leads to progressive atrophy of the distal limb muscles. It affects approximately 1 in 2500 persons and exists in several different forms. About 70% of patients who have the most common form (type 1A) display a 1.5 million-bp duplication on one copy of chromosome 17. As a result, they have three, rather than two, copies of the genes in this region. One of these genes, *PMP22*, encodes a component of peripheral myelin. The increased dosage of the gene product contributes to the demyelination that is characteristic of this form of the disorder. Interestingly, a deletion of this same region produces a different disease, hereditary neuropathy with liability to pressure palsies (paralysis). Because either a reduction (to 50%) or an increase (to 150%) in the gene product produces disease, this gene is said to display **dosage sensitivity**. Base-pair substitutions in *PMP22* itself can produce yet another disease: Dejerine-Sottas syndrome, which is characterized by distal muscle weakness, sensory alterations, muscular atrophy, and enlarged spinal nerve roots.

FIG 3-4 Frameshift mutations result from the addition or deletion of a number of bases that is not a multiple of three. This alters all of the codons downstream from the site of insertion or deletion.

Other types of mutation can alter the regulation of transcription or translation. A **promoter mutation** can decrease the affinity of RNA polymerase for a promoter site, often resulting in reduced production of mRNA and thus decreased production of a protein. Mutations of transcription factor genes or enhancer sequences can have similar effects.

Mutations can also interfere with the splicing of introns as mature mRNA is formed from the primary mRNA transcript. **Splice-site mutations,** those that occur at intron-exon boundaries, alter the splicing signal that is necessary for proper excision of an intron. Splice-site mutations can occur at the GT sequence that defines the 5′ splice site (the **donor site**) or at the AG sequence that defines the 3′ splice site (the **acceptor site**). They can also take place in the sequences that lie near the donor and acceptor sites. When such mutations occur, the excision is often made within the next exon, at a splice site located in the exon. These splice sites, whose DNA sequences differ slightly from those of normal splice sites, are ordinarily unused and hidden within the exon. They are thus termed **cryptic splice sites.** The use of a cryptic site for splicing results in partial deletion of the exon or, in other cases, the deletion of an entire exon. As Figure 3-5 shows, splice-site mutations can also result in the abnormal inclusion of part or all of an intron in the mature mRNA. Finally, a mutation can occur at a cryptic splice site, causing it to appear as a normal splice site and thus to compete with the normal splice site.

Several types of DNA sequences are capable of propagating copies of themselves; these copies are then inserted in other locations on chromosomes (examples include the LINE and *Alu* repeats, discussed in Chapter 2). Such insertions can cause frameshift mutations. The insertion of mobile elements has been shown to cause isolated cases of type 1 neurofibromatosis, Duchenne muscular dystrophy, β-thalassemia, familial breast cancer, familial polypo-

FIG 3-5 **A,** Normal splicing. **B,** Splice-site mutation. The donor sequence, GT, is replaced with AT. This results in an incorrect splice that leaves part of the intron in the mature mRNA transcript. In another example of splice-site mutation (**C**), a second GT donor site is created within the first intron, resulting in a combination of abnormally and normally spliced mRNA products.

sis (colon cancer), and hemophilia A and B (clotting disorders) in humans.

The final type of mutation to be considered here affects tandem repeated DNA sequences (see Chapter 2) that occur within or near certain disease-related genes. The repeat units are usually 3 bp long, so a typical example would be CAGCAGCAG. A normal person has a relatively small number of these tandem repeats (e.g., 10 to 30 CAG consecutive elements) at a specific chromosome location. Occasionally, the number of repeats increases during meiosis or possibly during early fetal development, so that a newborn might have hundreds or even thousands of tandem repeats. When this occurs in certain regions of the genome, it causes genetic disease. Like other mutations, these **expanded repeats** can be transmitted to the patient's offspring. More than 20 genetic diseases are now known to be caused by expanded repeats (see Chapter 4).

▶ Mutations are the ultimate source of genetic variation. Some mutations result in genetic disease, but most have no physical effects. The principal types of mutation are missense, nonsense, frameshift, promoter, and splice-site mutations. Mutations can also be caused by the random insertion of mobile elements, and some genetic diseases are known to be caused by expanded repeats.

Molecular Consequences of Mutation

It is useful to think of mutations in terms of their effects on the protein product. Broadly speaking, mutations can produce either a **gain of function** or a **loss of function** of the protein product (Fig. 3-6). Gain-of-function mutations occasionally result in a completely novel protein product. More commonly, they result in over-expression of the product or inappropriate expression (i.e., in the wrong tissue or in the wrong stage of development). Gain-of-function mutations produce dominant disorders. Charcot-Marie-Tooth disease can result from overexpression of the protein product, which is considered a gain-of-function mutation. Huntington disease, discussed in Chapter 4, is another example.

Loss-of-function mutations are often seen in recessive diseases, where the mutation results in the loss of 50% of the protein product (e.g., a metabolic enzyme) but the 50% that remains is sufficient for normal function. The heterozygote is thus unaffected, but the homozygote, having little or no protein prod-

Allele 1

Allele 2

Gain-of-function mutation produces novel
or excess protein product

A

Allele 1

Allele 2

Loss-of-function mutation reduces or
eliminates protein product

B

Allele 1

Allele 2

Dominant negative mutation (allele 2) produces
abnormal protein product that interferes with
normal protein produced by allele 1

C

FIG 3-6   A, Gain-of-function mutations produce a novel protein product or an increased amount of protein product. **B**, Loss-of-function mutations decrease the amount of protein product. **C**, Dominant negative mutations produce an abnormal protein product that interferes with the otherwise normal protein product of the normal allele in a heterozygote.

uct, is affected. In some cases, however, 50% of the gene's protein product is not sufficient for normal function (**haploinsufficiency**), and a dominant disorder can result. Haploinsufficiency is seen, for example, in the autosomal dominant disorder known as familial hypercholesterolemia (see Chapter 5). In this disease, a single copy of a mutation (heterozygosity) reduces the number of low-density lipoprotein (LDL) receptors by 50%. Cholesterol levels in heterozygotes are approximately double those of normal homozygotes, resulting in a substantial increase in the risk of heart disease. As with most disorders involving haploinsufficiency, the disease is more serious in affected homozygotes (who have few or no functional LDL receptors) than in heterozygotes.

A **dominant negative** mutation results in a protein product that not only is abnormal but also inhibits the function of the protein produced by the normal allele in the heterozygote. Typically, dominant negative mutations are seen in genes that encode multimeric proteins (i.e., proteins composed of two or more subunits). Type I collagen (see Chapter 2), which is composed of three helical subunits, is an example of such a protein. An abnormal helix created by a single mutation can combine with the other helices, distorting them and producing a seriously compromised triple-helix protein.

> Mutations can result in either a gain of function or a loss of function of the protein product. Gain-of-function mutations are sometimes seen in dominant diseases. Loss of function is seen in recessive diseases and in diseases involving haploinsufficiency, in which 50% of the gene product is insufficient for normal function. In dominant negative mutations, the abnormal protein product interferes with the normal protein product.

Clinical Consequences of Mutation: The Hemoglobin Disorders

Genetic disorders of human hemoglobin are the most common group of single-gene diseases (see Chapter 7). Almost all types of mutations are involved in hemoglobin disease. Sickle cell disease, which causes anemia, tissue infarctions, and multiple infections, is the result of a single missense mutation that produces an amino acid substitution in the β-globin chain. The α-thalassemia conditions are usually caused by deletions of α-globin genes. The loss of three of these genes leads to moderately severe anemia, and the loss of all four is fatal. Many different types of mutations can produce β-thalassemia. Nonsense, frameshift, and splice-site donor and acceptor mutations tend to produce more severe disease. Regulatory mutations and those involving splice-site consensus sequences and cryptic splice sites tend to produce less severe disease.

Causes of Mutation

A large number of agents are known to cause **induced mutations.** These mutations, which are attributed to known environmental causes, can be contrasted with **spontaneous mutations,** which arise naturally in cells, for example during DNA replication. Agents that cause induced mutations are known collectively as **mutagens.** Animal studies have shown that **radiation** is an important class of mutagen (Clinical Commentary 3-1). **Ionizing radiation,** such as that produced by X-rays and nuclear fallout, can eject electrons from atoms, forming electrically charged ions. When these ions are situated within or near the DNA molecule, they can promote chemical reactions that change DNA bases. Ionizing radiation can also break the bonds of double-stranded DNA. This form of radiation can reach all cells of the body, including the germline cells.

Nonionizing radiation does not form charged ions but can move electrons from inner to outer orbits within an atom. The atom becomes chemically unstable. Ultraviolet (UV) radiation, which occurs naturally in sunlight, is an example of nonionizing radiation. UV radiation causes the formation of covalent bonds between adjacent pyrimidine bases (i.e., cytosine or thymine). These **pyrimidine dimers** (a dimer is a molecule having two subunits) are unable to pair properly with purines during DNA

CLINICAL COMMENTARY 3-1
The Effects of Radiation on Mutation Rates

Because mutation is a rare event, it is difficult to measure directly in humans. The relationship between radiation exposure and mutation is similarly difficult to assess. For a person living in a developed country, a typical lifetime exposure to ionizing radiation is about 6 to 7 rem.* About one third to one half of this amount is thought to originate from medical and dental X-ray procedures.

Unfortunately, a few human populations have received much larger radiation doses. The most thoroughly studied such population consists of the survivors of the atomic bomb blasts that occurred in Hiroshima and Nagasaki, Japan, at the close of World War Ⅱ. Many of those who were exposed to high doses of radiation died from radiation sickness. Others survived, and many of the survivors produced offspring.

To study the effects of radiation exposure in this population, a large team of Japanese and American scientists conducted medical and genetic investigations of some of the survivors. A significant number developed cancers and chromosome abnormalities in their somatic cells, probably as a consequence of radiation exposure. To assess the effects of radiation exposure on the subjects' germlines, the scientists compared the offspring of those who suffered substantial radiation exposure with the offspring of those who did not. Although it is difficult to establish radiation doses with precision, there is no doubt that, in general, those who were situated closer to the blasts suffered much higher exposure levels. It is estimated that the exposed group received roughly 30 to 60 rem of radiation, many times the average lifetime radiation exposure.

In a sample of more than 76,000 offspring of these survivors, researchers assessed a large number of factors, including stillbirths, chromosome abnormalities, birth defects, cancer before 20 years of age, death before 26 years of age, and various measures of growth and development (e.g., intelligence quotient). There were no statistically significant differences between the offspring of persons who were exposed to radiation and the offspring of those who were not exposed. In addition, direct genetic studies of mutations have been carried out using minisatellite polymorphisms and protein electrophoresis,

a technique that detects mutations that lead to amino acid changes (discussed elsewhere in this chapter). Parents and offspring were compared to determine whether germline mutations had occurred at various loci. The numbers of mutations detected in the exposed and unexposed groups were statistically equivalent.

More recently, studies of those who were exposed to radiation from the Chernobyl nuclear power plant accident have demonstrated a significant increase in thyroid cancers among children exposed to radiation. This reflects the effects of somatic mutations. The evidence for increased frequencies of germline mutations in protein-coding DNA, however, remains unclear. A number of other studies of the effects of radiation on humans have been reported, including investigations of those who live near nuclear power plants. The radiation doses received by these persons are substantially smaller than those of the populations discussed previously, and the results of these studies are equivocal.

It is remarkable that even though there was substantial evidence for radiation effects on somatic cells in the Hiroshima and Nagasaki studies, no detectable effect could be seen for germline cells. What could account for this? Because large doses of radiation are lethal, many of those who would have been most strongly affected would not be included in these studies. Furthermore, because germline mutation rates are very small, even relatively large samples of radiation-exposed persons may be insufficient to detect increases in mutation rates. It is also possible that DNA repair compensated for some radiation-induced germline damage.

These results argue that radiation exposure, which is clearly associated with somatic mutations, should not be taken lightly. Above-ground nuclear testing in the American Southwest has produced increased rates of leukemia and thyroid cancer in a segment of the population. Radon, a radioactive gas that is produced by the decay of naturally occurring uranium, can be found at dangerously high levels in some homes and poses a risk for lung cancer. Any unnecessary exposure to radiation, particularly to the gonads or to developing fetuses, should be avoided.

*A rem is a standard unit for measuring radiation exposure. It is roughly equal to 0.01 joule of absorbed energy per kilogram of tissue.

---

replication; this results in a base-pair substitution (Fig. 3-7). Because UV radiation is absorbed by the skin, it does not reach the germline but can cause skin cancer (Clinical Commentary 3-2).

A variety of chemicals can also induce mutations, sometimes because of their chemical similarity to DNA bases. Because of this similarity, these **base analogs,** such as 5-bromouracil, can be substituted for a true DNA base during replication. The analog is not exactly the same as the base it replaces, so it can cause pairing errors during subsequent replications. Other chemi-

cal mutagens, such as acridine dyes, can physically insert themselves between existing bases, distorting the DNA helix and causing frameshift mutations. Still other mutagens can directly alter DNA bases, causing replication errors. An example of the latter is nitrous acid, which removes an amino group from cytosine, converting it to uracil. Although uracil is normally found in RNA, it mimics the pairing action of thymine in DNA. Thus, it pairs with adenine instead of guanine, as the original cytosine would have done. The end result is a base-pair substitution.

A

B

FIG 3-7 **A**, Pyrimidine dimers originate when covalent bonds form between adjacent pyrimidine (cytosine or thymine) bases. This deforms the DNA, interfering with normal base pairing. **B**, The defect is repaired by removal and replacement of the dimer and bases on either side of it, with the complementary DNA strand used as a template.

CLINICAL COMMENTARY 3-2
Xeroderma Pigmentosum: A Disease of Faulty DNA Repair

An inevitable consequence of exposure to UV radiation is the formation of potentially dangerous pyrimidine dimers in the DNA of skin cells. Fortunately, the highly efficient nucleotide excision repair (NER) system removes these dimers in normal persons. Among those affected with the rare autosomal recessive disease xeroderma pigmentosum (XP), this system does not work properly, and the resulting DNA replication errors lead to base-pair substitutions in skin cells. XP varies substantially in severity, but early symptoms are usually seen in the first 1 to 2 years of life. Patients develop dry, scaly skin (xeroderma) along with extensive freckling and abnormal skin pigmentation (pigmentosum). Skin tumors, which can be numerous, typically appear by 10 years of age. It is estimated that the risk of skin tumors in persons with XP is elevated approximately 1000-fold. These cancers are concentrated primarily in sun-exposed parts of the body. Patients are advised to avoid sources of UV light (e.g., sunlight), and cancerous growths are removed surgically. Neurological abnormalities are seen in about 30% of persons with XP. Severe, potentially lethal malignancies can occur before 20 years of age.

The NER system is encoded by at least 28 different genes, and inherited mutations in any of seven of these genes can give rise to XP. These genes encode helicases that unwind the double-stranded DNA helix; an endonuclease that cuts the DNA at the site of the dimer; an exonuclease that removes the dimer and nearby nucleotides; a polymerase that fills the gap with DNA bases (using the complementary DNA strand as a template); and a ligase that rejoins the corrected portion of DNA to the original strand.

It should be emphasized that the expression of XP requires inherited germline mutations of an NER gene as well as subsequent uncorrected somatic mutations of genes in skin cells. Some of these somatic mutations can affect genes that promote cancer (see Chapter 8), result-ing in tumor formation. The skin-cell mutations themselves are somatic and thus are not transmitted to future generations.

NER is but one type of DNA repair. The table below provides examples of a number of other diseases that result from defects in various types of DNA repair mechanisms (Fig. 3-8) (Table 3-1).

FIG 3-8 Xeroderma pigmentosum. This patient's skin has multiple hyperpigmented lesions, and skin tumors on the forehead have been marked for excision.

CLINICAL COMMENTARY 3-2
Xeroderma Pigmentosum: A Disease of Faulty DNA Repair (Continued)

TABLE 3-1	Examples of Diseases That Are Caused by a Defect in DNA Repair	
DISEASE	**FEATURES**	**TYPE OF REPAIR DEFECT**
Xeroderma pigmentosum	Skin tumors, photosensitivity, cataracts, neurological abnormalities	Nucleotide excision repair defects, including mutations in helicase and endonuclease genes
Cockayne syndrome	Reduced stature, skeletal abnormalities, optic atrophy, deafness, photosensitivity, mental retardation	Defective repair of UV-induced damage in transcriptionally active DNA; considerable etiological and symptomatic overlap with xeroderma pigmentosum and trichothiodystrophy
Fanconi anemia	Anemia; leukemia susceptibility; limb, kidney, and heart malformations; chromosome instability	As many as eight different genes may be involved, but their exact role in DNA repair is not yet known
Bloom syndrome	Growth deficiency, immunodeficiency, chromosome instability, increased cancer incidence	Mutations in the reqQ helicase family
Werner syndrome	Cataracts, osteoporosis, atherosclerosis, loss of skin elasticity, short stature, diabetes, increased cancer incidence; sometimes described as "premature aging"	Mutations in the reqQ helicase family
Ataxia-telangiectasia	Cerebellar ataxia, telangiectases,* immune deficiency, increased cancer incidence, chromosome instability	Normal gene product is likely to be involved in halting the cell cycle after DNA damage occurs
Hereditary nonpolyposis colorectal cancer	Proximal bowel tumors, increased susceptibility to several other types of cancer	Mutations in any of six DNA mismatch-repair genes

*Telangiectases are vascular lesions caused by the dilatation of small blood vessels. This typically produces discoloration of the skin.

Hundreds of chemicals are now known to be mutagenic in laboratory animals. Among these are nitrogen mustard, vinyl chloride, alkylating agents, formaldehyde, sodium nitrite, and saccharin. Some of these chemicals are much more potent mutagens than others. Nitrogen mustard, for example, is a powerful mutagen, whereas saccharin is a relatively weak one. Although some mutagenic chemicals are produced by humans, many occur naturally in the environment (e.g., aflatoxin B1, a common contaminant of foods).

 Many substances in the environment are known to be mutagenic, including ionizing and nonionizing radiation and hundreds of different chemicals. These mutagens are capable of causing base substitutions, deletions, and frameshifts. Ionizing radiation can induce double-stranded DNA breaks. Some mutagens occur naturally, and others are generated by humans.

DNA Repair

Considering that 3 billion DNA base pairs must be replicated in each cell division, and considering the large number of mutagens to which we are exposed, DNA replication is surprisingly accurate. A primary reason for this accuracy is the process of **DNA repair**, which takes place in all normal cells of higher organisms. Several dozen enzymes are involved in the repair of damaged DNA. They collectively recognize an altered base, excise it by cutting the DNA strand, replace it with the correct base (determined from the complementary strand), and reseal the DNA. These repair mechanisms are estimated to correct at least 99.9% of initial errors.

Because DNA repair is essential for the accurate replication of DNA, defects in DNA repair systems can lead to many types of disease. For example, inherited mutations in genes responsible for **DNA mismatch repair** result in the persistence of cells with replication errors (i.e., **mismatches**) and can lead to some types of cancer (see Chapter 8). A diminished capacity to repair **double-stranded DNA breaks** can lead to ovarian and/or breast cancer. **Nucleotide excision repair** is necessary for the removal of larger changes in the DNA helix (e.g., pyrimidine dimers); defects in excision repair lead to a number of diseases, of which xeroderma pigmentosum is an important example (see Clinical Commentary 3-2).

 DNA repair helps to ensure the accuracy of the DNA sequence by correcting replication errors (mismatches), repairing double-stranded DNA breaks, and excising damaged nucleotides.

Mutation Rates

How often do spontaneous mutations occur? At the nucleotide level, the mutation rate is estimated to be about 10^{-8} per base pair per generation (this figure represents mutations that have escaped the process of DNA repair). Thus, each gamete contains approximately 30 new mutations, the great majority of which occur in noncoding DNA. At the level of the gene, the mutation rate is quite variable, ranging from 10^{-4} to 10^{-7} per locus per cell division. There are at least two reasons for this large range of varia-

tion: the size of the gene and the susceptibility of certain nucleotide sequences.

First, genes vary tremendously in size. The somatostatin gene, for example, is quite small, containing 1480 bp. In contrast, the gene responsible for Duchenne muscular dystrophy (*DMD*) spans more than 2 million bp. As might be expected, larger genes present larger targets for mutation and usually experience mutation more often than do smaller genes. The *DMD* gene, as well as the genes responsible for hemophilia A and type 1 neurofibromatosis, are all very large and have high mutation rates.

Second, it is well established that certain nucleotide sequences are especially susceptible to mutation. These are termed **mutation hot spots**. The best-known example is the two-base (**dinucleotide**) sequence CG. In mammals, about 80% of CG dinucleotides are **methylated**: a methyl group is attached to the cytosine base (these dinucleotide sequences are also labeled CpG [cytosine-phosphate-guanine], to distinguish the two-base DNA sequence from a single pair of complementary bases, C and G). A methylated cytosine, 5-methylcytosine, easily loses an amino group, converting it to thymine. The end result is a mutation from cytosine to thymine (Fig. 3-9). Surveys of mutations in human genetic diseases have shown that the mutation rate at CG dinucleotides is about 12 times higher than at other dinucleotide sequences. Mutation hot spots, in the form of CG dinucleotides, have been identified in a number of important human disease genes, including the procollagen genes responsible for osteogenesis imperfecta (see Chapter 2). Other disease examples are

FIG 3-9 Cytosine methylation. The addition of a methyl group (CH₃) to a cytosine base forms 5-methylcytosine. The subsequent loss of an amino group (deamination) forms thymine. The result is a cytosine → thymine substitution.

discussed in Chapter 4.

Parental age is strongly correlated with the probability of transmitting a mutation to one's offspring. Some chromosome abnormalities increase dramatically with maternal age (see Chapter 6), and single-gene mutations increase with paternal age. The latter is seen in several single-gene disorders, including Marfan syndrome and achondroplasia. As Figure 3-10 shows, the risk of producing a child with Marfan syndrome is several times higher for a father older than 40 years than for a father in his 20s. This paternal age effect is usually attributed to the fact that the stem cells giving rise to sperm cells continue to divide throughout life, which allows a progressive buildup of DNA replication errors. Recent comparisons of whole genome sequences in parents and offspring estimate that approximately two additional mutations are transmitted with each additional year of paternal age.

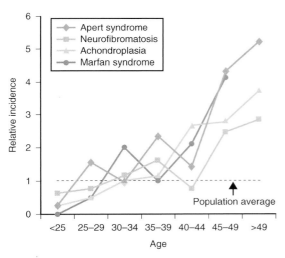

FIG 3-10 Paternal age effect. For some single-gene disorders, the risk of producing a child with the condition (*y-axis*) increases with the father's age (*x-axis*).

Large genes, because of their size, are generally more likely to experience mutations than are small genes. Mutation hot spots, particularly methylated CG dinucleotides, experience elevated mutation rates. For many single-gene disorders, there is a substantial increase in mutation risk with advanced paternal age.

DETECTION AND MEASUREMENT OF GENETIC VARIATION

For centuries, humans have been intrigued by the differences that can be seen among individuals. Attention was long focused on observable differences such as skin color or body shape and size. Only in the 20th century did it become possible to examine variation in genes, the consequence of mutations accumulated through time. The evaluation and measurement of this variation in populations and families are important for mapping genes to specific locations on chromosomes, a key step in determining gene function. The evaluation of genetic variation also provides the basis for genetic diagnosis, and it is highly useful in forensics. In this section, several key approaches to detecting genetic variation in humans are discussed in historical sequence.

Blood Groups

Several dozen **blood group** systems have been defined on the basis of antigens located on the surfaces of erythrocytes. Some are involved in determining whether a person can receive a blood transfusion from a specific donor. Because individuals differ extensively in terms of blood groups, these systems provided an important early means of assessing genetic variation.

Each of the blood group systems is determined by a different gene or set of genes. The various antigens that can be expressed within a system are the result of different DNA sequences in these genes. Two blood-group systems that have special medical significance—the ABO and Rh blood groups—are discussed here. The ABO and Rh systems are both important in determining the compatibility of blood transfusions and tissue grafts. Some combinations of these blood groups can produce maternal-fetal incompatibility, sometimes with serious results for the fetus. These issues are discussed in detail in Chapter 9.

The ABO Blood Group

Human blood transfusions were carried out as early as 1818, but they were often unsuccessful. After transfusion, some recipients suffered a massive, sometimes fatal, hemolytic reaction. In 1900 Karl Landsteiner discovered that this reaction was caused by the ABO antigens located on erythrocyte surfaces. The ABO system consists of two major antigens, labeled A and B. A person can have one of four major blood types: people with blood type A carry the A antigen on their erythrocytes, those with type B carry the B antigen, those with type AB carry both A and B, and those with type O carry neither antigen. Each individual has antibodies that react against any antigens that are not found on their own red blood cell surfaces. For example, a person with type A blood has anti-B antibodies, and transfusing type B blood into this person provokes a severe antibody reaction. It is straightforward to determine ABO blood type in the laboratory by mixing a small sample of a person's blood with solutions containing different antibodies and observing which combinations cause the observable clumping that is characteristic of an antibody-antigen interaction.

The ABO system, which is encoded by a single gene on chromosome 9, consists of three primary alleles, labeled I^A, I^B, and I^O. (There are also subtypes of both the I^A and I^B alleles, but they are not addressed here.) Persons with the I^A allele have the A antigen on their erythrocyte surfaces (blood type A), and those with I^B have the B antigen on their cell surfaces (blood type B). Those with both alleles express both antigens (blood type AB), and those with two copies of the I^O allele have neither antigen (type O blood). Because the I^O allele produces no antigen, persons who are $I^A I^O$ or $I^B I^O$ heterozygotes have blood types A and B, respectively (Table 3-2).

Because populations vary substantially in terms of the frequency with which the ABO alleles occur,

the ABO locus was the first blood group system to be used extensively in studies of genetic variation among individuals and populations. For example, early studies showed that the A antigen is relatively common in western European populations, and the B antigen is especially common among Asians. Neither antigen is common among native South American populations, the great majority of whom have blood type O.

The Rh System

Like the ABO system, the Rh system is defined on the basis of antigens that are present on erythrocyte surfaces. This system is named after the rhesus monkey, the experimental animal in which it was first isolated by Landsteiner in the late 1930s. It is typed in the laboratory by a procedure similar to the one described for the ABO system. Rh alleles vary considerably among individuals and populations and thus have been another highly useful tool for assessing genetic variation. The molecular basis of variation in both the ABO and the Rh systems has been elucidated (for further details, see the suggested readings at the end of this chapter), and it is becoming increasingly common to type these systems by directly examining an individual's DNA sequence rather than by assessing an antibody-antigen reaction.

The blood groups, of which the ABO and Rh systems are examples, have provided an important means of studying human genetic variation. Blood group variation is the result of antigens that occur on the surface of erythrocytes.

Protein Electrophoresis

Protein electrophoresis, developed first in the 1930s and applied widely to humans in the 1950s and 1960s, increased the number of detectable polymorphic loci considerably. This technique makes use of the fact that a single amino acid difference in a protein (the result of a mutation in the corresponding DNA sequence) can cause a slight difference in the electrical charge of the protein.

TABLE 3-2 Relationship between ABO Genotype and Blood Type		
GENOTYPE	**BLOOD TYPE**	**ANTIBODIES PRESENT**
$I^A I^A$	A	Anti-B
$I^A I^O$	A	Anti-B
$I^B I^B$	B	Anti-A
$I^B I^O$	B	Anti-A
$I^A I^B$	AB	None
$I^O I^O$	O	Anti-A and anti-B

An example is the common sickle cell disease mutation discussed earlier. The replacement of glutamic acid with valine in the β-globin chain produces a difference in electrical charge because glutamic acid has two carboxyl groups, whereas valine has only one carboxyl group. Electrophoresis can be used to determine whether a person has normal hemoglobin (HbA) or the mutation that causes sickle cell disease (HbS) (Fig. 3-11). The hemoglobin is placed in an electrically charged gel composed of starch, agarose, or polyacrylamide (see Fig. 3-11, A). The slight difference in charge resulting from the amino acid difference causes the HbA and HbS forms to migrate at different rates through the gel. The protein molecules are allowed to migrate for several hours and are then stained with chemical solutions so that their positions can be seen (see Fig. 3-11, B). From the resulting pattern it can be determined whether the person is an HbA homozygote, an HbS homozygote, or a heterozygote having HbA on one chromosome copy and HbS on the other.

Protein electrophoresis has been used to detect amino acid variation in hundreds of human proteins. However, silent substitutions, which do not alter amino acids, cannot be detected by this approach. In addition, some amino acid substitutions do not alter the electrical charge of the protein molecule. For these reasons, protein electrophoresis detects only about one third of the mutations that occur in coding DNA. In addition, single-base substitutions in noncoding DNA are not usually detected by protein electrophoresis.

> Protein electrophoresis detects variations in genes that encode certain serum proteins. These variations are observable because proteins with slight differences in their amino acid sequence migrate at different rates through electrically charged gels.

Detecting Variation at the DNA Level

Each human haploid DNA sequence (i.e., the sequence inherited from one parent) differs from

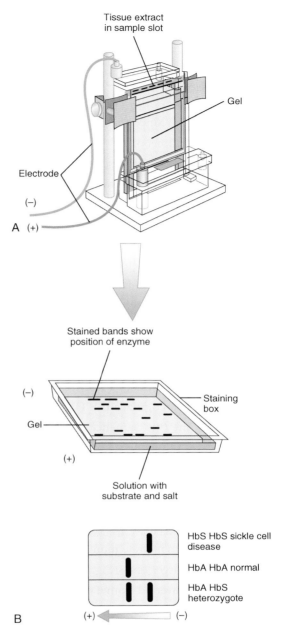

FIG 3-11   The process of protein electrophoresis. **A**, A tissue sample is loaded in the slot at the top of the gel, and an electrical current is run though the gel. After staining, distinct bands, representing molecules with different electrical charges and therefore different amino acid sequences, are visible. **B**, HbA homozygotes show a single band closer to the positive pole, whereas HbS homozygotes show a single band closer to the negative pole. Heterozygotes, having both alleles, show two bands.

any other human haploid sequence by at least three to four million DNA base pairs, which amounts to one single-base difference every 1000 base pairs. Because there are only a few hundred or so blood group and protein electrophoretic polymorphisms, these approaches have detected only a tiny fraction of human DNA variation. Yet the assessment of this variation is critical to gene identification and genetic diagnosis (see Chapters 10). Fortunately, molecular techniques developed since the 1980s have enabled the detection of millions of new polymorphisms at the DNA level. These techniques, which have revolutionized both the practice and the potential of medical genetics, are discussed next.

Southern Blotting and Restriction Fragment Analysis

An early approach to the detection of genetic variation at the DNA level took advantage of the existence of bacterial enzymes known as **restriction endonucleases,** or **restriction enzymes.** These enzymes cleave human DNA at specific sequences, termed restriction sites. For example, the intestinal bacterium *Escherichia coli* produces a restriction enzyme, called *Eco*RI, that recognizes the DNA sequence GAATTC. Each time this sequence is encountered, the enzyme cleaves the sequence between the G and the A (Fig. 3-12). A **restriction digest** of human DNA using this enzyme will produce more than 1 million DNA fragments (**restriction fragments**). These fragments are then subjected to gel electrophoresis, in which the smaller ones migrate more quickly through the gel than do the larger ones (Fig. 3-13). The DNA is denatured (i.e., converted from a double- stranded to a single-stranded form) by exposing it to alkaline chemical solutions. To fix their positions permanently, the DNA fragments are transferred from the gel to a solid membrane, such as nitrocellulose (this is a **Southern transfer,** after the man who invented the process in the mid-1970s). At this point, the solid membrane, often called a **Southern blot,** contains

FIG 3-13   Restriction enzyme digestion and Southern blotting. DNA is extracted from blood samples from subjects **A**, **B**, and **C**. The DNA is digested by a restriction enzyme and then loaded on a gel. Electrophoresis separates the DNA fragments according to their size. The DNA is denatured and transferred to a solid membrane (Southern blot), where it is hybridized with a radioactive probe. Exposure to X-ray film (autoradiography) reveals specific DNA fragments (bands) of different sizes in individuals **A**, **B**, and **C**.

FIG 3-12   Cleavage of DNA by the *Eco*RI restriction enzyme. In **B**, the enzyme cleaves the three GAATTC recognition sequences, producing two smaller fragments. In **A**, the middle sequence is GAATTT instead of GAATTC, so it cannot be cleaved by the enzyme. The result is a single, longer fragment.

many thousands of fragments arrayed according to their size. Because of their large number, the fragments are indistinguishable from one another.

To visualize only the fragments corresponding to a specific region of DNA, a **probe,** consisting of a small piece of single-stranded human DNA (a few kilobases [kb] in length), is constructed using recombinant DNA techniques (Box 3-1) (Fig. 3-14). The probe is labeled, often with a radioactive isotope, and then exposed to the Southern blot. The probe undergoes complementary base pairing only with the corresponding complementary single-stranded DNA fragments on the blot identifying one or a few fragments from a specific portion of the DNA. To visualize the position on the blot at which the probe hybridizes, the blot is exposed to X-ray film, which darkens at the probe's position due to the emission

of radioactive particles from the labeled probe. These darkened positions are usually referred to as **bands,** and the film is termed an **autoradiogram** (Fig. 3-15).

Southern blotting can be used in several ways. For example, it can detect insertions or deletions in DNA sequences, which cause specific fragments to become larger or smaller. If a disease-causing mutation alters a specific restriction site, as in the case of sickle cell disease (Fig. 3-16), this technique can be used as a cheap and efficient diagnostic tool. Because most disease-causing mutations do not affect restriction sites, this approach is somewhat limited, and other, newer techniques can be used. Finally, Southern blotting was instrumental in analyzing **restriction fragment length polymorphisms (RFLPs),** which are found throughout the human genome as a result of normal DNA sequence variation. These sequence

---

BOX 3-1   Genetic Engineering, Recombinant DNA, and Cloning

In the last two decades, most of the lay public has acquired at least a passing familiarity with the terms "recombinant DNA," "cloning," and "genetic engineering." Indeed, these techniques lie at the heart of what is often called the "new genetics."

Genetic engineering refers to the laboratory alteration of genes. An alteration that is of special importance in medical genetics is the creation of **clones.** Briefly, a clone is an identical copy of a DNA sequence. The following description outlines one approach to the cloning of human genes.

Our goal is to insert a human DNA sequence into a rapidly reproducing organism so that copies (clones) of the DNA can be made quickly. One system commonly used for this purpose is the **plasmid,** which is a small, circular, self-replicating piece of DNA that resides in many bacteria. Plasmids can be removed from bacteria or inserted into them without seriously disrupting bacterial growth or reproduction.

To insert human DNA into the plasmid, we need a way to cut DNA into pieces so that it can be manipulated. Restriction enzymes, discussed earlier in the text, perform this function efficiently. The DNA sequence recognized by the restriction enzyme *Eco*RI, GAATTC, has the convenient property that its complementary sequence, CTTAAG, is the same sequence, except backward. Such sequences are called **palindromes.** When plasmid or human DNA is cleaved with *Eco*RI, the resulting fragments have sticky ends. If human DNA and plasmid DNA are both cut with this enzyme, both types of DNA fragments contain exposed ends that can undergo complementary base pairing with each other. Then, when the human and plasmid DNA are mixed together, they recombine (hence the term **recombinant DNA**). The resulting plasmids contain human DNA **inserts.** The plasmids are

inserted back into bacteria, where they reproduce rapidly through natural cell division. The human DNA sequence, which is reproduced along with the other plasmid DNA, is thus cloned (Fig. 3-14).

The plasmid is referred to as a **vector.** Several other types of vectors may also be used as cloning vehicles, including **bacteriophages** (viruses that infect bacteria), **cosmids** (phage-plasmid hybrids capable of carrying relatively large DNA inserts), **yeast artificial chromosomes (YACs;** vectors that are inserted into yeast cells and that behave much like ordinary yeast chromosomes), **bacterial artificial chromosomes (BACs),** and **human artificial chromosomes** (see Chapters 10). Although plasmids and bacteriophages can accommodate only relatively small inserts (about 10 and 20 kb, respectively), cosmids can carry inserts of approximately 50 kb, and YACs can carry inserts up to 1000 kb in length.

Cloning can be used to create the thousands of copies of human DNA needed for Southern blotting and other experimental applications. In addition, this approach is now used to produce genetically engineered therapeutic products, such as insulin, interferon, human growth hormone, clotting factor VIII (used in the treatment of hemophilia A, a coagulation disorder), and tissue plasminogen activator (a blood clot-dissolving protein that helps to prevent heart attacks and strokes). When these genes are cloned into bacteria or other organisms, the organism produces the human gene product along with its own gene products. In the past, these products were obtained from donor blood or from other animals. The processes of obtaining and purifying them were slow and costly, and the resulting products sometimes contained contaminants. Genetically engineered gene products are rapidly becoming a cheaper, purer, and more efficient alternative.

BOX 3-1   Genetic Engineering, Recombinant DNA, and Cloning (Continued)

FIG 3-14 Recombinant DNA technology. Human and circular plasmid DNA are both cleaved by a restriction enzyme, producing sticky ends (*1-3*). This allows the human DNA to anneal and recombine with the plasmid DNA. Inserted into the plasmid DNA, the human DNA is now replicated when the plasmid is inserted into the *Escherichia coli* bacterium (*4*).

variants were used to localize many important disease-causing genes, including those responsible for cystic fibrosis, Huntington disease, and type 1 neurofibromatosis.

 Restriction enzymes can cut DNA into fragments, which are sorted according to their length by electrophoresis, transferred to a solid membrane (Southern blotting), and visualized through the use of labeled probes. This process can detect deletions or duplications of DNA, as well as RFLPs.

Tandem Repeat Polymorphisms

The approach just described can detect polymorphisms that reflect the presence or absence of a restriction site. These polymorphisms have only two possible alleles, placing a limit on the amount of genetic diversity that can be seen. More diversity

FIG 3-15 An autoradiogram, showing the positions of a 4.1-kb band and a 3.3-kb band. Each lane represents DNA from a subject in the family whose pedigree is shown above the autoradiogram.

could be observed if a polymorphic system had many alleles, rather than just two. One such system exploits the microsatellites and minisatellites that exist throughout the genome. As discussed in Chapter 2, these are regions in which the same DNA sequence is repeated over and over, in tandem (Fig. 3-17). Microsatellites are typically composed of units that are only 2 to 5 bp long, whereas minisatellites contain longer repeat units. The genetic variation measured is the number of repeats in a given region, which varies substantially from individual to individual: a specific region could have as few as two or three repeats or as many as 20 or more. These polymorphisms can therefore reveal a high degree of genetic variation. Minisatellite polymorphisms are termed **variable**

FIG 3-16 Cleavage of β-globin DNA by the *Mst*II restriction enzyme. Normal individuals have glutamic acid at position 6 of the β-globin polypeptide. Glutamic acid is encoded by the DNA sequence GAG. The sickle cell mutation results in the sequence GTG at this site instead of GAG, causing valine to be substituted for glutamic acid. The restriction enzyme *Mst*II recognizes the DNA sequence CCTNAGG (the *N* signifies that the enzyme will recognize any DNA base, including G, in this position). Thus, *Mst*II recognizes and cleaves the DNA sequence of the normal chromosome at this site as well as at the restriction sites on either side of it. The sickle cell mutation removes an *Mst*II recognition site, producing a longer, 1.3-kb fragment. The normal DNA sequence includes the restriction site (i.e., the sequence CCTGAG instead of CCT-GTG), so a shorter, 1.1-kb fragment is produced. Therefore, on the autoradiogram, sickle cell homozygotes have a single 1.3-kb band, normal homozygotes have a single 1.1-kb band, and heterozygotes have both the 1.1-kb and the 1.3-kb bands. Because shorter fragments migrate farther on a gel, the two fragment sizes can easily be distinguished after hybridization of the blot with a probe containing DNA from the β-globin gene. Note that the banding pattern here, based on DNA sequence differences, resembles the banding pattern shown in Figure 3-11, which is based on hemoglobin amino acid sequences detected by protein electrophoresis.

FIG 3-17 Tandem repeat polymorphisms. Bands of differing length **(A and B)** are created by different numbers of tandem repeats in the DNA on the two copies of a chromosome. Following amplification and labeling of the region that contains the polymorphism, different fragment lengths are separated by electrophoresis and visualized on an autoradiogram.

number of tandem repeats (VNTR), and microsatellite polymorphisms are termed **short tandem repeats (STRs)**. The latter are especially easy to assay, and tens of thousands of them are distributed throughout the human genome. These properties make them useful for mapping genes by the process of linkage analysis, discussed in Chapter 8. Both types of polymorphisms are useful in forensic applications, such as paternity testing and the identification of criminal suspects (Box 3-2) (Fig. 3-18).

BOX 3-2   DNA Profiles in the Forensic Setting

Because of the large number of polymorphisms observed in the human genome, it is virtually certain that each of us is genetically unique (with the exception of identical twins, whose DNA sequences are nearly always identical). It follows that genetic variation could be used to identify individuals, much as a conventional fingerprint does. Because DNA can be found in any tissue sample, including blood, semen, and hair,* genetic variation has substantial potential in forensic applications (e.g., criminal cases, paternity suits, identification of accident victims). STRs, with their many alleles, are very useful in establishing a highly specific **DNA profile.**

The principle underlying a DNA profile is quite simple. If we examine enough polymorphisms in a given individual, the probability that any other individual in the population has the same allele at each examined locus becomes extremely small. DNA left at the scene of a crime in the form of blood or semen, for example, can be typed for a series of STRs. Because of the extreme sensitivity of the PCR approach, even a tiny sample several years old can yield enough DNA for laboratory analysis (although extreme care must be taken to avoid contamination when using PCR with such samples). The detected alleles are then compared with the alleles of a suspect. If the alleles in the two samples match, the suspect is implicated (Fig. 3-18).

A key question is whether another person in the general population might have the same alleles as the suspect. Could the DNA profile then falsely implicate the wrong person? In criminal cases, the probability of obtaining an allele match with a random member of the population is calculated. Because of the high degree of allelic variation in STRs, this probability is usually very small. The use of 13 STRs, which is now common practice, yields random match or more probabilities in the neighborhood of 1 in 1 trillion. Provided that a large enough number of loci are used under well-controlled laboratory conditions, and provided that the data are collected and evaluated carefully, DNA profiles can furnish highly useful forensic evidence. DNA profiles are now used in many thousands of criminal court cases each year.

Although we tend to think of such evidence in terms of identifying the guilty party, it should be kept in mind that when a match is not obtained, a suspect may be exonerated. In addition, postconviction DNA testing has resulted in the release of hundreds of persons who were wrongly imprisoned. Thus, DNA profiles can also benefit the innocent.

FIG 3-18   DNA profiles. **A,** An autoradiogram shows that the band pattern of DNA from suspect 1 does not match the DNA taken from the crime scene (3), whereas the band pattern from suspect 2 does match. In practice, multiple STRs are assayed to reduce the possibility of a false match. **B,** STRs are now commonly assayed using a capillary gel apparatus. The resulting STR profile is displayed as an electropherogram, in which the locations of peaks indicate the lengths (in base pairs) of each STR allele. (Panel **A** courtesy Jay Henry, Criminalistics Laboratory, Department of Public Safety, State of Utah.)

---

*Even fingerprints left at a crime scene sometimes contain enough DNA for PCR amplification and DNA profiling.

VNTRs are a type of polymorphism that results from varying numbers of minisatellite repeats in a specific DNA region. STRs are a similar type of polymorphism that results from varying numbers of smaller, microsatellite repeats. Because VNTRs and STRs can have many different alleles in a population, they are especially useful in medical genetics and forensics.

Single Nucleotide Polymorphisms

The most numerous type of polymorphism in the human genome consists of variants at single nucleotide positions on a chromosome, or **single nucleotide polymorphisms (SNPs).** RFLPs, which are usually caused by single-base differences that occur only at restriction sites, are a subset of the more general set of SNPs. These polymorphisms, when they occur in functional DNA sequences, can cause inherited diseases, although most are harmless. Increasingly, they are being detected by microarray and direct sequencing methods, which are discussed later in this chapter.

Copy Number Variants

Throughout the human genome, there are sections of DNA that vary in their number of copies from one individual to another. These **copy number variants (CNVs),** typically defined as DNA sequences larger than 1000 base pairs, may be present in zero to more than a dozen copies in a haploid genome. Each human is heterozygous for at least 100 CNVs (i.e., he or she inherited a different number of copies from the mother than from the father). Although CNVs are much less numerous than SNPs, their large individual size means that they account for several million total base pair differences between any pair of haploid DNA sequences (roughly the same amount as SNPs). Some CNVs have been shown to be associated with inherited diseases, and some are associated with response to specific therapeutic drugs. Figure 3-19 highlights the differences among RFLPs, tandem repeats, SNPs, and CNVs.

SNPs are the most common type of variation in the human genome. CNVs consist of differences in the number of repeated DNA sequences longer than 1000 bp.

FIG 3-19   A, Restriction fragment length polymorphisms (RFLPs) result from DNA sequence differences that occur at restriction sites in the human genome. The locations of these sites are identified by hybridizing restriction fragments with cloned probes. **B,** Tandem repeats consist of short segments of DNA (microsatellites) or somewhat longer segments (minisatellites whose lengths can be 14 to 500 bp) that are repeated over and over, in tandem. **C,** Copy number variants (CNVs) represent differences in the numbers of larger repeated segments of DNA (>1000 bp to 2 million bp). **D,** Single nucleotide polymorphisms (SNPs) are single-base variations in the genome.

DNA Amplification Using the Polymerase Chain Reaction

Because the DNA molecule is tiny, it is not possible to visualize DNA variation (i.e., different base pairs) directly. All methods of assessing DNA variation involve indirect assessment, as in the use of labeled probes to bind to specific DNA regions in Southern blotting.

Nearly all methods of visualizing DNA variation require indirect labeling of DNA. To observe the labels, multiple copies must be made. For example, bacteria can be used to make thousands of cloned copies of the labeled probes used in Southern blotting. However, this process (see Box 3-1) is time-consuming, often requiring several days or more, and it typically requires a relatively large amount of DNA from the subject (several micrograms). An alternative process, the **polymerase chain reaction (PCR),** was developed in the mid-1980s and has made the detection of genetic variation at the DNA level much more efficient. Essentially, PCR is an artificial means of replicating a short, specific **DNA sequence** (several kb or less) very quickly, so that millions of copies of the sequence are made.

The PCR process, summarized in Figure 3-20, requires four components:

- Two **primers,** each consisting of 15 to 20 bases of DNA. These small DNA sequences are termed **oligonucleotides** (*oligo* means "a few"). The primers correspond to the DNA sequences immediately adjacent to the sequence of interest (such as a sequence that contains a tandem repeat polymorphism or a mutation that causes disease). The oligonucleotide primers are synthesized using a laboratory instrument.
- DNA polymerase. A thermally stable form of this enzyme, initially derived from the bacterium *Thermus aquaticus*, performs the vital process of DNA replication (here termed **primer extension**).
- A large number of free DNA nucleotides.
- Genomic DNA from an individual. Because of the extreme sensitivity of PCR, the quantity of this DNA can be very small.

The genomic DNA is first heated to a relatively high temperature (approximately 95℃) so that

it denatures and becomes single-stranded. As the single-stranded DNA is then cooled to a temperature of approximately 35℃ to 65℃, it is exposed to large quantities of single-stranded primers, which hybridize, or anneal, to a specific location in the genomic

FIG 3-20   The polymerase chain reaction process. Genomic DNA is first heated and denatured to form single strands. In the annealing phase, the DNA is cooled, allowing hybridization with primer sequences that flank the region of interest. Then the reaction is heated to an intermediate primer extension temperature, and in this step the DNA polymerase adds free bases in the 3′ direction along each single strand, starting at the primer. Blunt-ended DNA fragments are formed, and these provide a template for the next cycle of heating and cooling. Repeated cycling produces a large number of DNA fragments bounded on each end by the primer sequence.

DNA that contains the appropriate complementary bases. The DNA is then heated to an intermediate temperature (70℃ to 75℃). In the presence of a large number of free DNA bases, a new DNA strand is synthesized by the DNA polymerase at this temperature, extending from the primer sequence. The newly synthesized DNA consists of a double strand that has the 5′ end of the primer at one end, followed by the bases added through primer extension by DNA polymerase. This double-stranded DNA is heated to a high temperature again, causing it to denature. The heating-and- cooling cycle is then repeated. Now, the newly synthesized DNA serves as the template for further synthesis. As the cooling-and-heating cycles are repeated, the primer-bounded DNA products are amplified geometrically: the number of copies doubles in each cycle (i.e., 2, 4, 8, 16, etc.). This is why the process is termed a *chain reaction*. Typically, the cycles are repeated 20 to 30 times, producing millions of copies of the original DNA. In summary, the PCR process consists of three basic steps: DNA denaturing at high temperature, primer hybridization at a low temperature, and primer extension at an intermediate temperature. The result is a product that consists almost entirely of a specific DNA sequence.

Because each heating-and-cooling cycle requires only a few minutes or less, a single molecule of DNA can be amplified to make millions of copies in only a few hours. Because the procedure is simple and entirely self-contained, inexpensive machines have been developed to automate it completely. Once the DNA is amplified, it can be analyzed in a variety of ways.

PCR has several advantages over older techniques. First, it can be used with extremely small quantities of DNA (usually nanogram amounts, as opposed to the micrograms required for cloning). The amount of DNA in a several-year-old blood stain, a single hair, or even the back of a licked postage stamp is often sufficient for analysis. Second, because it does not require cloning, the procedure is much faster than older techniques. Genetic testing for sickle cell disease, for example, can be done in a single day with

PCR. Finally, because PCR can make large quantities of very pure DNA, it is less often necessary to use radioactive probes to detect specific DNA sequences or mutations. Instead, safer, nonradioactive substances, such as biotin, can be used.

PCR does have some disadvantages. First, primer synthesis requires identification of the DNA sequence flanking the DNA of interest. If this sequence is ambiguous, other techniques must be used. Second, the extreme sensitivity of PCR makes it susceptible to contamination in the laboratory. A number of precautions are commonly taken to guard against contamination. Finally, because it can be difficult to apply PCR to sequences longer than a few kilobases, it is not typically useful for detecting larger deletions (i.e., it is difficult or impossible to amplify the longer, normal sequence). Southern blotting or other techniques are used instead.

Because PCR is such a powerful and versatile technique, it is now used extensively in genetic disease diagnosis, forensic medicine, and evolutionary genetics. PCR is so sensitive that it has been used to analyze DNA from ancient mummies and even from Neanderthal specimens more than 30,000 years old. Analysis of these specimens showed that modern humans are genetically distinct from Neanderthals but that most modern humans have a small amount of Neanderthal DNA (1%-3%) in their genomes.

PCR provides a convenient and efficient means of making millions of copies of a short DNA sequence. Heating-and-cooling cycles are used to denature DNA and then build new copies of a specific, primer-bounded sequence. Because of its speed and ease of use, this technique is now widely used for assessing genetic variation, for diagnosing genetic diseases, and for performing forensic investigations.

DNA Sequencing

In many genetic studies, a primary goal is to determine the actual array of DNA base pairs that makes up a gene or part of a gene. Such a **DNA sequence** can indicate a great deal about the nature of a specific mutation, the function of a gene, and the gene's degree of similarity to other known genes. We first discuss a technique that has been widely used to determine DNA sequences.

The **dideoxy method** of DNA sequencing, invented by Frederick Sanger, makes use of chain-terminating dideoxynucleotides. These are chemically quite similar to ordinary deoxynucleotides, except that they are missing one hydroxyl group. This prevents the subsequent formation of phosphodiester bonds with free DNA bases. Thus, although dideoxynucleotides can be incorporated into a growing DNA helix, no additional nucleotides can be added once they are included.

Four different dideoxynucleotides are used, each corresponding to one of the four nucleotides (A, C, G, and T). The single-stranded DNA whose sequence we wish to determine is mixed with labeled primers, DNA polymerase, ordinary nucleotides, and one type of dideoxynucleotide (Fig. 3-21). The primer hybridizes to the appropriate complementary position in the single-stranded DNA, and DNA polymerase adds free bases to the growing DNA molecule, as in the PCR process. At any given position, either an ordinary nucleotide or the corresponding dideoxynucleotide may be incorporated into the chain; this is a

FIG 3-21 DNA sequencing by the dideoxy (Sanger) method. Labeled primer is added to the single-stranded DNA whose sequence is unknown. DNA polymerase adds free bases to the single strand, using complementary base pairing. Four different reactions are carried out, corresponding to the four dideoxynucleotides (ddATP, ddCTP, ddGTP, and ddTTP). Each of these terminates the DNA sequence whenever it is incorporated in place of the normal deoxynucleotide (dATP, dCTP, dGTP, and dTTP, corresponding to the bases A, C, G, and T, respectively). The process results in fragments of varying length, which can be separated by electrophoresis. The position of each fragment is indicated by the emission of radioactive particles from the label, which allows the DNA sequence to be read directly.

random process. However, once a dideoxynucleotide is incorporated, the chain is terminated. The procedure thus yields DNA fragments of varying length, each ending with the same dideoxynucleotide.

The DNA fragments can be separated according to length by electrophoresis, as discussed previously. Four different sequencing reactions are run, one for each base. The fragments obtained from each reaction are electrophoresed side by side on the same gel, so that the position of each fragment can be compared. Because each band corresponds to a DNA chain that terminates with a unique base, the DNA sequence can be read by observing the order of the bands on the gel after autoradiography or other detection methods. Several hundred base pairs can usually be sequenced in one reaction series.

▶ DNA sequencing can be accomplished using the dideoxy method. This method depends on the fact that dideoxynucleotides behave in a fashion similar to ordinary deoxynucleotides, except that once they are incorporated into the DNA chain, they terminate the chain. They thus mark the positions of specific bases.

It should be apparent that this method of sequencing DNA is a relatively slow, laborious, and error-prone process. Nowadays, most strategies for DNA sequencing are automated and use fluorescent, chemiluminescent, or colorimetric detection systems. The use of fluorochrome-labeled primers or dideoxynucleotides is the most popular method, partly because it was easily adapted for rapid automation.

Typically, a DNA template is sequenced using a method similar to the primer extension step in PCR. Each of the four different nucleotides can be labeled with a fluorochrome that emits a distinct spectrum of light. The fluorochrome-labeled reaction products are electrophoresed through a very thin polyacrylamide gel or through a thin capillary tube; as they migrate past a window, they are excited by a beam of light from a laser. The emitted light is captured by a digital camera for translation into an electronic

signal, and a composite gel image is generated. This gel image is analyzed to produce a graph in which each of the four different nucleotides is depicted by a different-colored peak (Fig. 3-22). Automated sequencers can also be adapted to assay STRs, single-nucleotide polymorphisms, and other types of polymorphisms.

FIG 3-22 Analyzed data from a single DNA template sequenced on an automated DNA sequencer. Peaks of different colors represent the identity and relative location of different nucleotides in the DNA sequence. For example, the leftmost peak is blue and identifies the position of a cytosine. The next peak is red, indicating the presence of a thymine. This base-calling continues until the end of the DNA template is reached (typically a few hundred base pairs).

By using computers and advanced automated technology, approaches such as these have greatly increased the potential speed of DNA sequencing. These techniques have permitted the completion of the entire 3-billion-bp human DNA sequence.

▶ Automated DNA sequencing, using fluorescent labels and laser detection, greatly increases the speed and efficiency of the sequencing process.

High-Throughput DNA Sequencing

During the past several years, the development of new **high-throughput DNA sequencing** technology has decreased the cost of DNA sequencing by many orders of magnitude (this technology is also sometimes termed "next generation" or "massively parallel" sequencing). In one common approach, genomic DNA is chopped at random into small segments, typically 100 to several hundred bp in size (Fig. 3-23). Short synthetic DNA sequences, termed adapters, are joined to the ends of the genomic DNA fragments. These double-stranded DNA fragments are separated into single strands and then attached to a solid surface, such as a glass slide. Each individual DNA fragment is amplified by PCR into a cluster of thousands of identical copies, using the adapters as primer sequences (the multiple copies provide a signal strong enough to be visualized by a camera, as described below). A sequencing reaction then occurs, in which these fragment clusters serve as templates for synthesizing complementary sequences. Similar to the Sanger sequencing process described previously, new complementary bases (to which a base-specific fluorescent label is attached) are added one at a time. The fluorescent signal from each cluster is recorded by a camera, revealing the base-pair sequence of each fragment. The key advantage of this approach is that millions of different DNA fragments are sequenced simultaneously, in contrast to older methods in which only a few dozen fragments are sequenced at a time.

When the sequencing reactions are completed, millions of short DNA sequences must be stitched together to form a completed assembly. Each short sequence is compared (aligned) to a fully assembled reference sequence, typically the first published human genome or a consensus sequence of multiple genomes. Each base pair of the reference genome is covered by multiple short sequences ("reads") so that it is sequenced 30 to 60 or more times. A consensus base call is made from the short sequences. Since sequencing errors will appear in very few reads, they will be removed, and true mutations and polymorphisms will remain as differences from the reference sequence. Genomic regions that are present in many copies (like mobile elements) or have repeated sequences within them (like STRs) can be a challenge for this method.

There are many variations on this theme, including techniques in which single DNA molecules are sequenced, rather than clusters of copies. In many applications (see Chapter 10), the protein-coding exons are of primary interest, so DNA probes can be used to "pull down" only this portion of the genome (termed the **exome**) for sequencing. These approaches have been adapted to sequence RNA and to assess methylation patterns in the genome.

Because of this new technology, the sequencing of a human genome, which required months of time

FIG 3-23 High-throughput DNA sequencing. In one commonly used approach, whole genomic DNA, typically obtained from a blood or saliva sample, is mechanically sheared into small fragments (100 to several hundred bp). Standard adapter sequences are attached (ligated) to the ends of the DNA fragments, which are then converted from double-stranded to single-stranded form and attached to a glass slide. The attached adapter sequences serve as primers for PCR amplification, creating thousands of copies of each DNA fragment. Clusters of identical single-stranded fragments are templates for a sequencing reaction in which complementary bases are added one at a time. These complementary bases are labeled by a fluorescent dye specific for A, C, G, or T, allowing the bases to be visualized by a camera. The sequencing reactions occur in parallel, rapidly creating millions of short sequence "reads." The sequence reads, which typically cover each base 40 to 50 times, are aligned to a reference genome sequence (shown at the bottom of the figure in orange) to recreate the individual's genome sequence.

and millions of dollars just a few years ago, can now be completed in several hours at a cost of one to several thousand dollars. Many thousands of human genomes have been sequenced using high-through-put sequencing, leading to the discovery of disease-causing genes and to more effective genetic testing (see Chapters10).

Detection of Mutations at the DNA Level

The detection of mutations or polymorphisms in DNA sequences is often a critical step in under-standing how a gene causes a specific disease. New molecular methods have spawned a number of techniques for detecting DNA sequence variation. Many of the techniques summarized in Table 3-3 can provide rapid and efficient screening for the presence of mutations. These methods can indirectly indicate the existence and location of a mutation, after which the DNA in the indicated region can be sequenced to identify the specific mutation. Direct sequencing of DNA is a useful and accurate means of detecting

mutations and is regarded as the definitive method of identifying and verifying mutations. As it becomes less expensive, direct DNA sequencing is being used with increasing frequency.

A great deal of progress has been made in fabricating **DNA microarrays** (also known as **DNA chips**) and using them for detection of DNA variation (Fig. 3-24). To make a DNA microarray, robots place single-stranded oligonucleotides on a small glass slide. A single slide ($1cm^2$) can contain millions of different oligonucleotides. These oligonucleotides consist of normal DNA sequences as well as DNA sequences that contain known disease-causing mutations. Fluo-rescently labeled single-stranded DNA from a subject is hybridized with the oligonucleotides on the slide to determine whether the DNA hybridizes with the normal or with the mutation-containing oligonucle-otides, and the pattern of hybridization signals is analyzed by a computer. With current technology, enough probes can be placed on a single microar-ray to analyze variation in one to several million

TABLE 3-3 Methods of Mutation Detection

TECHNIQUE	BRIEF DESCRIPTION	APPLICATION
Southern blotting	Digestion of test DNA with restriction enzyme; resolution of fragments with agarose gel electrophoresis; transfer of DNA to nylon membrane and hybridization of labeled probe to DNA fragments	Detection of insertions, deletions, rearrangements; ordering of DNA fragments into physical map
Analysis of PCR product size	PCR products are sorted by size using electrophoresis on an agarose or polyacrylamide gel	Detection of small insertions and deletions and triplet repeat expansions
Direct DNA sequencing	Determination of linear order of nucleotides of test DNA; specific nucleotide detected by chemical cleavage, dideoxy-chain termination, or fluorochrome dye	Detection of insertions, deletions, point mutations, rearrangements
DNA mismatch cleavage	Hybridization of a labeled probe to test DNA; cleavage of DNA at site of base pairing mismatch	Detection of small insertions or deletions, point mutations
Allele-specific oligonu-cleotide (ASO) hybridization	Preferential hybridization of labeled probe to test DNA with uniquely complementary base composition	Detection of alleles of known composition
Multiplex ligation-dependent probe amplification (MLPA)	Ligation of DNA fragments after hybridization of probes specific to a region	Detection of deletions and duplications of exons or whole genes
Mass spectrometry	Detection of physical mass of sense and antisense strands of test DNA	Detection of small insertions or deletions, point mutations
DNA microarray hybridization	Hybridization of test DNA to arrays of oligonucleotides ordered on silicone chip or glass slide	Detection of SNPs, CNVs, expression differences
Protein truncation	Test DNA used to make complementary DNA (**cDNA**) by RT-PCR with 5' primer containing T7 promoter; cDNA translated and product resolved by SDS-PAGE	Detection of frameshift, splice-site, or nonsense mutations that truncate the protein product

RT-PCR, Reverse transcriptase-polymerase chain reaction; *SDS-PAGE*, sodium dodecyl sulfate polyacrylamide gel electrophoresis.

SNPs in an individual. Microarrays are also used to examine copy number variants, methylation patterns in a person's genome, and genetic variation in various pathogenic organisms. A key difference between microarrays and the methods summarized in the preceding paragraph is that microarrays typically test for known mutations that are incorporated in oligonucleotide probes. A rare, previously unidentified mutation cannot be detected by conventional microarrays.

Still another application of DNA microarrays is to determine which genes are being expressed (i.e., transcribed) in a given tissue sample (e.g., from a tumor). mRNA from the tissue is extracted and

FIG 3-24 **A,** Schematic diagram of a microarray. Oligonucleotides are placed or synthesized on a chip. They are then exposed to labeled DNA from a subject. Hybridization occurs only if the oligonucleotide contains a DNA sequence that is complementary to that of the subject's DNA. The fluorescent label marks the location of the complementary oligonucleotide sequence on the chip. **B,** A microarray containing 36,000 oligonucleotides. This microarray was exposed to DNA from normal fibroblasts (*red*, see *arrows*) and fibroblasts from a patient with Niemann-Pick disease, type C (*green*). Arrows point to regions in which there was a strong hybridization signal with either normal or disease DNA. This microarray was used to search for genes that are highly expressed in the fibroblasts of patients.

used as a template to form a complementary DNA sequence, which is then hybridized on the slide with oligonucleotides representing many different genes. The pattern of positive hybridization signals indicates which genes are expressed in the tissue sample. The DNA microarray approach offers the extraordinary speed, miniaturization, and accuracy of computer-based mutation analysis. Tests for specific mutations, an important aspect of genetic diagnosis, are discussed further in Chapter 10.

 Many techniques can be used to detect mutations at the DNA sequence level. These include Southern blotting, direct DNA sequencing, and microarray analysis. Microarrays are used in mutation detection, gene expression analysis, and a wide variety of other applications.

GENETIC VARIATION IN POPULATIONS

Although mutation is the ultimate source of genetic variation, it cannot alone account for the substantial differences in the incidence of many genetic diseases among different human populations. Why, for example, is sickle cell disease seen in approximately 1 of every 600 African Americans, but seldom in northern Europeans? Why is cystic fibrosis 40 times more common in Europeans than in Asians? In this section, concepts are introduced that explain these differences. The study of genetic variation in populations is an important focus of **population genetics**.

Basic Concepts of Probability

Probability plays a central role in genetics because it helps us to understand the transmission of genes through generations, and it helps to explain and analyze genetic variation in populations. It also aids in risk assessment, an important part of medical genetics. For example, the physician or genetic counsel or commonly informs couples about their risk of producing a child with a genetic disorder. A **probability** is defined as the proportion of times that a specific outcome occurs in a series of events. Thus, we may

speak of the probability of obtaining a 4 when a die is tossed, or the probability that a couple will produce a son rather than a daughter. Because probabilities are proportions, they lie between 0 and 1, inclusive.

During meiosis, one member of a chromosome pair is transmitted to each sperm or egg cell. The probability that a given member of the pair will be transmitted is 1/2, and the probability that the other member of the pair will be transmitted is also 1/2. (Note that the probabilities of all possible events must add to 1 for any given experiment.) Because this situation is directly analogous to coin tossing, in which the probabilities of obtaining heads or tails are each 1/2, we will use coin tossing as our illustrative example.

When a coin is tossed repeatedly, the outcome of each toss has no effect on subsequent outcomes. Each event (toss) is said to be **independent.** Even if we have obtained 10 heads in a row, the probability of obtaining heads or tails on the next toss remains 1/2. Similarly, the probability that a parent will transmit one of the two alleles at a locus is independent from one reproductive event to the next.

The independence principle allows us to deduce two fundamental concepts of probability, the **multiplication rule** and the **addition rule.** The multiplication rule states that if two trials are independent, then the probability of obtaining a given outcome in both trials is the product of the probabilities of each outcome. For example, we may wish to know the probability of obtaining heads on both tosses of a fair coin. Because the tosses are independent events, this probability is given by the product of the probabilities of obtaining heads in each individual toss: $1/2 \times 1/2 = 1/4$. Similarly, the probability of obtaining two tails in a row is $1/2 \times 1/2 = 1/4$.

The multiplication rule can be extended for any number of trials. Suppose a couple wants to know the probability that all three of their planned children will be girls. Because the probability of producing a girl is approximately 1/2, and because reproductive events are independent of one another, the probability of producing three girls is $1/2 \times 1/2 \times 1/2 = 1/8$. However, if the couple has already produced two girls and then wants to know the probability of producing a third girl, it is simply 1/2. This is because the previous two events are no longer probabilities; they have actually occurred. Because of independence, these past events have no effect on the outcome of the third event.

The addition rule states that if we want to know the probability of either one outcome or another, we can simply add the respective probabilities together. For example, the probability of getting two heads in a row is 1/2 × 1/2, or 1/4, and the probability of getting two tails in a row is the same. The probability of getting either two heads or two tails in a total of two tosses is the sum of the probabilities: 1/4 + 1/4 = 1/2. As another example, imagine that a couple plans to have three children, and they have a strong aversion to having three children all of the same sex. They can be reassured somewhat by knowing that the probability of producing three girls or three boys is only 1/8 + 1/8, or 1/4. The probability that they will have some combination of boys and girls is 3/4 because the sum of the probabilities of all possible outcomes must add up to 1.

▶ Basic probability enables us to understand and estimate genetic risks and to understand genetic variation among populations. The multiplication rule is used to estimate the probability that two events will occur together. The addition rule is used to estimate the probability that one event or another will occur.

Gene and Genotype Frequencies

The prevalence of many genetic diseases varies considerably from one population to another. The concepts of **genotype frequency** and **gene frequency** help us to measure and understand population variation in the incidence of genetic disease.

Imagine that we have typed 200 persons in a population for the MN blood group. This blood group, which is encoded by a locus on chromosome 2, has two major alleles, labeled M and N. In the MN system, the effects of both alleles can be observed in the heterozygote. M and N are therefore said to be **codominant:** The heterozygote can be distinguished from both homozygotes. Any individual in the population can have one of three possible genotypes (recall that the genotype is one's genetic makeup at a locus): He or she could be homozygous for M (genotype MM), heterozygous (MN), or homozygous for N (NN). After typing each person in our sample, we find the following distribution of genotypes: MM, 64; MN, 120; NN, 16. The genotype frequency is obtained simply by dividing each genotype count by the total number of subjects. The frequency of MM is 64/200, or 0.32; the frequency of MN is 120/200, or 0.60; and the frequency of NN is 16/200, or 0.08. The sum of these frequencies must equal 1.

The gene frequency for each allele, M and N, can be obtained here by the process of gene counting. Each MM homozygote has two M alleles, and each heterozygote has one M allele. Similarly, NN homozygotes have two N alleles, and heterozygotes have one N allele. In the example described, there are

$(64 \times 2) + 120 = 248$ M alleles

$(16 \times 2) + 120 = 152$ N alleles

In total, there are 400 alleles at the MN locus (i.e., twice the number of subjects, because each subject has two alleles). To obtain the frequency of M, we divide the number of M alleles by the total number of alleles at that locus: 248/400 = 0.62. Likewise, the frequency of N is 152/400, or 0.38. The sum of the two frequencies must equal 1.

▶ Gene and genotype frequencies specify the proportions of each allele and each genotype, respectively, in a population. Under simple conditions these frequencies can be estimated by direct counting.

The Hardy-Weinberg Principle

The example given for the MN locus presents an ideal situation for gene frequency estimation because, owing to co-dominance, the three genotypes can easily be distinguished and counted. What happens when one of the homozygotes is indistinguishable from the heterozygote (i.e., when there is dominance)? Here the basic concepts of probability can be used to specify a predictable relationship between gene frequencies and genotype frequencies.

Imagine a locus that has two alleles, labeled A and a. Suppose that, in a population, we know the frequency of allele A, which we will call p, and the frequency of allele a, which we will call q. From these data, we wish to determine the expected population frequencies of each genotype, AA, Aa, and aa. We will assume that individuals in the population mate at random with regard to their genotype at this locus (**random mating** is also referred to as **panmixia**). Thus, the genotype has no effect on mate selection. If men and women mate at random, then the assumption of independence is fulfilled. This allows us to apply the addition and multiplication rules to estimate genotype frequencies.

Suppose that the frequency, p, of allele A in our population is 0.7. This means that 70% of the sperm cells in the population must have allele A, as must 70% of the egg cells. Because the sum of the frequencies p and q must be 1, 30% of the egg and sperm cells must carry allele a (i.e., $q = 0.30$). Under panmixia, the probability that a sperm cell carrying A will unite with an egg cell carrying A is given by the product of the gene frequencies: $p \times p = p^2 = 0.49$ (multiplication rule). This is the probability of producing an offspring with the AA genotype. Using the same reasoning, the probability of producing an offspring with the aa genotype is given by $q \times q = q^2 = 0.09$.

What about the frequency of heterozygotes in the population? There are two ways a heterozygote can be formed. Either a sperm cell carrying A can unite with an egg carrying a, or a sperm cell carrying a can unite with an egg carrying A. The probability of each of these two outcomes is given by the product of the gene frequencies, pq. Because we want to know the overall probability of obtaining a heterozygote (i.e., the first event or the second), we can apply the addition rule, adding the probabilities to obtain a heterozygote frequency of $2pq$. These operations are summarized in Figure 3-25. The relationship between gene frequencies and genotype frequencies was established independently by Godfrey Hardy

and Wilhelm Weinberg and is termed the **Hardy-Weinberg principle.**

FIG 3-25   The Hardy-Weinberg principle. The population frequencies of genotypes AA, Aa, and aa are predicted on the basis of gene frequencies (p and q). It is assumed that the gene frequencies are the same in males and females.

As already mentioned, this principle can be used to estimate gene and genotype frequencies when dominant homozygotes and heterozygotes are indistinguishable. This is often the case for recessive diseases such as cystic fibrosis. Only the affected homozygotes, with genotype aa, are distinguishable. The Hardy-Weinberg principle tells us that the frequency of aa should be q^2. For cystic fibrosis in the European population, $q^2 = 1/2500$ (i.e., the prevalence of the disease among newborns). To estimate q, we take the square root of both sides of this equation: $q = \sqrt{1/2500} = 1/50 = 0.02$. Because $p + q = 1$, $p = 0.98$. We can then estimate the genotype frequencies of AA and Aa. The latter genotype, which represents heterozygous carriers of the disease allele, is of particular interest. Because p is almost 1.0, we can simplify the calculation by rounding p up to 1.0 without a significant loss of accuracy. We then find that the frequency of heterozygotes is $2pq = 2q = 2/50 = 1/25$. This tells us something rather remarkable about cystic fibrosis and about recessive diseases in general. Whereas the incidence of affected homozygotes is only 1 in 2500, heterozygous **carrier**s of the disease gene are much more common (1 in 25 individuals). The vast majority of recessive disease alleles, then, are effectively "hidden" in the genomes of heterozygotes.

Under panmixia, the Hardy-Weinberg principle specifies the relationship between gene frequencies and genotype frequencies. It is useful in estimating gene frequencies from disease prevalence data and in estimating the incidence of heterozygous carriers of recessive disease genes.

Causes of Genetic Variation

Mutation is the source of all genetic variation, and new genetic variants can be harmful, can be beneficial, or can have no effect whatsoever. **Natural selection** is often described as the "editor" of genetic variation. It increases the population frequency of favorable mutations (i.e., those who carry the mutation will produce more surviving offspring), and it decreases the frequency of variants that are unfavorable in a given environment (i.e., gene carriers produce fewer surviving offspring). Typically, disease-causing mutations are continually introduced into a population through the error processes described earlier. At the same time, natural selection removes these mutations.

Certain environments, however, can confer a selective advantage for a disease mutation. Sickle cell disease again provides an example. As discussed previously, persons who are homozygous for the sickle cell mutation are much more likely to die early. Heterozygotes ordinarily have no particular advantage or disadvantage.

However, it has been shown that sickle cell heterozygotes have a distinct survival advantage in environments in which *Plasmodium falciparum* malaria is common (e.g., west-central Africa) (Fig. 3-26). Because the malaria parasite does not survive well in the erythrocytes of sickle cell heterozygotes, these persons are less likely to succumb to malaria than are normal homozygotes, conferring a selective advantage on the sickle cell mutation in this environment. Although there is selection against the mutation in sickle cell homozygotes, there is selection for the mutation in heterozygotes. The result is that the disease-causing mutation persists at a relatively high frequency in many African and Mediterranean populations. In nonmalarial environments (e.g., northern Europe), the sickle cell mutation has no advantage, so natural selection acts strongly against it by eliminating homozygotes. This example illustrates the concept that variation in genetic disease incidence among populations can be caused by natural selection operating differentially in different environments.

As environments change, or as human populations occupy new environments, natural selection can act to increase the frequencies of variants that permit more successful adaptation. For example, natural selection has acted on several loci that affect skin pigmentation as humans moved from lower tropical latitudes to higher latitudes. As human populations in northern Europe and parts of Africa began to drink cow's milk through adulthood, natural selec-

10%–20%
5%–10%
1%–5%

**Frequency of
sickle cell gene**

**Distribution of
falciparum malaria**

FIG 3-26   Correspondence between the frequency of the sickle cell allele and the distribution of *Plasmodium falciparum* malaria.

tion increased the frequency of hereditary lactase persistence, allowing adults to effectively metabolize lactose (in most populations, lactase levels decline after weaning). Natural selection has acted on components of the hypoxia-inducing factor pathway, allowing some human populations to adapt successfully to oxygen-deficient high-altitude environments such as the Tibetan plateau and the Andean mountains.

▶ Natural selection is the evolutionary process in which alleles that confer survival or reproductive advantages in a specific environment are selected positively to increase in frequency, and alleles that confer lower survival or reproductive disadvantages are selected negatively so that they decrease in frequency.

Genetic drift is another force that can cause disease genes to vary in frequency among populations. To understand the process of genetic drift, consider a coin-tossing exercise in which 10 coins are tossed. Because heads and tails are equally likely, the expected number of heads and tails in this exercise would be 5 each. However, it is intuitively clear that, by chance, a substantial departure from this expectation could be observed. It would not be surprising to see 7 heads and 3 tails in 10 throws, for example. However, if 1000 coins are tossed, the degree of departure from the expected ratio of 50% heads and 50% tails is much smaller. A reasonable outcome of 1000 throws might be 470 heads and 530 tails, but it would be quite unlikely to obtain 700 heads and 300 tails. Therefore, there is less random fluctuation in larger samples.

The same principle applies to gene frequencies in populations. In a very small population, a gene frequency can deviate substantially from one generation to the next, but this is unlikely in a large population. Thus, genetic drift is greater in smaller populations. As a result, genetic diseases that are otherwise uncommon may be seen fairly frequently in a small population. For example, Ellis-van Creveld syndrome, a rare disorder that involves reduced

stature, polydactyly (extra digits), and congenital heart defects, is seen with greatly elevated frequency among the Old Order Amish population of Pennsylvania. The Amish population was founded in the United States by about 50 couples. Because of this small population size, there was great potential for genetic drift, resulting in increased frequencies of certain disease-causing alleles.

It is common to observe the effect of genetic drift in small, isolated populations throughout the world. Even relatively large populations might have experienced drift effects in the recent past if they underwent severe population bottlenecks or were established by a small number of founders (**founder effect**). For example, more than 30 otherwise rare genetic diseases are found with elevated frequency in Finland's population, which is thought to have been founded primarily by a small number of individuals some 100 generations ago. Phenylketonuria and cystic fibrosis, which are common in other Western European populations, are relatively rare in Finland, illustrating the fact that genetic drift can both increase and decrease the frequency of disease genes. Several genetic diseases (e.g., torsion dystonia, Tay-Sachs disease, Gaucher disease) occur with increased frequency in the Ashkenazi Jewish population (see Chapter 7); this may be the result of population bottlenecks that have occurred in the history of this population.

▶ Genetic drift is a random evolutionary process that produces larger changes in gene frequencies in smaller populations. Founder effect, in which small founder populations can experience large changes in gene frequency because of their small size, is a special case of genetic drift.

Gene flow occurs when populations exchange migrants who mate with one another. Through time, gene flow between populations tends to make them genetically more similar to each other. One reason sickle cell disease is less common in African Americans than in many African populations is because of gene flow between African Americans and European Americans (this same process is likely to have increased the frequency of cystic fibrosis in the African American population). In addition, because *P. falciparum* malaria is not found in North America, natural selection does not favor the sickle cell mutation.

The forces of mutation, natural selection, genetic drift, and gene flow interact in complex and sometimes unexpected ways to influence the distribution and prevalence of genetic diseases in populations. The interplay of mutation, which constantly introduces new variants, and natural selection, which often eliminates them, is an important and medically relevant example of such an interaction. A simple analysis of the relationship between mutation and selection helps us to understand variation in gene frequencies. Consider, for example, a dominant disease that results in death before the person can reproduce. This is termed a **genetic lethal mutation** because, even though the individual might survive for some time, he or she contributes no genes to the next generation. Each time mutation introduces a new copy of the lethal dominant disease allele into a population, natural selection eliminates it. In this case, p, the gene frequency of the lethal allele in the population, is equal to μ, the mutation rate ($p = \mu$). Now, suppose that those who inherit the allele can survive into their reproductive years, but, on average, they produce 30% fewer children than those who do not inherit the allele. This reduction in offspring represents the **selection coefficient**, s, of the allele. In this case, $s = 0.30$. When the allele is completely lethal, $s = 1$ (i.e., no children are produced). We can now estimate the gene frequency for this allele as $p = \mu/s$. As we would expect, the predicted frequency of an allele that merely reduces the number of offspring is higher (given the mutation rate) than the frequency of an allele that is completely lethal, where $p = \mu/s = \mu$. This predictable relationship between the effects of mutation and selection on gene frequencies is termed **mutation-selection balance.**

We can use the same principles to predict the relationship between mutation and selection against recessive alleles. The Hardy-Weinberg principle shows that most copies of harmful recessive alleles

are found in heterozygotes and are thus protected from the effects of natural selection. We would therefore expect their gene frequencies to be higher than those of harmful dominant alleles that have the same mutation rate. Indeed, under mutation-selection balance, the predicted frequency of a recessive allele, q, that is lethal in homozygotes is $q = \sqrt{\mu}$ (because $\mu < 1$, $\sqrt{\mu} > \mu$, which results in a relatively higher allele frequency for lethal recessive alleles). If the allele is not lethal in homozygotes, then $q = \sqrt{\mu/s}$, where s is again the selection coefficient for those who have a homozygous affected genotype. Thus, understanding the principle of mutation-selection balance helps to explain why, in general, the gene frequencies for recessive disease-causing alleles are higher than are the frequencies of dominant disease-causing alleles.

▶ Mutation-selection balance predicts a relatively constant gene frequency when new mutations introduce harmful alleles, whereas natural selection removes them. This process predicts that the gene frequencies should be lower for dominant diseases, in which most alleles are exposed to natural selection, than in recessive diseases, where most alleles are found in heterozygotes and are thus protected from natural selection.

The techniques described earlier in this chapter (e.g., SNP microarrays and high-throughput DNA sequencing) have now been used extensively to assay variation among individuals and populations. Because these technologies provide information about millions of genetic variants in each individual, they offer unprecedented opportunities to investigate important questions about the origins of modern humans and the differences and similarities among individuals and populations. In addition, they allow investigators to test hypotheses about the ways in which evolutionary processes such as natural selection, gene flow, and genetic drift have influenced the distribution of genetic diseases in human populations.

SUMMARY

Human genetic variation originates as a result of mutations and polymorphisms. The term mutation is often reserved to describe DNA sequence changes that cause genetic disease and are consequently relatively rare, with a population frequency of less than 1%. The principal types of mutation include missense, nonsense, frameshift, promoter, and splice-site mutations. Mutations can also be caused by the random insertion of mobile elements, and some genetic diseases are known to be caused by expanded repeats. Mutations can result in either a gain of function or a loss of function of the protein product. Gain-of-function mutations are sometimes seen in dominant diseases; dominant-negative mutations can result in gain of function. Loss-of-function mutations are usually seen in recessive diseases. Haploinsufficiency can result in loss of function. Certain nucleotide sequences are especially susceptible to mutation; these are termed mutation hot spots (eg, CpG dinucleotides, most of which are methylated and cause mutation). Ionizing and nonionizing radiation as well as many chemicals are powerful mutagens.

Polymorphisms are common in populations. The evaluation of genetic variation can provide the basis for genetic diagnosis and is highly useful in forensic analysis. Types of polymorphism at the DNA level include variable number of tandem repeats (VNTRs), short tandem repeats (STRs), single nucleotide polymorphisms (SNPs), and copy number variations (CNVs). Restriction fragment length polymorphism (RFLP) can reflect deletions or duplications of DNA. Many techniques can be used to detect mutations at the DNA sequence level. These include Southern blotting, direct DNA sequencing, high-throughput DNA sequencing, and microarray analysis. Protein variation can be detected by protein electrophoresis. In addition, various antigens are expressed by ABO and Rh blood type.

Under the concept of random mating, or panmixia, the Hardy-Weinberg principle specifies the relation between gene frequency and genotype frequency. Mutation, natural selection, genetic drift, and founder effect can affect gene frequency and genotype frequency in a population.

IMPORTANT TERMINOLOGY

genetic variation   遗传变异

allele   等位基因

homozygote   纯合子

heterozygote   杂合子

genotype   基因型

dominant   显性

recessive   隐性

silent substitution   沉默替换

point mutation   点突变

frameshift mutation   移码突变

duplication   重复

gain of function   功能获得

haploinsufficiency   单倍剂量不足

dominant negative   显性负效应

mutation hot spots   突变热区

genotype frequency   基因型频率

gene frequency   基因频率

codominant   共显性

genetic drift   遗传漂变

founder effect   奠基者效应

gene flow   基因流

selection coefficient   选择系数

REVIEW QUESTIONS

1. In the following list, the normal amino acid sequence is given first, followed by sequences that are produced by different types of mutations. Identify the type of mutation most likely to cause each altered amino acid sequence.

    Normal: Phe-Asn-Pro-Thr-Arg

    Mutation 1: Phe-Asn-Pro

    Mutation 2: Phe-Asn-Ala-His-Thr

    Mutation 3: Phe-His-Pro-Thr-Arg

2. Missense and transcription (promoter, enhancer,

transcription factor) mutations often produce milder disease conditions than do frameshift, donor/acceptor site, and nonsense mutations. Using the globin genes as examples, explain why this is so.

3. Persons who have mutations that lower their production of both α- and β-globin often present with milder disease symptoms than do those who have mutations lowering the production of only one type of chain. Why?

4. Outline the major differences between SNPs, VNTRs, and STRs. Which of these three types of polymorphism is represented in the autoradiogram in Figure 3-27?

5. α₁-Antitrypsin deficiency is a disease that arises when both copies of the α_1-antitrypsin gene are altered by mutations. Liver disease, chronic emphysema, and pulmonary failure can result. One of the mutations that causes α_1-antitrypsin deficiency occurs in exon 3 of the gene and destroys a recognition site for the restriction enzyme BstE Ⅱ. RFLP analysis was performed on three members of a family, producing the autoradiogram in Figure 3-28. Determine the disease status of each individual.

6. Using protein electrophoresis, 100 members of a population were studied to determine whether they carry genes for normal hemoglobin (HbA) or sickle hemoglobin (HbS). The following genotypes were observed:

HbA/HbA: 88
HbA/HbS: 10
Hbs/Hbs: 2

What are the gene frequencies of HbA and HbS? What are the observed genotype frequencies? Assuming Hardy-Weinberg proportions, what are the expected genotype frequencies?

7. Approximately 1 in 10,000 Europeans is born with phenylketonuria. What is the frequency of the disease-causing allele? What is the frequency of heterozygous carriers in the population?

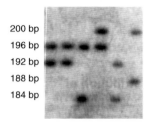

FIG 3-27 Autoradiogram for study question 4.

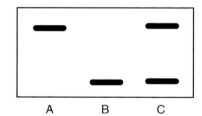

A   B   C

FIG 3-28 Autoradiogram for study question 5.

SUGGESTED READINGS AND WEBSITES

1. Campbell CD, Eichler EE. Properties and rates of germline mutations in humans. *Trends Genet.* 2013; 29(10): 575-584.

2. Fu W, Akey JM. Selection and adaptation in the human genome. *Annu Rev Genomics Hum Genet.* 2013; 14: 467-489.

3. Gill P. DNA as evidence—the technology of identification. *N Engl J Med.* 2005; 352: 2669-2671.

4. Gonzaga-Jauregui C, Lupski JR, Gibbs RA. Human genome sequencing in health and disease. *Annu Rev Med.* 2012; 63: 35-61.

5. Higgs DR, Engel JD, Stamatoyannopoulos G. Thalassaemia. *Lancet.* 2012; 379(9813): 373-383.

6. Jorde LB. Human genetic variation and disease. In: Meyers RA, ed. *Encyclopedia of Molecular Biology and Molecular Medicine.* 2nd ed. Weinheim, Germany: Wiley-VCH; 2005: 323-337.

7. Kayser M, de Knijff P. Improving human forensics through advances in genetics, genomics and molecular biology. *Nat Rev Genet.* 2011; 12(3): 179-192.

8. Mardis ER. Next-generation sequencing platforms. *Annu Rev Anal Chem (Palo Alto Calif).* 2013; 6: 287-303.

9. Mouro I, Colin Y, Cherif-Zahar B. Molecular genetic basis of the human Rhesus blood group system. *Nat Genet.* 1993; 5: 62-65.

10. Nakamura N, Suyama A, Noda A, Kodama Y. Radiation effects on human heredity. *Annu Rev Genet.* 2013; 47: 33-50.

11. Neel JV. New approaches to evaluating the genetic effects of the atomic bombs. *Am J Hum Genet.* 1995; 57: 1263-1266.

12. Piel FB, Weatherall DJ. The α-thalassemias. *N Engl J Med.* 2014; 371: 1908-1916.

13. Rees DC, Williams TN, Gladwin MT. Sickle-cell disease. *Lancet.* 2010; 376(9757): 2018-2031.

14. Strachan T, Read AP. *Human Molecular Genetics.* 4th ed. New York: Garland Science; 2010.

15. Trevino V, Falciani F, Barrera-Saldana HA. DNA microarrays: a powerful genomic tool for biomedical and clinical research. *Mol Med.* 2007; 13(9-10): 527-541.

16. Webb S. Xeroderma pigmentosum. *BMJ.* 2008; 336(7641): 444-446.

17. Yamamoto F, Clausen H, White T, et al. Molecular genetic basis of the histo-blood group ABO system. *Nature.* 1990; 345: 229-233.

18. Genetic Science Learning Center (tutorials on PCR, microarrays, PCR, and SNPs): http://learn.genetics.utah.edu/

19. Sickle Cell Information Center: http://www.scinfo.org/

20. Thalassemia (information on thalassemias and their management): http://sickle.bwh.harvard.edu/menu_thal.html

(Dan Wu)

4 | Chapter

Single Gene Disorders

Many important and well-understood genetic diseases are the result of a mutation in a single gene. The online edition of McKusick's *Mendelian Inheritance in Man* (http://www.ncbi.nlm.nih.gov/Omim/) lists nearly 15,000 single genes and nearly 8000 **single-gene**, or **monogenic**, traits defined thus far in humans. Of these 23,000 genes and traits, nearly 21,000 are located on autosomes, more than 1200 are located on the X chromosome, and 59 are located on the Y chromosome. The identification of genes that cause monogenic traits has led to new and exciting insights not only in genetics but also in the basic pathophysiology of disease.

In this chapter we first focus on single-gene disorders caused by mutations on the autosomes. We discuss the patterns of inheritance of these diseases in families, as well as factors that complicate these patterns. We also discuss the risks of transmitting single-gene diseases to one's offspring, because this is usually an important concern for at-risk couples. Then we discuss disease-causing mutations that are inherited in ways that are unknown to Mendel and are thus sometimes termed **nonmendelian**. The first mutations to be discussed are DNA variants of the sex chromosomes (X and Y), known as **sex-linked** mutations. The human X chromosome is large, containing about 5% of the nuclear genome's DNA (approximately 155 million base pairs [155 megabases, 155 Mb]). More than 1,200 genes have been localized to the X chromosome, and the diseases caused by these genes are said to be **X-linked**. In contrast to the X chromosome, the Y chromosome is quite small (60 Mb) and contains only a few dozen genes.

Another group of disease-causing mutations is located in the mitochondrial genome, which is inherited only from one's mother. Mitochondrial diseases thus display a unique pattern of inheritance in families. Extensive analyses have revealed a growing number of disease-causing mutations in the mitochondrial genome.

Finally, we discuss two processes that have been elucidated only in the past 2 to 3 decades: anticipation and imprinting. **Anticipation** refers to earlier age-of-onset of some genetic diseases in more recent generations of families. **Imprinting** refers to the fact that some genes are expressed only on paternally transmitted chromosomes and others are expressed only on maternally transmitted chromosomes. Our understanding of both of these processes has been greatly enhanced by detailed molecular analyses of humans and model organisms.

BASIC CONCEPTS OF FORMAL GENETICS

Gregor Mendel's Contributions

Monogenic traits are also known as mendelian traits, after Gregor Mendel, the 19th-century Austrian monk who deduced several important genetic principles from his well-designed experiments with garden peas. Mendel studied seven traits in the pea, each of which is determined by a single gene. These traits included attributes such as height (tall versus short plants) and seed shape (smooth versus wrinkled). The variation in each of these traits is caused by the presence of different alleles at individual loci.

Several important principles emerged from Mendel's work. The first, the principle of dominant and recessive inheritance, was discussed in Chapter 3. Mendel also discovered the **principle of segregation,**

68

which states that sexually reproducing organisms possess genes that occur in pairs and that only one member of this pair is transmitted to the offspring (i.e., it segregates). The prevalent thinking during Mendel's time was that hereditary factors from the two parents are blended in the offspring. In contrast, the principle of segregation states that genes remain intact and distinct. An allele for "smooth" seed shape can be transmitted to an offspring in the next generation, which can, in turn, transmit the same allele to its own offspring. If, instead of remaining distinct, genes were somehow blended in offspring, it would be impossible to trace genetic inheritance from one generation to the next. Thus, the principle of segregation was a key development in modern genetics.

Mendel's **principle of independent assortment** was another significant contribution to genetics. This principle states that genes at different loci are transmitted independently. Consider the two loci mentioned previously. One locus can have either the "smooth" or the "wrinkled" allele, and the other can have either the "tall" or the "short" allele. In a reproductive event, a parent transmits one allele from each locus to its offspring. The principle of independent assortment dictates that the transmission of a specific allele at one locus ("smooth" or "wrinkled") has no effect on which allele is transmitted at the other locus ("tall" or "short").

The principle of segregation describes the behavior of chromosomes in meiosis. The genes on chromosomes segregate during meiosis, and they are transmitted as distinct entities from one generation to the next. When Mendel performed his critical experiments, he had no direct knowledge of chromosomes, meiosis, or genes (indeed, the last term was not coined until 1909, long after Mendel's death). Although his work was published in 1865 and cited occasionally, its fundamental significance was unrecognized for several decades. Yet Mendel's research, which was eventually replicated by other researchers at the turn of the 20th century, forms the foundation of much of modern genetics.

 Mendel's key contributions were the principles of dominance and recessiveness, segregation, and independent assortment.

The Concept of Phenotype

The term **genotype** has been defined as an individual's genetic constitution at a locus. The **phenotype** is what is actually observed physically or clinically. Genotypes do not uniquely correspond to phenotypes. Individuals with two different genotypes, a dominant homozygote and a heterozygote, can have the same phenotype. An example is cystic fibrosis (Clinical Commentary 4-1), an autosomal recessive condition in which only the recessive homozygote is affected. Conversely, the same genotype can produce different phenotypes in different environments. An example is the recessive disease phenylketonuria (PKU, see Chapter 7), which is seen in approximately 1 of every 10,000 European births. Mutations at the locus encoding the metabolic enzyme phenylalanine hydroxylase render the homozygote unable to metabolize the amino acid phenylalanine. Although babies with PKU are unaffected at birth, their metabolic deficiency produces a buildup of phenylalanine and its toxic metabolites. This process is highly destructive to the central nervous system, and it eventually produces severe mental impairment. It has been estimated that babies with untreated PKU lose, on average, 1 to 2 IQ points per week during the first year of life. Thus, the PKU genotype can produce a severe disease phenotype. However, it is straight forward to screen for PKU at birth (see Chapter 10), and damage to the brain can be avoided by initiating a low-phenylalanine diet within 1 month after birth. The child still has the PKU genotype, but the phenotype has been profoundly altered by environmental modification.

This example shows that the phenotype is the result of the interaction of genotype and environmental factors. It should be emphasized that "environment" can include the genetic environment (i.e., genes at other loci whose products can interact with a specific gene or its product).

CLINICAL COMMENTARY 4-1

Cystic Fibrosis

Cystic fibrosis (CF) is one of the most common single-gene disorders in North America, affecting approximately 1 in 2000 to 1 in 4000 European American newborns. The prevalence among African Americans is about 1 in 15,000 births, and it is less than 1 in 30,000 among Asian Americans. Approximately 30,000 Americans have this disease.

CF was first identified as a distinct disease entity in 1938 and was termed "cystic fibrosis of the pancreas." This refers to the fibrotic lesions that develop in the pancreas, one of the principal organs affected by this disorder (Fig. 4-1). Approximately 85% of CF patients have pancreatic insufficiency, in which the pancreas is unable to secrete digestive enzymes, contributing to chronic malabsorption of nutrients. The intestinal tract is also affected, and approximately 15% to 20% of newborns with CF have meconium ileus (thickened, obstructive intestinal matter). The sweat glands of CF patients are abnormal, resulting in high levels of chloride in the sweat. This is the basis for the sweat chloride test, commonly used in the diagnosis of this disease. More than 95% of males with CF are sterile due to absence or obstruction of the vas deferens.

The major cause of morbidity and mortality in CF patients is pulmonary disease. Patients with CF have lower airway inflammation and chronic bronchial infection, progressing to end-stage lung disease characterized by extensive airway damage and fibrosis of lung tissue. Airway obstruction and lung injury are thought to be caused by a dehydrated airway surface and reduced clearance, resulting in thick airway mucus. This is associated with infection by bacteria such as *Staphylococcus aureus* and *Pseudomonas aeruginosa*. The combination of airway obstruction, inflammation, and infection leads to destruction of the airways and lung tissue, resulting eventually in death from pulmonary disease in more than 90% of CF patients.

As a result of improved nutrition, airway clearance techniques, and antibiotic therapies, the survival rate of CF patients has improved substantially during the past 3 decades. Median survival time is now nearly 40 years. CF has highly variable expression, with some patients experiencing only mild respiratory difficulty and nearly normal survival. Others have much more severe respiratory problems and may survive less than 2 decades.

CF is caused by mutations in a gene, *CFTR*, that encodes the cystic fibrosis transmembrane conductance regulator (Fig. 4-2). *CFTR* encodes cyclic AMP-regulated chloride ion channels that span the membranes of specialized epithelial cells, such as those that line the bowel and lung.

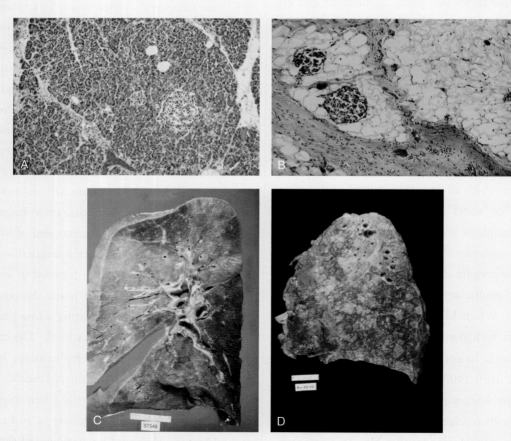

FIG 4-1   A, Normal pancreas. **B,** Pancreas from a cystic fibrosis patient, showing infiltration of fat and fibrotic lesions. **C,** Normal lung tissue. **D,** Lung tissue from a cystic fibrosis patient, which shows extensive destruction as a result of obstruction and infection. (Courtesy Dr. Edward Klatt, Florida State University School of Medicine.)

CLINICAL COMMENTARY 4-1
Cystic Fibrosis (Continued)

In addition, CFTR is involved in regulating the transport of sodium ions across epithelial cell membranes. The role of CFTR in sodium and chloride transport helps us to understand the multiple effects of mutations at the CF locus. Defective ion transport results in salt imbalances, depleting the airway of water and producing the thick, obstructive secretions seen in the lungs. The pancreas is also obstructed by thick secretions, leading to fibrosis and pancreatic insufficiency. The chloride ion transport defect explains the abnormally high concentration of chloride in the sweat secretions of CF patients: chloride cannot be reabsorbed from the lumen of the sweat duct.

DNA sequence analysis has revealed nearly 2,000 different mutations at the *CFTR* locus. The most common of these, labeled F508del, is a three-base deletion that results in the loss of a phenylalanine residue (F) at position 508 of the CFTR protein. F508del accounts for nearly 70% of all CF mutations. This mutation, along with several dozen other relatively common ones, is assayed in the genetic diagnosis of CF (see Chapter 10).

Identification of the specific mutation or mutations that are responsible for CF in a patient can help to predict the severity of the disease. For example, the most severe classes of mutations (of which F508del is an example) result in a complete lack of chloride ion channel production or in channels that cannot migrate to the cell membrane. Patients homozygous for these mutations nearly always have pancreatic insufficiency. In contrast, other mutations (e.g., R117H, a missense mutation) result in ion channels that do proceed to the cell membrane but respond poorly to cyclic AMP and consequently do not remain open as long as they should. The phenotype is thus milder, and patients who have this mutation are less likely to have pancreatic insufficiency. Some males with mild *CFTR* mutations have only congenital bilateral absence of the vas deferens (CBAVD) but little, if any, lung or gastrointestinal disease. The correlation between genotype and phenotype is far from perfect, however, indicating that modifier loci and environmental factors must also influence expression of the disease (see text). In general, there is a reasonably good correlation between genotype and pancreatic function and a more variable relationship between genotype and pulmonary function.

The ability to identify *CFTR* mutations has led to surveys of persons who have one (heterozygous) or two (homozygous) *CFTR* mutations but who do not have cystic fibrosis. They have increased risks for a number of disease conditions, including CBAVD, bronchiectasis (chronic dilatation of the bronchi and abnormal mucus production), and pancreatitis (pancreatic inflammation).

By enhancing our understanding of the pathophysiology of CF, identification of *CFTR* has opened the possibility of new treatments for this disease. Examples include administration of drugs that cause ribosomes to read through the premature stop codons that account for approximately 7% of *CFTR* mutations. Other drugs can increase the activity of chloride channels in patients with class III or IV mutations. The first FDA-approved drug for CF treatment, ivacaftor, increases CFTR channel activity in response to ATP. Clinical trials have demonstrated that this drug significantly improves lung function in patients with the class III G551D mutation seen in approximately 4% of CF patients. Gene therapy, in which the normal *CFTR* gene is placed in viral or other vectors that are then introduced to the patient's airway (see Chapter 10), is also being actively investigated. This strategy, however, has encountered difficulties because viral vectors often induce an inflammatory immune response.

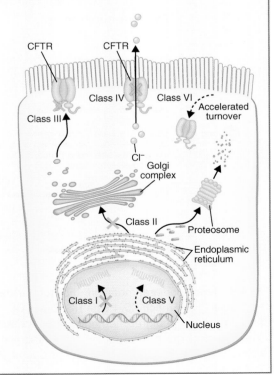

FIG 4-2 Classes of mutations in the *CFTR* gene and their effects in cells. Class I mutations result in no synthesis of the gene product. Class II mutations produce a defective protein product that is destroyed in proteasomes. Class III mutations produce a protein that gets to the cell surface but is abnormally regulated. Class IV mutations result in defective chloride ion conductance. Class V mutations are typically promoter or intron-exon splicing mutations that reduce the number of mRNA transcripts, allowing some normal protein products. Class VI mutations result in increased rates of turnover of the chloride channel at the cell surface.

> The phenotype, which is physically observable, results from the interaction of genotype and environment.

Basic Pedigree Structure

The **pedigree** is one of the most commonly used tools in medical genetics. It illustrates the relationships among family members, and it shows which family members are affected or unaffected by a genetic disease. Typically, an arrow denotes the **proband,** the first person in whom the disease is diag-nosed in the pedigree. The proband is sometimes also referred to as the **index case** or **propositus** (proposita for a female). Figure 4-3 describes the features of pedigree notation.

When discussing relatives in families, one often refers to degrees of relationship. First-degree relatives are those who are related at the parent-offspring or sibling (brother and sister) level. Second-degree relatives are those who are removed by one additional generational step (e.g., grandparents and their grandchildren, uncles or aunts and their nieces or nephews). Continuing this logic, third-degree relatives would include, for example, one's first cousins and great-grandchildren.

AUTOSOMAL DOMINANT INHERITANCE

Characteristics of Autosomal Dominant Inheritance

Autosomal dominant diseases are seen in roughly 1 of every 200 individuals (see Table 1-3 in Chapter 1). Individually, each autosomal dominant disease is rather rare in populations, however, with the most common ones having gene frequencies of about 0.001. For this reason, matings between two individuals who are both affected by the same autosomal dominant disease are uncommon. Most often, affected offspring are produced by the union of an unaffected parent with an affected heterozygote. The **Punnett square** in Figure 4-4 illustrates such a mating. The affected par-

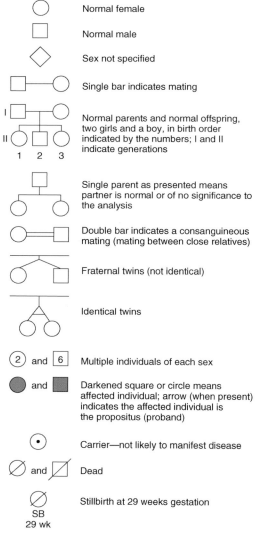

FIG 4-3 Basic pedigree notation. (For further details, see Bennett RL, French KS, Resta RG, Doyle DL. Standardized human pedigree nomenclature: update and assessment of the recommendations of the National Society of Genetic Counselors. *J Genet Couns.* 2008; 17: 424-433.)

FIG 4-4 Punnett square illustrating the mating of an unaffected individual (*aa*) with an individual who is heterozygous for an autosomal dominant disease gene (*Aa*). The genotypes of affected offspring are shaded.

ent can pass either a disease allele or a normal allele to his or her children. Each event has a probability of 0.5. Thus, on the average, half of the children will be heterozygotes and will express the disease, and half will be unaffected homozygotes.

Postaxial polydactyly, the presence of an extra digit next to the fifth digit (Fig. 4-5), can be inherited as an autosomal dominant trait. An idealized pedigree for this disease, shown in Figure 4-6, illustrates several important characteristics of autosomal dominant inheritance. First, the two sexes exhibit the trait in approximately equal ratios, and males and females are equally likely to transmit the trait to their offspring. This is because postaxial polydactyly is an autosomal disease (as opposed to a disease caused by an X chromosome mutation, in which these ratios typically differ). Second, there is no skipping of generations: if an individual has polydactyly, one parent must also have it. This leads to a vertical transmission pattern, in which the disease phenotype is usu-

ally seen in one generation after another. If neither parent has the trait, none of the children will have it. Third, father-to-son transmission of the disease gene is observed. Although father-to-son transmission is not required to establish autosomal dominant inheritance, its presence in a pedigree rules out some other modes of inheritance (particularly X-linked inheritance). Finally, as we have already seen, an affected heterozygote transmits the disease-causing allele to approximately half of his or her children. However, because gamete transmission, like coin tossing, is subject to chance fluctuations, it is possible that all or none of the children of an affected parent will have the trait. When large numbers of matings of this type are studied, the ratio of affected children closely approximates 1/2.

▶ Autosomal dominant inheritance is characterized by vertical transmission of the disease phenotype, a lack of skipped generations, and roughly equal numbers of affected males and females. Father-to-son transmission may be observed.

Recurrence Risks

Parents at risk for producing children with a genetic disease typically want to know the risk, or probability, that their future children will be affected. This probability is termed the **recurrence risk**. If one parent is affected by an autosomal dominant disease and the other is unaffected, the recurrence risk for each child is 1/2 (assuming that the affected parent is a heterozygote, which is nearly always the case). It is important to keep in mind that each birth is an independent event, as in the coin-tossing examples. Thus, even if the parents have already had a child with the disease, their recurrence risk remains 1/2. Even if they have had several children, all affected (or all unaffected) by the disease, the law of independence dictates that the probability that their next child will have the disease is still 1/2. Although this concept seems intuitively obvious, it is commonly misunderstood by the lay population. Further aspects of communicating risks to families are discussed in Chapter 12.

FIG 4-5 Postaxial polydactyly. An extra digit is located next to the fifth digit.

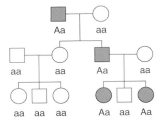

FIG 4-6 Pedigree illustrating the inheritance pattern of post-axial polydactyly, an autosomal dominant disorder. Affected individuals are represented by shading.

> The recurrence risk for an autosomal dominant disorder is 50%. Because of independence, this risk remains constant no matter how many affected or unaffected children are born.

AUTOSOMAL RECESSIVE INHERITANCE

Like autosomal dominant diseases, autosomal recessive diseases are fairly rare in populations. As shown previously, heterozygous carriers for recessive disease alleles are much more common than affected homozygotes. Consequently, the parents of individuals affected with autosomal recessive diseases are usually both heterozygous carriers. As the Punnett square in Figure 4-7 demonstrates, one fourth of the offspring of two heterozygotes will be unaffected homozygotes, half will be phenotypically unaffected heterozygous carriers, and one fourth will be homozygotes affected with the disease (on average).

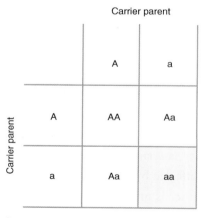

FIG 4-7 Punnett square illustrating the mating of two heterozygous carriers of an autosomal recessive gene. The genotype of the affected offspring is shaded.

Characteristics of Autosomal Recessive Inheritance

Figure 4-8 is a pedigree showing the inheritance pattern of an autosomal recessive form of albinism that results from mutations in the gene that encodes tyrosinase, a tyrosine-metabolizing enzyme. This form of albinism, termed *tyrosinase-negative* oculo-cutaneous albinism (OCA1), is distinguished from

a second, milder form termed *tyrosinase-positive* oculocutaneous albinism (OCA2). OCA2 is typically caused by mutations in a gene on chromosome 15 whose protein product is thought to be involved in the transport and processing of tyrosinase. The resulting tyrosinase deficiency (OCA1) creates a block in the metabolic pathway that normally leads to the synthesis of melanin pigment. Consequently, the affected individual has very little pigment in the skin, hair, and eyes (Fig. 4-9). Because melanin is also required for the normal development of the optic fibers, persons with albinism can also display nystagmus (rapid uncontrolled eye movement), strabismus (deviation of the eye from its normal axis), and reduced visual acuity. The pedigree demonstrates most of the important criteria for distinguishing **autosomal recessive inheritance** (Table 4-1). First, unlike autosomal dominant diseases, in which the disease phenotype is seen in one generation after another, autosomal recessive diseases are usually observed in one or more siblings but not in earlier generations. Second, as in autosomal dominant inheritance, males and females are affected in equal proportions. Third, on average, one fourth of the offspring of two

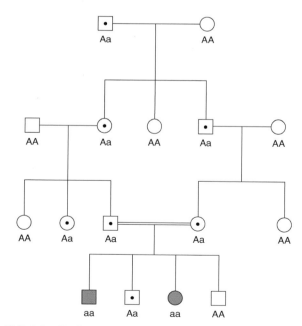

FIG 4-8 Pedigree showing the inheritance pattern of tyrosinase-negative albinism, an autosomal recessive disease. Consanguinity in this pedigree is denoted by a double bar connecting the parents of the affected individuals.

heterozygous carriers will be affected with the disorder. Finally, **consanguinity** is present more often in pedigrees involving autosomal recessive diseases than in those involving other types of inheritance (see Fig. 4-8). The term consanguinity (Latin, "with blood") refers to the mating of related persons. It is sometimes a factor in recessive disease because related persons are more likely to share the same disease-causing alleles. Consanguinity is discussed in greater detail later in this chapter.

> Autosomal recessive inheritance is characterized by clustering of the disease phenotype among siblings, but the disease is not usually seen among parents or other ancestors. Equal numbers of affected males and females are usually seen, and consanguinity may be present.

Recurrence Risks

As already discussed, the most common mating type seen in recessive disease involves two heterozygous carrier parents. This reflects the relative commonness of heterozygous carriers and the fact that many autosomal recessive diseases are severe enough that affected individuals are less likely to become parents.

The Punnett square in Figure 4-7 demonstrates that one fourth of the offspring from this mating will be homozygous for the disease gene and therefore affected. The recurrence risk for the offspring of carrier parents is then 25%. As before, these are *average* figures. In any given family chance fluctuations are likely, but a study of a large number of families would yield a figure quite close to this fraction.

Occasionally, a carrier of a recessive disease-causing allele mates with a person who is homozygous for this allele. In this case, roughly half of their children will be affected, and half will be heterozygous carriers. The recurrence risk is 50%. Because this pattern of inheritance mimics that of an autosomal dominant trait, it is sometimes referred to as **quasidominant** inheritance. With studies of extended pedigrees in which matings of heterozygotes are observed, quasidominant inheritance can be distinguished from true dominant inheritance.

When two persons affected by a recessive disease mate, all of their children must also be affected. This observation helps to distinguish recessive from dominant inheritance because two parents who are both

FIG 4-9 An African woman with oculocutaneous albinism, illustrating a lack of pigmentation in the hair and skin. She is looking away from the camera because her eyes are more sensitive to light than are those of persons with normally pigmented retinas. (Courtesy Dr. Phil Fischer, Mayo Clinic.)

TABLE 4-1	**A Comparison of the Major Attributes of Autosomal Dominant and Autosomal Recessive Inheritance Patterns**	
ATTRIBUTE	**AUTOSOMAL DOMINANT**	**AUTOSOMAL RECESSIVE**
Usual recurrence risk	50%	25%
Transmission pattern	Vertical; disease phenotype seen in generation after generation	Disease phenotype may be seen in multiple siblings, but usually not in earlier generations
Sex ratio	Equal number of affected males and females (usually)	Equal number of affected males and females (usually)
Other	Father-to-son transmission of disease gene is possible	Consanguinity is sometimes seen, especially for rare recessive diseases

affected by a dominant disease are almost always both heterozygotes and one fourth of their children, on average, will be unaffected.

 The recurrence risk for autosomal recessive diseases is usually 25%. Quasidominant inheritance, with a recurrence risk of 50%, is seen when an affected homozygote mates with a heterozygote.

"Dominant" Versus "Recessive": Some Cautions

The preceding discussion has treated dominant and recessive disorders as though they belong in rigid categories. However, these distinctions are becoming less strict as our understanding of these diseases increases. Most dominant diseases are actually more severe in affected homozygotes than in heterozygotes. An example is achondroplasia, an autosomal dominant disorder in which heterozygotes have reduced stature (Fig. 4-10). Heterozygotes have a nearly normal life span, estimated to be about 10 years less

FIG 4-10   Achondroplasia. This girl has short limbs relative to trunk length. She also has a prominent forehead, low nasal root, and redundant skinfolds in the arms and legs.

than average. Affected homozygotes are much more severely affected and usually die in infancy from respiratory failure.

Although heterozygous carriers of recessive disease genes are clinically normal, the effects of recessive genes can often be detected in heterozygotes because they result, for example, in reduced levels of enzyme activity. This is usually the basis for biochemical carrier detection tests (see Chapter 10). A useful and valid way to distinguish dominant and recessive disorders is that heterozygotes are clinically affected in most cases of dominant disorders, whereas they are almost always clinically unaffected in recessive disorders.

 Although the distinction between dominant and recessive diseases is not rigid, a dominant disease allele will produce disease in a heterozygote, whereas a recessive disease allele will not.

Another caution is that a disease may be inherited in autosomal dominant fashion in some cases and in autosomal recessive fashion in others. Familial isolated growth hormone deficiency (IGHD), another disorder that causes reduced stature, is one such disease. DNA sequencing of a pituitary growth hormone gene on chromosome 17 (*GH1*) has revealed a number of different mutations that can produce IGHD. *Recessive* IGHD can be caused by nonsense, frameshift, or splice-site mutations that have a loss-of-function effect in which a mature protein product is not synthesized. Because they have one normal copy of *GH1*, heterozygotes still produce half of the normal amount of growth hormone. This is sufficient for normal stature. Homozygotes for these mutations produce no GH1 product and have reduced stature.

Dominant IGHD can result from dominant negative mutations (see Chapter 3) in *GH1*. In one form of dominantly inherited IGHD, a splice-site mutation deletes the third exon of *GH1*, producing an abnormal protein that proceeds to the secretory granules. Here, the abnormal GH1 product interacts with the normal protein encoded by the normal *GH1* allele.

The abnormal molecules disable the normal growth hormone molecules, resulting in greatly reduced production of GH1 product and thus reduced stature.

Another example is given by β-thalassemia, a condition discussed in Chapter 3. Although the great majority of β-thalassemia cases occur as a result of autosomal recessive alleles, a small fraction of cases are inherited in autosomal dominant fashion. Some of these are caused by nonsense or frameshift mutations that terminate translation in exon 3 of the β-globin gene or in downstream exons. The resulting messenger RNA (mRNA) proceeds to the cytoplasm and produces unstable β-globin chains. In heterozygotes, these abnormal chains exert a dominant negative effect on the normal β-globin chains produced by the normal allele. In contrast, frameshift or nonsense mutations that result in termination of translation in exons 1 or 2 of the gene result in very little abnormal mRNA in the cytoplasm, leaving the product of the normal allele intact. In these cases, the heterozygote is unaffected.

These examples illustrate some of the complexities involved in applying the terms "dominant" and "recessive." They also show how molecular analysis of a gene can help to explain important disease features.

> In some cases, a disease may be inherited in either autosomal dominant or autosomal recessive fashion, depending on the nature of the mutation that alters the gene product.

A final caution is that the terms dominant and recessive, strictly speaking, apply to traits, not genes. To see why, consider the sickle cell mutation, discussed in Chapter 3. Homozygotes for this mutation develop sickle cell disease. Heterozygotes, who are said to have sickle cell *trait*, are usually clinically normal. However, a heterozygote has an increased risk for splenic infarctions at very high altitude. Is the mutant gene then dominant or recessive? Clearly, it makes more sense to refer to sickle cell *disease* as recessive and sickle cell *trait* as dominant. Nonetheless, it is common (and often convenient) to apply the terms dominant and recessive to genes.

FACTORS THAT AFFECT EXPRESSION OF DISEASE-CAUSING GENES

The inheritance patterns described previously for conditions like postaxial polydactyly, cystic fibrosis, and albinism are quite straightforward. However, most genetic diseases vary in their degree of expression, and sometimes a person has a disease-causing genotype but never manifests the phenotype. Genetic diseases are sometimes seen in the absence of any previous family history. These phenomena, and the factors responsible for them, are discussed next.

New Mutation

If a child has been born with a genetic disease that has not occurred previously in the family, it is possible that the disease is the product of a **new** (or **de novo**) **mutation.** That is, the gene transmitted by one of the parents underwent a change in DNA sequence, resulting in a mutation from a normal to a disease-causing allele. The alleles at this locus in the parent's other germ cells would still be normal. In this case the recurrence risk for the parents' subsequent offspring would not be elevated above that of the general population. However, the offspring of the affected child might have a substantially elevated risk (e.g., it would be 50% for an autosomal dominant disease). A large fraction of the observed cases of many autosomal dominant diseases are the result of new mutations. For example, approximately 7/8 of all cases of achondroplasia are caused by new mutations, and only 1/8 are inherited from an affected parent. This is primarily because the disease tends to limit the potential for reproduction. To provide accurate risk estimates, it is essential to know whether a patient's disease is due to an inherited mutation or a new mutation. This can be done only if an adequate family history has been taken.

> New mutations are a common cause of the appearance of a genetic disease in a person with no previous family history of the disorder. The recurrence risk for the person's siblings is very low, but the recurrence risk for the person's offspring may be substantially increased.

Germline Mosaicism

Occasionally, two or more offspring present with an autosomal dominant or X-linked disease when there is no family history of the disease. Because mutation is a rare event, it is unlikely that this would be due to multiple new mutations in the same family. The mechanism most likely to be responsible is termed **germline mosaicism** (mosaicism describes the presence of more than one genetically distinct cell line in the body). During the embryonic development of one of the parents, a mutation occurred that affected all or part of the germline but few or none of the somatic cells of the embryo (Fig. 4-11). Thus, the parent carries the mutation in his or her germline but does not actually express the disease because the mutation is absent in other cells of the body. As a result, the parent can transmit the mutation to multiple offspring. Although this phenomenon is relatively rare, it can have significant effects on recurrence risks when it does occur.

Germline mosaicism has been studied extensively in the lethal perinatal form of osteogenesis imperfecta (OI type II; see Chapter 2), which is caused by mutations in the type 1 procollagen genes. The fact that unaffected parents sometimes produced multiple offspring affected with this disease led to the conclusion that type II OI was an autosomal recessive trait. This was disputed by studies in which the polymerase chain reaction (PCR) technique was used to amplify DNA from the sperm of a father of two children with type II OI. This DNA was compared with DNA extracted from his somatic cells (skin fibroblasts). Although procollagen mutations were not detected in the fibroblast DNA, they were found in approximately one of every eight sperm cells. This was a direct demonstration of germline mosaicism in this man. Although germline mosaicism has been demonstrated for type II OI, most noninherited cases (approximately 95%) are thought to be caused by new mutations. Some cases of true autosomal recessive inheritance have also been documented, and genes that can cause autosomal recessive OI have been identified (Clinical Commentary 2-1, Chapter 2).

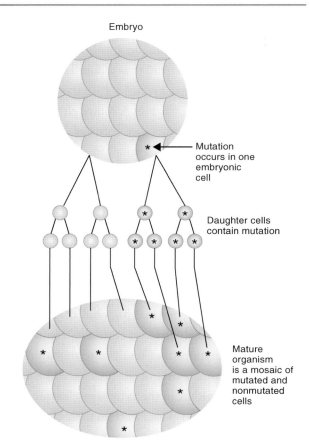

FIG 4-11   A mutation occurs in one cell of the developing embryo. All descendants of that cell have the same mutation, resulting in mosaicism. If the first mutated cell is part of the germline lineage, then germline mosaicism results.

Other diseases in which germline mosaicism has been observed include achondroplasia, neurofibromatosis type 1, hemophilia A and Duchenne muscular dystrophy (the latter two diseases are discussed in Clinical Commentary 4-6 and Clinical Commentary 4-7). It has been estimated that germline mosaicism accounts for up to 15% of Duchenne muscular dystrophy cases and 20% of hemophilia A cases in which there is no previous family history.

 Germline mosaicism occurs when all or part of a parent's germline is affected by a disease-causing mutation but the somatic cells are not. It elevates the recurrence risk for offspring of the mosaic parent.

Reduced Penetrance

Another important characteristic of many genetic diseases is reduced (or incomplete) **penetrance**: a person who has a disease-causing genotype might not exhibit the disease phenotype at all, even though he or she can transmit the disease-causing allele to the next generation. Retinoblastoma, a malignant eye tumor (Clinical Commentary 4-2), is a good example of an autosomal dominant disorder in which reduced penetrance is seen. The transmission pattern of this disorder is illustrated in Figure 4-12. Family studies have shown that about 10% of the **obligate carriers** of a retinoblastoma-causing allele (i.e., those who have an affected parent and affected children and therefore must themselves carry the allele) do not have the disease. The penetrance of the disease-causing genotype is then said to be 90%. Penetrance rates are usually estimated by examining a large number of families and determining what percentage of the obligate carriers (or obligate homozygotes, in the case of recessive disorders) develop the disease phenotype.

Age-Dependent Penetrance

Although some genetic diseases are expressed at birth or shortly afterward, many others do not become apparent until well into adulthood. A delay in the age of onset of a genetic disease is known as **age-dependent penetrance.** One of the best-known examples is Huntington disease, a neurological disorder whose main features are progressive dementia and increasingly uncontrollable movements of the limbs (Clinical Commentary 4-3). The latter feature is known as *chorea* (from the Greek word for "dance," *khoreia*), and the disease is sometimes called Huntington chorea. This autosomal dominant disorder is named after Dr. George Huntington, who first described the disease in 1872. Symptoms are not usually seen until age 30 years or later (Fig. 4-13). Thus, those who develop the disease often have children before they are aware that they carry the disease-causing allele. If the disease were present at birth, nearly all affected persons would die before reaching reproductive age, and the frequency of the disease in the population would be much lower. Delaying the age of onset of the disease thus reduces natural selection against a disease-causing allele, increasing its frequency in a population.

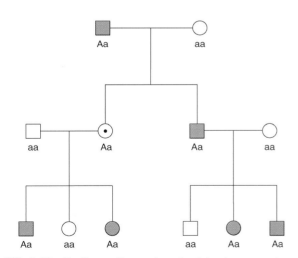

FIG 4-12 Pedigree illustrating the inheritance pattern of retinoblastoma, a disorder with reduced penetrance. The unaffected obligate carrier, denoted by a dot, has the same genotype as the affected pedigree members.

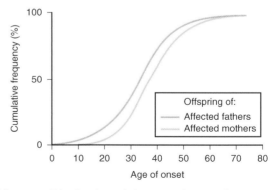

FIG 4-13 Distribution of the age of onset for Huntington disease. The age of onset tends to be somewhat earlier when the affected parent is the father. (Data from Conneally PM. Huntington disease: genetics and epidemiology. *Am J Hum Genet.* 1984; 36: 520.)

 Reduced penetrance describes the situation in which persons who have a disease-causing genotype do not develop the disease phenotype.

A person whose parent has Huntington disease has a 50% chance of inheriting the disease allele. Until recently, this person would be confronted with a torturous question: Should I have children, know-

CLINICAL COMMENTARY 4-2
Retinoblastoma

Retinoblastoma is the most common childhood eye tumor, affecting approximately 1 in 20,000 children. The tumor typically initiates between 3 months after conception and 4 years of age, when retinal cells are actively dividing and proliferating. It nearly always presents clinically by the age of 5 years.

Approximately 60% of retinoblastoma cases are caused by somatic mutations that occur in early development and are therefore not transmitted to the affected individual's offspring. The remaining 40% are caused by inherited mutations: About 3/4 of these (30% of total cases) are the result of new mutations, most often transmitted by the father. The other 1/4 of inherited cases (10% of the total) are inherited from a parent who carries a retinoblastoma-causing mutation in all of his or her cells. About 10% of those who have inherited a disease-causing mutation never develop a tumor (reduced penetrance).

The analysis of changes in DNA in and near the disease-causing gene, *RB1*, has explained the mechanism responsible for reduced penetrance. Briefly, an individual who has inherited a disease-causing *RB1* mutation carries the mutation in every cell of his or her body. However, this is not sufficient to cause tumor formation (if it were, every cell in the body would give rise to a tumor). In any cell, the presence of one normal *RB1* allele is sufficient to prevent tumor formation. To initiate a tumor in a developing retinal cell, a second somatic event must occur that disables the other, normal *RB1* allele (this "two-hit" process is discussed further in Chapter 8). The second event, which can be considered a somatic mutation, has a relatively low probability of occurring in any given cell. However, there are at least 1 million retinal cells in the developing fetus, each representing a potential target for the event. Usually, an individual who has inherited one disease-causing mutation will experience a second somatic mutation in several different retinal cells, giving rise to several tumors. Inherited retinoblastoma is thus usually multifocal (consisting of several tumor foci) and bilateral (affecting both eyes). Because the second mutations are random events, a small fraction of persons who inherit the disease-causing allele never experience a second mutation in any retinal cell and they do not develop a retinoblastoma. The requirement for a second somatic mutation thus explains the reduced penetrance seen in this disorder.

The retinoblastoma gene, *RB1*, encodes a protein product, pRb, that plays a key role in cell cycle control. A major function of pRb, when hypophosphorylated, is to bind and inactivate members of the E2F family of nuclear transcription factors. The cell requires active E2F to proceed from the G1 to the S phase of mitosis. By inactivating E2F, pRb applies a brake to the cell cycle. When cell division is required, pRb is phosphorylated by cyclin-dependent kinase complexes (see Chapter 2) and E2F is released by pRb and activated. A loss-of-function mutation in pRb can cause a permanent loss of E2F-binding capacity. The cell, having lost its brake, will undergo repeated, uncontrolled mitosis,

potentially leading to a tumor. Because of its controlling effect on the cell cycle, the *RB1* gene belongs to a class of genes known as tumor suppressors (see Chapter 8).

If untreated, retinoblastomas can grow to considerable size and can metastasize to the central nervous system or other organ systems. Fortunately, these tumors are now usually detected and treated before they progress. If found early enough through ophthalmological examination, the tumor may be treated successfully with cryotherapy (freezing) or laser photocoagulation. In more advanced cases, radiation, chemotherapy, or enucleation (removal) of the eye may be necessary. Currently, the 5-year survival rate for retinoblastoma patients in the United States is nearly 95%.

Because persons with familial retinoblastoma have inherited an *RB1* mutation in all cells of their body, they are also susceptible to other types of cancer later in life. In particular, about 15% of those who inherit an *RB1* mutation later develop osteosarcomas (malignant bone tumors). Other common second cancers include soft tissue sarcomas and cutaneous melanomas. Careful monitoring for subsequent tumors and avoidance of agents that could produce a second mutation (e.g., X-rays) are thus important aspects of management for the patient with inherited retinoblastoma (Fig. 4-14).

FIG 4-14   A, A white reflex (leukocoria) can be seen in the right eye of this individual on ophthalmoscopic examination. **B,** Bilateral retinoblastoma, showing presence of neoplastic tissue. (From Rosai J. *Ackerman's Surgical Pathology*. 8th ed. St Louis: Mosby; 1996.)

CLINICAL COMMENTARY 4-3

Huntington Disease

Huntington disease (HD) affects approximately 1 in 20,000 persons of European descent but is substantially less common in most other populations The disorder usually manifests between the ages of 30 and 50 years, although it has been observed as early as 1 year of age and as late as 80 years of age.

HD is characterized by a progressive loss of motor control, dementia, and psychiatric disorders. There is a substantial loss of neurons in the brain, which is detectable by techniques such as magnetic resonance imaging (MRI). Decreased glucose uptake in the brain, an early sign of the disorder, can be detected by positron-emission tomography (PET). (These techniques, however, are not specific enough to diagnose the disorder accurately.) Although many parts of the brain are affected, the area most noticeably damaged is the corpus striatum. In some patients, the disease leads to a loss of 25% or more of total brain weight.

The clinical course of HD is protracted, and the interval from initial diagnosis to death is typically 15 to 20 years. As in many neurological disorders, patients with HD experience difficulties in swallowing; aspiration pneumonia is the most common cause of death. Cardiorespiratory failure and subdural hematoma (due to head trauma) are other frequent causes of death. The suicide rate among HD patients is 5 to 10 times higher than in the general population. Treatment includes drugs such as benzodiazepines to help control the choreic movements. Affective disturbances, which are seen in nearly half of the patients, are sometimes controlled with antipsychotic drugs and antidepressants. Although these drugs help to control some of the symptoms of HD, there is currently no way to alter the outcome of the disease.

HD has the distinction of being the first genetic disease mapped to a specific chromosome using an RFLP marker, in 1983. Subsequent sequencing of the disease-causing gene showed that the great majority of HD cases are caused by a CAG expanded repeat (see Chapter 3) located in exon 1. In 90% to 95% of cases, the mutation is inherited from an affected parent. In the general population, the number of CAG tandem repeats ranges from 10 to 26. Persons with 27 to 35 repeats are unaffected but are more likely to transmit a still larger number of repeats to their offspring. The inheritance of 36 or more copies of the repeat can produce disease, although incomplete penetrance of the disease phenotype is seen in those who have 36 to 40 repeats. As in many disorders caused by trinucleotide repeat expansion, a larger number of repeats is correlated with earlier age of onset of the disorder. About 60% to 70% of the variation in age of onset of HD can be predicted by repeat number. There is a tendency for greater repeat expansion when the father, rather than the mother, transmits the disease-causing mutation, which helps to explain the difference in ages of onset for maternally and paternally transmitted disease seen in Figure 4-13. In particular, 80% of cases with onset before 20 years of age (juvenile Huntington disease) are due to paternal transmission, and these cases are characterized by especially large repeat expansions. It remains unknown why the degree of repeat instability in the HD gene is greater in paternal transmission than in maternal transmission (Fig. 4-15).

The protein product, termed huntingtin, is involved in the transport of vesicles in cellular secretory pathways. In addition, there is evidence that huntingtin is necessary for the normal production of brain-derived neurotrophic factor. The CAG repeat expansion produces a lengthened series of glutamine residues near huntingtin's amino terminal. Although the precise role of the expanded glutamine tract in disease causation is unclear, it is correlated with a buildup of toxic protein aggregates within and near neuronal nuclei. These aggregates are thought to be toxic and are associated with early neuronal death. HD is notable in that affected homozygotes appear to display a clinical course very similar to that of heterozygotes (in contrast to most dominant disorders, in which homozygotes are more severely affected). This attribute, and the fact that mouse models in which one copy of the gene is inactivated are perfectly normal, supports the hypothesis that the mutation causes a harmful gain of function (see Chapter 3).

FIG 4-15 Two cross sections of the brain of an adult with Huntington disease, which illustrate severe caudate atrophy and enlarged lateral ventricles. (Courtesy Dr. Thomas Bird, University of Washington.)

ing that there is a 50% chance that I have inherited this mutation and pass it to half of my children? With the identification of the gene responsible for Huntington disease, it is now possible for at-risk persons to know with a high degree of certainty whether they carry a disease-causing allele.

As mentioned previously, a number of important genetic diseases exhibit age-dependent penetrance. These include hemochromatosis, a recessive disorder of iron storage (see Chapter 7); familial Alzheimer disease (see Chapter 5); and many inherited cancers, including autosomal dominant breast cancer (See Chapters 5 and 8 for further discussion).

 Age-dependent penetrance is observed in many genetic diseases. It complicates the interpretation of inheritance patterns in families.

Variable Expression

Penetrance and expression are distinct entities. Penetrance is an all-or-none phenomenon: one either has the disease phenotype or does not. **Variable expression** refers to the degree of severity of the disease phenotype.

The severity of expression of many genetic diseases can vary greatly. A well-studied example of variable expression in an autosomal dominant disease is neu-

rofibromatosis type 1 (Clinical Commentary 4-4). A parent with mild expression of the disease—so mild that he or she is not aware of it—can transmit the disease-causing allele to a child, who may have severe expression. Many factors can affect the expression of a genetic disease, including environmental (i.e., nongenetic) influences such as diet, exercise, or exposure to harmful agents such as tobacco smoke. In the absence of a certain environmental factor, the disease-causing gene is expressed with diminished severity or not at all (e.g., the diminished expression of PKU under a low-phenylalanine diet). Another factor that can influence disease expression is the interaction of other genes, called **modifier genes,** with the disease-causing gene. Finally, variable expression can result from different types of mutations (i.e., different alleles) at the same disease locus. This is termed **allelic heterogeneity.** Efforts are often made to establish **genotype-phenotype correlations** to better predict the severity of a genetic disease, given the patient's genotype. In some cases, clinically distinct diseases may be the result of allelic heterogeneity, as in the β-globin mutations that can cause either sickle cell disease or various forms of β-thalassemia.

Cystic fibrosis, discussed in Clinical Commentary 4-1, illustrates ways these factors can influence disease severity. *CFTR* mutations that result in a com-

---

CLINICAL COMMENTARY 4-4

Neurofibromatosis: A Disease with Highly Variable Expression

Neurofibromatosis type 1 (NF1) is also known as von Recklinghausen disease, recognizing the German physician who first described this condition in 1882. It is one of the more common autosomal dominant disorders, affecting approximately 1 in 3000 individuals in all studied populations. NF1 provides a good example of variable expression in a genetic disease. Some patients have only *café-au-lait* spots (French for "coffee with milk," describing the color of the hyperpigmented skin patches), Lisch nodules (benign growths on the iris), and a few neurofibromas (nonmalignant peripheral nerve tumors). These persons are sometimes unaware that they have the condition. Other patients have a much more severe expression of the disorder, including hundreds to thousands of neurofibromas, plexiform neurofibromas, optic pathway gliomas (benign tumors of the optic nerve), learning disabilities, hypertension, scoliosis (lateral curvature of the spine), and malignancies. About two thirds of patients have only a mild cutaneous involve-

ment. Approximately 10% develop malignant peripheral nerve sheath tumors (MPNSTs), which typically arise from plexiform neurofibromas. Expression can vary significantly within the same family: a mildly affected parent can produce a severely affected offspring.

A standard set of diagnostic criteria for NF1 has been developed. Two or more of the following must be present:

1. Six or more *café-au-lait* spots greater than 5 mm in diameter in prepubertal patients and greater than 15 mm in postpubertal patients
2. Freckling in the armpits or groin area
3. Two or more neurofibromas of any type or one plexiform neurofibroma (i.e., an extensive growth that occurs along a large nerve sheath)
4. Two or more Lisch nodules
5. Optic glioma
6. Distinctive bone lesions, particularly an abnormally formed sphenoid bone or tibial pseudarthrosis*

CLINICAL COMMENTARY 4-4
Neurofibromatosis: A Disease with Highly Variable Expression (Continued)

7. A first-degree relative with neurofibromatosis diagnosed using the previous six criteria

Although NF1 has highly variable expression, the penetrance of disease-causing mutations is virtually 100%. Approximately 50% of patients with NF1 have the condition because of a new mutation. In fact, the *NF1* gene has one of the highest known locus-specific mutation rates, about 1 in 10,000 per generation. This is due in part to the large size of the *NF1* gene (approximately 350 kb), making it a large target for mutation. The gene product, neurofibromin, acts as a tumor suppressor (see Chapter 8 for further details). *NF1* mutations can be detected in more than 90% of cases, using a combination of detection methods including DNA sequencing, cytogenetic analysis, and analysis of abnormal (truncated) products. Persons in whom the entire *NF1* gene is deleted tend to be severely affected, with large numbers of neurofibromas and an increased risk of developing MPNSTs.

An *NF1* mutation that occurs during embryonic development will affect only some cells of the individual, resulting in somatic mosaicism. In this case, the disease features may be confined to only one part of the body (segmental neurofibromatosis).

Neurofibromatosis type 2 (NF2) is much rarer than NF1 and is characterized by vestibular schwannomas (tumors that arise in Schwann cells and affect the eighth cranial nerve) and, occasionally, *café-au-lait* spots. Patients who have NF2 do not, however, have true neurofibromas, so the term "neurofibromatosis type 2" is a misnomer. The *NF2* gene encodes a tumor suppressor protein called merlin or schwannomin.

Mild cases of neurofibromatosis can require very little clinical management. However, surgery may be required if malignancies develop or if benign tumors interfere with normal function. Scoliosis, tibial pseudarthrosis, and/or tibial bowing, seen in less than 5% of cases, can require orthopedic management. Hypertension can develop and is often secondary to a pheochromocytoma or a stenosis (narrowing) of the renal artery. The most common clinical problems in children are learning disabilities (seen in about 50% of persons with NF1), short stature, and optic gliomas (which can lead to vision loss). Close follow-up can help to detect these problems and minimize their effects. Recent clinical trials designed to reduce or eliminate the tumors seen in patients with NF1 have provided hope for better treatment options (Fig. 4-16).

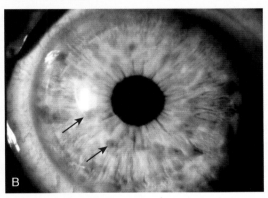

FIG 4-16   Neurofibromatosis type 1 (NF1). **A,** Multiple neurofibromas in an adult with type 1 neurofibromatosis. **B,** Lisch nodules (benign hamartomas of the iris) visible on a slit-lamp examination of an individual with type 1 neurofibromatosis. (**A** from Habif T, Campbell J, Chapman M, et al. *Skin Disease: Diagnosis and Treatment.* 2nd ed. St. Louis: Mosby; 2005; **B** from Jones KL. *Smith's Recognizable Patterns of Human Malformation.* 6th ed. Philadelphia: Mosby; 2006.)

*pseudarthrosis can occur when a long bone, such as the tibia, undergoes a loss of bone cortex, leading to weakening and fracture. Abnormal callus formation causes a false joint in the bone, leading to the term (*arthron* = "joint").

plete absence of chloride channels on cell surfaces tend to produce more-severe disease than do mutations that result in partially active chloride ion channels (allelic heterogeneity). Some of the variation in severity of lung disease among CF patients with identical *CFTR* genotypes can be explained by variation in the *TGFB1* gene (transforming growth factor β), a modifier gene whose increased expression is also associated with asthma and chronic obstructive pulmonary disease. Mutations in another modifier gene, *DCTN4*, appear to reduce the effectiveness of the dynactin protein in clearing *Pseudomonas aeruginosa* from the airway. Patients with CF who suffer from more frequent and severe bacterial infections experience accelerated lung damage. This disease thus provides examples of all three major causes of variable expression: allelic heterogeneity, modifier genes, and nongenetic environmental factors (bacterial infections).

Because of the many factors that can influence the expression of a genetic disease, it should be apparent that the commonly used term "single-gene disease" is an oversimplification. Although a mutation in a single gene may be sufficient to cause such a disease, its severity—always an important concern for clinicians—is typically influenced by many genetic and nongenetic factors.

 Variable expression of a genetic disease may be caused by environmental effects, modifier genes, or allelic heterogeneity.

Locus Heterogeneity

Quite commonly, a single disease phenotype can be caused by mutations at different loci in different families, which is termed **locus heterogeneity** (compare with allelic heterogeneity, discussed in the previous section, in which different mutations are seen within the same disease locus). A good example is adult polycystic kidney disease (APKD), an autosomal dominant disorder in which a progressive accumulation of renal cysts is seen. Patients can also develop liver cysts, hypertension, cerebral aneurysms, and cardiac valvular defects. Occurring in about 1 of every 1000 persons of European descent, this disorder is responsible for 8% to 10% of end-stage renal disease in North America. APKD can be caused by mutations in genes on either chromosome 16 (*PKD1*) or chromosome 4 (*PKD2*). Both of these genes encode membrane-spanning glycoproteins that interact with one another and may be involved in cellular signaling. (When this signaling goes awry, it is thought that cellular growth regulation is compromised, resulting in cyst formation.) In one family, the disease may be caused by a *PKD1* mutation, whereas in another family it may be caused by a *PKD2* mutation. The disease states produced by mutations in these two genes may be clinically indistinguishable.

Osteogenesis imperfecta provides a second example of locus heterogeneity. Recall from Chapter 2 that the subunits of the procollagen triple helix are encoded by two genes, one on chromosome 17 and the other on chromosome 7 (Fig. 4-17). A mutation occurring in either of these genes can alter the normal structure of the triple helix, resulting ultimately in osteogenesis imperfecta. Locus heterogeneity is seen in many other genetic diseases, including familial forms of Alzheimer disease, breast cancer, colon cancer, and melanoma.

FIG 4-17 Structure of the triple helix type 1 collagen protein. The two α_1 chains are encoded by a gene on chromosome 17, and the α_2 chain is encoded by a gene on chromosome 7.

 A disease that can be caused by mutations at different loci in different families is said to exhibit locus heterogeneity.

Pleiotropy

Genes that have more than one discernible effect on the body are said to be **pleiotropic.** A good example of a gene with pleiotropic effects is given by Marfan syndrome. First described in 1896 by Antoine Marfan, a French pediatrician, this autosomal dominant disorder affects the eye, the skeleton, and the cardiovascular system (Clinical Commentary 4-5). Most of the observed features of Marfan syndrome are caused by unusually stretchable connective tissue. The great majority of Marfan syndrome cases are caused by mutations in the gene that encodes fibrillin, a component of connective tissue that is expressed in most of the tissues and organs affected by Marfan syndrome (see Clinical Commentary 4-5). We have already discussed several other single-gene diseases in which **pleiotropy** is seen, including cystic fibrosis, in which sweat glands, lungs, and pancreas can be affected; osteogenesis imperfecta, in which bones, teeth, and sclerae can be affected; and albinism, in which pigmentation and optic fiber development are affected.

> Genes that exert effects on multiple aspects of physiology or anatomy are pleiotropic. Pleiotropy is a common feature of human genes.

CLINICAL COMMENTARY 4-5
Marfan Syndrome: An example of Pleiotropy

Marfan syndrome is an autosomal dominant condition seen in approximately 1 of every 10,000 North Americans. It is characterized by defects in three major systems: ocular, skeletal, and cardiovascular. The ocular defects include myopia, which is present in most patients with Marfan syndrome, and displaced lens (ectopia lentis), which is observed in about half of Marfan syndrome patients. The skeletal defects include dolichostenomelia (unusually long and slender limbs), pectus excavatum ("hollow chest"), pectus carinatum ("pigeon chest"), scoliosis, and arachnodactyly (literally "spider fingers," denoting the characteristically long, slender fingers) (Fig. 4-18). Marfan patients also typically exhibit joint hypermobility.

The cardiovascular features of Marfan syndrome can be life-threatening. Most patients with Marfan syndrome develop prolapse of the mitral valve, a condition in which the cusps of the mitral valve protrude upward into the left atrium during systole, which can result in mitral regurgitation (leakage of blood back into the left atrium from the left ventricle). Mitral valve prolapse, however, is seen in 1% to 3% of the general population and is often of little consequence. A more serious complication is dilatation (widening) of the ascending aorta, which is seen in 90% of Marfan patients. As dilatation increases, the aorta becomes susceptible to dissection or rupture, particularly when cardiac output is high (as in heavy exercise or pregnancy). As the aorta widens, the left ventricle enlarges, and cardiomyopathy (damage to the heart muscle) ensues. The end result is congestive heart failure, a common cause of death among Marfan syndrome patients.

Most cases of Marfan syndrome are caused by mutations in a gene, *FBN1*, that is expressed in the aorta, the periosteum, and the suspensory ligament of the lens. Because *FBN1* encodes a connective tissue protein, fibrillin, mutations of this gene alter the structure of connective tissue. This helps to explain some of the cardiovascular and ocular features of this disorder. Hundreds of different *FBN1* mutations have been identified in Marfan syndrome patients. Most of these are missense mutations, but frameshifts and nonsense mutations producing a truncated fibrillin protein are also seen. In many cases, the missense mutations produce a more severe disease phenotype because of a dominant negative effect (i.e., the abnormal fibrillin proteins bind to and disable many of the normal fibrillin proteins produced by the normal allele in a heterozygote). A severe neonatal form of the disease is produced by mutations in exons 24 to 32. At least one Marfan syndrome compound heterozygote has been reported. This infant, who inherited a disease-causing

FIG 4-18 **A,** A young man with Marfan syndrome. Note characteristically long limbs and narrow face. **B,** Arachnodactyly in an 8-year-old girl with Marfan syndrome. Note projection of the thumb well beyond the edge of the palm (Steinberg thumb sign). (**A** from Jones KL. *Smith's Recognizable Patterns of Human Malformation.* 6th ed. Philadelphia: Saunders; 2006:549. **B** from Jones KL. *Smith's Recognizable Patterns of Human Malformation.* 6th ed. Philadelphia: Mosby; 2006.)

CLINICAL COMMENTARY 4-5
Marfan Syndrome: An example of Pleiotropy (Continued)

allele from each of its affected heterozygous parents, had severe congestive heart failure and died from cardiac arrest at 4 months of age.

Specific mutations in *FBN1* can cause familial arachnodactyly (with no other symptoms of Marfan syndrome), whereas others can cause familial ectopia lentis. A disease called *congenital contractural arachnodactyly* exhibits many of the skeletal features of Marfan syndrome but does not involve cardiac or ocular defects. This disease is caused by mutations in a second gene, *FBN2*, that encodes another form of fibrillin.

A small percentage of persons with Marfan syndrome do not have mutations in *FBN1* or *FBN2* but instead have mutations in the gene that encodes transforming growth factor β receptor 2 (*TGFBR2*). These mutations increase the signaling activity of transforming growth factor β (TGF-β), which contributes to aortic dilatation and abnormal bone growth. It is interesting that the fibrillin protein contains a domain that binds TGF-β, and mutations that disrupt fibrillin increase TGF-β signaling. Thus, *FBN1* mutations can produce structural connective tissue abnormalities as well as abnormal TGF-β activity, accounting for the pleiotropic features of this disorder.

Treatment for Marfan syndrome includes regular ophthalmological examinations and, for individuals with aortic dilatation, the avoidance of heavy exercise and contact sports. In addition, β-adrenergic blockers (e.g., atenolol)

can be administered to decrease the strength and abruptness of heart contractions. This reduces stress on the aorta, although it is unclear whether these drugs reduce aortic dilatation. In some cases, the aorta and aortic valve are surgically replaced with a synthetic tube and artificial valve. With such treatment, persons with Marfan syndrome can achieve nearly normal life spans.

Another possible avenue for treatment has been opened by the discovery of elevated TGF-β signaling in Marfan syndrome. In mouse models of this disorder, administration of TGF-β antagonists has been shown to prevent aortic dilatation. One of these agents, losartan, is an angiotensin II type 1 receptor antagonist and is commonly used to treat high blood pressure. This drug has been evaluated in clinical trials and has been shown to cause a significant reduction in aortic dilatation in patients with Marfan syndrome.

A number of historical figures might have had Marfan syndrome, including Niccolo Paganini, the violinist, and Sergei Rachmaninoff, the composer and pianist, and U.S. President Abraham Lincoln. Some of Lincoln's skeletal features are seen in Marfan syndrome, and examination of his medical records has shown that he had features consistent with aortic dilatation. It has been suggested that he was in congestive heart failure at the time of his death and that, had he not been assassinated, he still would not have survived his second term of office.

CONSANGUINITY IN HUMAN POPULATIONS

Although consanguinity is relatively rare in Western populations, it is common in many populations of the world. For example, first-cousin unions are seen in 20% to 50% of marriages in many countries of the Middle East, and uncle-niece and first-cousin marriages occur in some parts of India. Because relatives more often share disease genes inherited from a common ancestor, consanguineous unions are more likely to produce offspring affected by autosomal recessive disorders. It is possible to quantify the percentage of DNA sequence shared by a pair of relatives by estimating the **coefficient of relationship** (Box 4-1). Estimation of this quantity shows, for example, that siblings share 1/2 of their DNA sequences, on average, because they share two parents. Uncles and nieces share 1/4 of their DNA sequences because of common ancestry, first cousins share 1/8, first cousins once removed share 1/16, second cousins share 1/32, and so on. (First cousins are the offspring of

two siblings and thus share a set of grandparents. A first cousin once removed is the offspring of one's first cousin. Second cousins are the offspring of two different first cousins and thus share a set of great-grandparents.)

Consanguinity and the Frequency of Recessive Diseases

Recall that about 1 in 25 whites is a heterozygous carrier of a mutation that causes cystic fibrosis. A man who carries this allele thus has a 1 in 25 chance of meeting another carrier if he mates with somebody in the general population. He only triples his chance of meeting another carrier if he mates with a first cousin, who has a 1/8 chance of carrying the same gene. In contrast, a carrier of a relatively rare recessive disease, such as classic galactosemia (a metabolic disorder discussed in Chapter 7), has only a 1/170 chance of meeting another carrier in the general population. Because he shares 1/8 of his DNA with his first cousin, the chance that his first cousin

BOX 4-1   Measurement of Consanguinity: The Coefficient of Relationship

To determine the possible consequences of a consanguineous mating, it is useful to know what percentage of DNA is shared by two related individuals because of their descent from a common ancestor. The coefficient of relationship is a measure of this percentage. Clearly, individuals who are more closely related must share a greater percentage of their genes. To begin with a simple example, an individual receives half of his or her genes from each parent. Thus, the coefficient of relationship between a parent and offspring is 1/2. This also means that the probability that the parent and offspring share a given DNA sequence (e.g., a disease allele) is 1/2.

To continue with a more complex example, suppose that a man is known to be a heterozygous carrier for galactosemia, a relatively rare autosomal recessive metabolic disorder. If he mates with his first cousin, what is the probability that she also carries this disease-causing allele? We know that this probability must be higher than that of the general population, because first cousins share one set of grandparents. There is thus a possibility that the grandparent who transmitted the galactosemia allele to the known carrier also transmitted it to the carrier's cousin. The coefficient of relationship specifies this probability. A pedigree for a first-cousin mating is shown below in panel A on the left. The male carrier is labeled A, and his female cousin is labeled E. Because we are interested only in the family members who are related to both the man and his cousin, the pedigree is condensed, in panel B on the right, to include only those individuals who form a path between the man and his cousin.

To estimate the coefficient of relationship, we begin with the carrier and ascend the pedigree. We know that there is a probability of 1/2 that the known carrier inherited the gene from the parent in the path (labeled B). There is also a probability of 1/2 that he inherited the gene from his other parent, who is not related to his cousin and is thus not included in the diagram. By similar reasoning, the probability that individual B inherited the disease gene from his parent, individual C, is also 1/2. The probability that individual C in turn passed on the disease gene to his offspring, D, is 1/2, and the probability that D passed the disease gene to E is also 1/2. Thus, for E to share a disease-causing allele with A, each of these four events must have taken place. The multiplication rule dictates that, to find the probability that all four events have taken place, we take the product of all four probabilities. Because each of these probabilities is 1/2, the result is $(1/2)^4 = 1/16$.

If individuals A and E shared only one grandparent, the coefficient of relationship would be 1/16. But, as with most first cousins, they share a common grandfather and grandmother. Thus, there are two paths through which the disease gene could have passed. To obtain the probability that the gene passed through the second path, we use the same procedure as in the previous paragraph and obtain a probability of 1/16. Now we need to estimate the probability that the gene went through either the first path or the second (i.e., through one grandparent or the other). The addition rule states that we can add these two probabilities together to get the overall probability that A and E share a disease gene: $1/16 + 1/16 = 1/8$. The probability that the carrier's cousin shares his disease allele, as a result of their descent from a common set of grandparents, is thus 1/8. This is the coefficient of relationship for first cousins.[*]

It should be recognized that individual E could also inherit a disease allele from an ancestor not included in either of these paths. However, for disease alleles that are relatively rare in populations, this probability is small and can usually be disregarded.

The rules for calculating the coefficient of relationship can be summarized as follows:

1. Each individual can appear in a route only once.
2. Always begin with one individual, proceed up the pedigree to the common ancestor, then down the pedigree to the other individual.
3. The coefficient of relationship for one route is given by $(1/2)^{n-1}$, where n is the number of individuals in the route.
4. If there are multiple routes (i.e., multiple common ancestors), the probabilities estimated for each route are added together.

A, Pedigree for a first-cousin mating.
B, The pedigree is condensed to show only those individuals who are related to both of the first cousins.

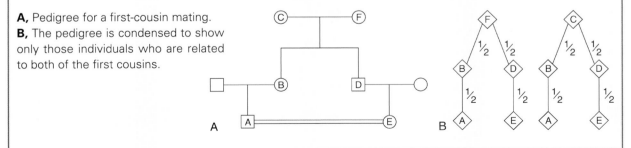

*A related quantity, often used in population genetics, is the **inbreeding coefficient**. This coefficient is the probability that an individual is homozygous at a locus as a result of consanguinity in his or her parents. For a given type of mating, the inbreeding coefficient of an individual always equals the parents' coefficient of relationship multiplied by 1/2 (e.g., the inbreeding coefficient for the offspring of a first-cousin mating is 1/16).

also has a galactosemia mutation is still 1/8. With this rarer disease, a carrier is 21 times more likely to mate with another carrier in a first-cousin marriage than in a marriage with an unrelated individual. This illustrates an important principle: the rarer the recessive disease, the more likely that the parents of an affected individual are consanguineous.

This principle has been substantiated empirically. A French study showed that the frequency of first-cousin marriages in that country was less than 0.2%. Among patients with cystic fibrosis, a relatively common recessive disorder, 1.4% were the offspring of first-cousin matings. This percentage rose to 7.1% for cystinosis and 12.5% for achromatopsia, both of which are less-common recessive disorders.

> Consanguinity increases the chance that a mating couple will both carry the same disease-causing mutation. It is seen more often in pedigrees involving rare recessive diseases than in those involving common recessive diseases.

Health Consequences of Consanguinity

It has been estimated that each person carries the equivalent of one to five recessive mutations that would be lethal to offspring if matched with another copy of the mutation (i.e., homozygosity). It would therefore be expected that matings between relatives would more often produce offspring with genetic diseases. In fact, most empirical studies do show that mortality rates among the offspring of first-cousin marriages are substantially greater than those of the general population (Table 4-2). Similarly, the prevalence of genetic disease is roughly twice as high among the offspring of first-cousin marriages as among the offspring of unrelated persons. First-cousin marriages are illegal in most states of the United States, and marriages between closer relatives (except double first cousins, who share both sets of grandparents) are prohibited throughout the United States.

Very few data exist for matings between siblings or parents and offspring (defined as **incest**). The limited data indicate that between 1/4 and 1/2 of incestuous matings result in offspring affected by serious disease, with mental impairment as one of the most common consequences. Because of small sample sizes in these studies, it is difficult to separate the effects of genetics from those of a substandard environment. It is likely that the problems experienced by the offspring of incestuous matings are caused by both genetic and environmental influences.

> At the population level, consanguinity increases the frequency of genetic disease and mortality. The closer the degree of consanguinity, the greater the increase.

TABLE 4-2	Mortality Levels among Cousin and Unrelated Control Marriages in Selected Human Populations								
POPULATION	MORTALITY TYPE	1.0 COUSIN %	1.0 COUSIN N	1.5 COUSIN* %	1.5 COUSIN* N	2.0 COUSIN %	2.0 COUSIN N	UNRELATED %	UNRELATED N
Amish (Old Order)	Prereproductive	14.4	1218†	—	—	13.3	6064	8.2	17,200
Bombay, India	Perinatal	4.8	3309	2.8	176	0	30	2.8	35,620
France (Loir-et-Cher)	Prereproductive	17.7	282	6.7	105	11.7	240	8.6	1117
Fukuoka, Japan	0 to 6 yr	10.0	3442	8.3	1048	9.2	1066	6.4	5224
Hirado, Japan	Prereproductive	18.9	2301	15.3	764	14.7	1209	14.3	28,569
Kerala, India	Prereproductive	18.6	391	—	—	11.8	34	8.7	770
Punjab, Pakistan	Prereproductive	22.1	3532	22.9	1114	20.1	57	16.4	4731
Sweden	Prereproductive	14.1	185	13.7	227	11.4	79	8.6	625
Utah Mormons	Prereproductive	22.4	1048	15.3	517	12.2	1129	13.2	302,454

Modified from Jorde LB. Inbreeding in human populations. In: Dulbecco R, ed. *Encyclopedia of Human Biology.* Vol. 5. New York: Academic Press; 1997:1-13.
*First cousins once removed.
†Includes 1.5 cousins.

X INACTIVATION

The X chromosome contains many important protein-coding genes, and it has long been known that human females have two X chromosomes and males have only one. Thus, females have two copies of each X-linked gene, and males have only one copy. Yet males and females do not differ in terms of the amounts of protein products (e.g., enzyme levels) encoded by most of these genes. What could account for this?

In the early 1960s Mary Lyon hypothesized that one X chromosome in each somatic cell of the female is inactivated. This would result in **dosage compensation,** an equalization of the amount of X-linked gene products in males and females. The **Lyon hypothesis** stated that **X inactivation** occurs early in female embryonic development and that the X chromosome contributed by the father is inactivated in some cells, whereas in other cells the X chromosome contributed by the mother is inactivated. In each cell, one of the two X chromosomes is chosen at random for inactivation, so the maternally and paternally transmitted X chromosomes are each inactivated in about half of the embryo's cells. Thus,

inactivation, like gamete transmission, is analogous to a cointossing experiment. Once an X chromosome is inactivated in a cell, it will remain inactive in all descendants of that cell. X inactivation is therefore a randomly determined, but *fixed* (or permanent), process. As a result of X inactivation, all normal females have two distinct populations of cells: one population has an active paternally derived X chromosome, and the other has an active maternally derived X chromosome. (Fig. 4-19 provides a summary of this process.) Because they have two populations of cells, females are mosaics for X chromosome activity. Males, having only one copy of the X chromosome, are not mosaics but are **hemizygous** for the X chromosome (*hemi* means "half").

The Lyon hypothesis states that one X chromosome in each cell is randomly inactivated early in the embryonic development of females. This ensures that females, who have two copies of the X chromosome, will produce X-linked gene products in quantities roughly similar to those produced in males (dosage compensation).

The Lyon hypothesis relied on several pieces of evidence, most of which were derived from animal studies. First, it was known that females are typically mosaics for some X-linked traits and males are not. For example, female "calico" cats have alternating black and orange patches of fur that correspond to two populations of cells: one that contains X chromosomes in which an "orange" allele is active and one that contains X chromosomes in which a "black" allele is active. Male cats of this breed do not exhibit alternating colors and have either black or orange patches of fur. Another example, seen in humans, is X-linked ocular albinism. This is an X-linked recessive condition characterized by a lack of melanin production in the retina and by ocular problems such as nystagmus (rapid involuntary eye movements) and decreased visual acuity. Males who inherit the mutation show a relatively uniform lack of melanin in their retinas, whereas female heterozygotes exhibit

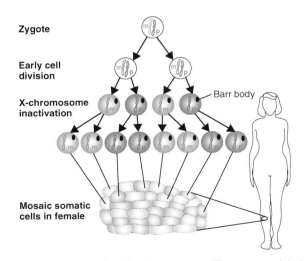

FIG 4-19   The X inactivation process. The maternal (*m*) and paternal (*p*) X chromosomes are both active in the zygote and in early embryonic cells. X inactivation then takes place, resulting in cells having either an active paternal X or an active maternal X chromosome. Females are thus X chromosome mosaics, as shown in the tissue sample at the bottom of the figure.

FIG 4-20   Fundus photos of X-linked ocular albinism. **A,** Fundus photograph of a female heterozygous carrier for X-linked ocular albinism. The pigmented and nonpigmented patches demonstrate mosaicism of the X chromosome as a result of random X inactivation. **B,** Fundus photograph of the heterozygous carrier's son, showing a much greater lack of melanin pigment. (Courtesy Dr. Donnell J. Creel, University of Utah Health Sciences Center.)

alternating patches of pigmented and nonpigmented tissue (Fig. 4-20).

The Lyon hypothesis was also supported by biochemical evidence. The enzyme glucose-6-phosphate dehydrogenase (G6PD) is encoded by a gene on the X chromosome and is present in equal quantities in males and females (dosage compensation). In females who are heterozygous for two common G6PD alleles (labeled A and B), some skin cells produce only the A variant of the enzyme and others produce only the B variant. This is further proof of X chromosome mosaicism in females.

Finally, cytogenetic studies in the 1940s showed that interphase cells of female cats often contained a densely staining chromatin mass in their nuclei. These masses were not seen in males. They were termed **Barr bodies**, after Murray Barr, one of the scientists who described them. Barr and his colleague Ewart Bertram hypothesized that the **Barr body** represented a highly condensed X chromosome. It is now known that Barr and Bertram were correct and that the inactive X chromosome is observable as a Barr body in the somatic cells of normal females. Its condensed state is correlated with reduced transcriptional activity, and its DNA is replicated later in the S phase than that of other chromosomes.

▶ The Lyon hypothesis is supported by cytogenetic evidence: Barr bodies, which are inactive X chromosomes, are seen only in cells with two or more X chromosomes. It is also supported by biochemical and animal studies that reveal mosaicism of X-linked traits in female heterozygotes.

Further study has largely verified the Lyon hypothesis. Messenger RNA (mRNA) is transcribed from only one X chromosome in each somatic cell of a normal female. The inactivation process takes place within approximately 7 to 10 days after fertilization, when the embryonic inner-cell mass contains no more than a few dozen cells. Inactivation is initiated in a single 1-Mb region on the X chromosome long arm, the **X inactivation center,** and then spreads along the chromosome. Although inactivation is random among cells that make up the embryo itself, only the paternally derived X chromosome is inactivated in cells that will become extraembryonic tissue (e.g., the placenta). X inactivation is permanent for all somatic cells in the female, but the inactive X chromosome must later become reactivated in the female's germline so that each of her egg cells will receive one active copy of the X chromosome.

An important implication of the Lyon hypothesis is that the number of Barr bodies in somatic cells is always one less than the number of X chromosomes. Normal females have one Barr body in each somatic cell, and normal males have none. Females with Turner syndrome (see Chapter 6), having only one X chromosome, have no Barr bodies. Males with Klinefelter syndrome (two X chromosomes and a Y chromosome) have one Barr body in their somatic cells, and females who have three X chromosomes per cell have two Barr bodies in each somatic cell. This pattern leads to another question: if the extra X chromosomes are inactivated, why aren't people with extra (or missing) X chromosomes phenotypically unaffected?

The answer to this question is that X inactivation is *incomplete*. Some regions of the X chromosome remain active in all copies. For example, the tips of the short and long arms of the X chromosome do not undergo inactivation. The tip of the short arm of the X chromosome is homologous to the distal short arm of the Y chromosome (see Chapter 6). In total, about 15% of the genes on the human X chromosome escape inactivation, and relatively more genes on the short arm escape inactivation than on the long arm. Some of the X-linked genes that remain active on both copies of the X chromosome have homologs on the Y chromosome, preserving equal gene dosage in males and females. Thus, having extra (or missing) copies of active portions of the X chromosome contributes to a disease phenotype.

 X inactivation is random, fixed, and incomplete. The last feature helps to explain why, despite X inactivation, most persons with abnormal numbers of sex chromosomes have a disease phenotype.

The X inactivation center contains a gene, *XIST*, that is transcribed only on the inactive X chromosome; its 17-kb mRNA transcripts are detected in normal females but not in normal males. The RNA transcript, however, is not translated into a pro-

tein and is an example of a **long noncoding RNA (lncRNA;** compare with miRNA in Chapter 2). The *XIST* RNA transcript remains in the nucleus and coats the inactive X chromosome. This process acts as a signal that leads to other aspects of inactivation, including late replication and condensation of the inactive X chromosome.

Methylation and histone deacetylation are additional features of the inactive X chromosome. Many CG dinucleotides in the 5′ regions of genes on the inactive X are heavily methylated, and the administration of demethylating agents, such as 5-azacytidine, can partially reactivate an inactive X chromosome in vitro. However, methylation does not appear to be involved in spreading the inactivation signal from the inactivation center to the remainder of the X chromosome. It is more likely to be responsible for maintaining the inactivation of a specific X chromosome in a cell and all of its descendants.

The *XIST* gene is located in the X inactivation center and is required for X inactivation. It encodes a lncRNA product that coats the inactive X chromosome. X inactivation is also associated with methylation of the inactive X chromosome, a process that might help to ensure the long-term stability of inactivation.

SEX-LINKED INHERITANCE

Sex-linked genes are those that are located on either the X or the Y chromosome. Because only a few dozen genes are known to be located on the human Y chromosome, our attention will be focused mostly on X-linked diseases. These have traditionally been grouped into X-linked recessive and X-linked dominant categories, and these categories are used here for consistency with other literature. However, because of variable expression, incomplete penetrance, and the effects of random X inactivation, the distinction between **X-linked dominant** and **X-linked recessive inheritance** is sometimes ambiguous.

X-Linked Recessive Inheritance

A number of well-known diseases and traits are caused by X-linked recessive genes. These include hemophilia A (Clinical Commentary 4-6), Duchenne muscular dystrophy (Clinical Commentary 4-7), and red-green colorblindness (Box 4-2). Additional X-linked diseases are listed in Table 4-3. The inheritance patterns and recurrence risks for X-linked recessive diseases differ substantially from those for diseases caused by autosomal genes.

Because females inherit two copies of the X chromosome, they can be homozygous for a disease-causing allele at a given locus, heterozygous at the locus, or homozygous for the normal allele at the locus. In this way, X-linked loci in females are much like autosomal loci. However, for most X-linked loci, there is only one copy of the allele in an individual somatic cell because of X inactivation. This means that about half of the cells in a heterozygous female will express the disease allele and half will express the normal allele.

CLINICAL COMMENTARY 4-6

Hemophilia A

Hemophilia A is caused by mutations in the gene that encodes clotting factor VIII and affects approximately 1 in 5000 to 1 in 10,000 males worldwide. It is the most common of the severe bleeding disorders and has been recognized as a familial disorder for centuries. The Talmud states that boys whose brothers or cousins bled to death during circumcision are exempt from the procedure (this may well be the first recorded example of genetic counseling).

Hemophilia A is caused by deficient or defective factor VIII, a key component of the clotting cascade. Fibrin formation is affected, resulting in prolonged and often severe bleeding from wounds and hemorrhages in the joints and muscles (Fig. 4-21). Bruising is often seen. Hemarthroses (bleeding into the joints) are common in the ankles, knees, hips, and elbows. These events are often painful, and repeated episodes can lead to destruction of the synovium and diminished joint function. Intracranial hemorrhages can occur and are a leading cause of death. Platelet activity is normal in hemophiliacs, so minor lacerations and abrasions do not usually lead to excessive bleeding.

Hemophilia A varies considerably in its severity, and this variation is correlated directly with the level of factor VIII. About half of hemophilia A patients fall into the severe category, with factor VIII levels that are less than 1% of normal. These persons experience relatively frequent bleeding episodes, often several per month. Patients with moderate hemophilia (1%-5% of normal factor VIII) generally have bleeding episodes only after mild trauma and typically experience one to several episodes per year. Persons with mild hemophilia have 5% to 30% of the normal factor VIII level and usually experience bleeding episodes only after surgery or relatively severe trauma.

Historically, hemophilia A was often fatal before 20 years of age, but a major advance in treatment came in the early 1960s with the ability to purify factor VIII from donor plasma. Factor VIII is usually administered at the first sign of a bleeding episode and is a highly effective treatment. Prophylactic factor VIII administration in severe hemophiliacs is effective in preventing loss of joint function. By the 1970s, the median age at death of persons with hemophilia had increased to 68 years.

FIG 4-21   A, The enlarged right knee joint of a patient with hemophilia A, demonstrating the effects of hemarthrosis. **B,** Extensive bruising of the right outer thigh. (From Hoffbrand VA. *Color Atlas of Clinical Hematology.* 3rd ed. Philadelphia: Mosby; 2000:281-283.)

CLINICAL COMMENTARY 4-6
Hemophilia A (Continued)

The major drawback of donor-derived factor VIII was the fact that, because a typical infusion contained plasma products from hundreds or thousands of different donors, it was often contaminated by viruses. Consequently, patients often suffered from hepatitis B and C infections. More seriously, human immunodeficiency virus (HIV) can be transmitted in this manner, and it is estimated that half of American hemophilia patients treated with donor-derived factor VIII between 1978 and 1985 became infected with HIV. From 1979 to 1998, acquired immune deficiency syndrome (AIDS) accounted for nearly half of deaths among Americans with hemophilia A, which resulted in a decrease in the median age at death to 49 years in the 1980s. Donor blood has been screened for HIV since 1985, and heat treatment of donor-derived factor VIII kills HIV and hepatitis B virus, nearly eliminating the threat of infection. Consequently, AIDS mortality among those with hemophilia A has decreased markedly since 1995.

Cloning and sequencing of the factor VIII gene has led to a number of insights. Patients with nonsense or frameshift mutations usually develop severe hemophilia, and those with missense mutations usually have mild to moderate disease. This is expected because nonsense and frameshift mutations typically produce a truncated protein that is degraded and lost. Missense mutations produce a single amino acid substitution without a dominant negative effect, usually resulting in an altered but partially functional protein product. Many of the point mutations take place at methylated CG sequences, which are hot spots for mutation (see Chapter 3). About 45% of severe cases of hemophilia A are caused by a chromosome inversion (see Chapter 6) that disrupts the factor VIII gene. An additional 5% of patients have deletions, which usually lead to relatively severe disease. About 10% of female heterozygotes have factor VIII levels less than 35%, and some of these are manifesting heterozygotes, with mild symptoms of hemophilia A.

Cloning of the factor VIII gene has enabled the production of human factor VIII using recombinant DNA techniques. Extensive clinical testing showed that recombinant factor VIII works as effectively as the donor-derived form, and it was approved for commercial use in 1994. Recombinant factor VIII has, of course, the advantage that there is no possibility of viral contamination. However, as with other forms of factor VIII, recombinant factor VIII generates antifactor VIII antibody production in approximately 10% to 15% of patients. (This response is most common in patients who have no native factor VIII production.)

Two other major bleeding disorders are hemophilia B and von Willebrand disease. Hemophilia B, sometimes called Christmas disease (Christmas was the last name of the first reported patient), is also an X-linked recessive disorder and is caused by a deficiency of clotting factor IX. This condition is about one fifth as common as hemophilia A and can be treated with donor-derived or recombinant factor IX. Von Willebrand disease is an autosomal dominant disorder that is highly variable in expression. Although it can affect as many as 1% of individuals of European descent, it reaches severe expression in fewer than 1 in 10,000. The von Willebrand factor, which is encoded by a gene on chromosome 12, acts as a carrier protein for factor VIII. In addition, it binds to platelets and to damaged blood vessel endothelium, thus promoting the adhesion of platelets to damaged vessel walls.

Hemophilia is of historical interest because it affected members of the royal families of Germany, Spain, England, and Russia (Fig. 4-22). Among these families, Queen Victoria of England was the first known heterozygous hemophilia carrier. She had one affected son, and two of her daughters had affected sons, making them presumptive carriers. One of her affected great-grandsons was the Tsarevitch Alexei of Russia, the son of Tsar Nicholas II and Alexandra. Grigori Rasputin, called the "mad monk," had an unusual ability to calm the Tsarevitch during bleed-

FIG 4-22   A pedigree showing the inheritance of hemophilia B in the European royal families. The first known carrier in the family was Queen Victoria. Note that all of the affected individuals are male. (Modified from McCance K, Huether S. *Pathophysiology: The Biologic Basis for Disease in Adults and Children*. 5th ed. St. Louis: Mosby; 2005.)

CLINICAL COMMENTARY 4-6
Hemophilia A (Continued)

ing episodes, probably through hypnosis. As a result, he came to have considerable influence in the royal court, and some historians believe that his destabilizing effect helped to bring about the 1917 Bolshevik revolution. Recently, the Russian royal family was again touched by genetics. Using the polymerase chain reaction, autosomal DNA microsatellites and mitochondrial DNA sequences were assayed in the remains of several bodies exhumed near Yekaterinburg, the reputed murder site of the royal family. Analysis of this genetic variation and comparison with living maternal relatives showed that the bodies were indeed those of the Russian royal family. Further analysis demonstrated that Alexei had a pathogenic mutation in the gene that encodes factor IX, establishing that the royal families were affected by hemophilia B (rather than the more common hemophilia A).

CLINICAL COMMENTARY 4-7
Duchenne Muscular Dystrophy

Muscular dystrophy, defined as a progressive weakness and loss of muscle, exists in dozens of different forms. Of these, Duchenne muscular dystrophy (DMD), named after the French neurologist who provided the first comprehensive description in 1868, is one of the most severe and common forms. It affects approximately 1 of every 4,000 males, a prevalence figure that is similar among all ethnic groups studied thus far.

The symptoms of DMD are usually seen before the age of 5 years, when parents begin to notice unusual clumsiness and muscle weakness. Pseudohypertrophy of the calves, the result of infiltration of muscle by fat and connective tissue, is often seen early in the course of the disease. All skeletal muscle degenerates eventually, and most patients with DMD are confined to a wheelchair by 11 years of age. The heart and respiratory musculature become impaired, and death usually results from respiratory or cardiac failure. Survival beyond age 25 years is uncommon; little can be done to alter the ultimate course of this disease.

As muscle cells die, the enzyme creatine kinase (CK) leaks into the blood stream. In DMD patients, serum CK is elevated at least 20 times above the upper limit of the normal range. This elevation can be observed presymptomatically, before clinical symptoms such as muscle wasting are seen. Other traditional diagnostic tools include electromyography, which reveals reduced action potentials, and muscle biopsy.

Female heterozygous carriers of the DMD-causing mutations are usually free of disease, although 8% to 10% have some degree of muscle weakness. In addition, serum CK exceeds the 95th percentile in approximately two thirds of heterozygotes.

Until the gene responsible for DMD was identified in 1986, little was known about the mechanism responsible for muscle deterioration. The *DMD* gene covers approximately 2.5 Mb of DNA, making it by far the largest gene known in the human. It contains 79 exons that produce a 14-kb mRNA transcript. Because of this gene's huge size, transcription of an mRNA molecule can take as long as 24 hours. The protein product, named dystrophin, was unknown before the identification of *DMD*. Dystrophin accounts for only about 0.002% of a striated muscle cell's protein mass and is localized on the cytoplasmic side of the cell membrane. Its amino terminus binds F-actin, a key cytoskeletal protein. The carboxyl terminus of dystrophin binds a complex of glycoproteins, known as the dystroglycan-sarcoglycan complex, that spans the cell membrane and binds to extracellular proteins. Dystrophin thus links these two cellular components and plays a key role in maintaining the structural integrity of the muscle cell. Lacking dystrophin, the muscle cells of the DMD patient gradually die as they are stressed by muscle contractions.

The large size of *DMD* helps to explain its high mutation rate, about 10^{-4} per locus per generation. As with the gene responsible for neurofibromatosis type 1, the *DMD* gene presents a large target for mutation. A slightly altered form of the *DMD* gene product is normally found in brain cells, in which the transcription initiation site is farther downstream in the gene and a different promoter is used. Thus, the mRNA transcript and the resulting gene product differ from the gene product found in muscle cells. Dystrophin's expression in the brain helps to explain why approximately 25% of DMD patients have some degree of intellectual disability. Several additional promoters have also been found, providing a good example of a single gene that can produce different gene products as a result of modified transcription.

Becker muscular dystrophy (BMD), another X-linked recessive dystrophic condition, is less severe than the Duchenne form. The progression is also much slower, with onset at 11 years of age, on average. One study showed that whereas 95% of DMD patients are confined to a wheelchair before 12 years of age, 95% of those with BMD become wheelchair bound after 12 years of age. Some never lose their ability to walk. BMD is less common than DMD, affecting about 1 in 18,000 male births.

For some time it was unclear whether BMD and DMD are caused by distinct X-linked loci or by different mutations at the same locus. Identification of *DMD* showed the latter to be the case. Both diseases usually result from deletions (65% of DMD cases and 85% of BMD cases) or duplications (6% to 7% of DMD and BMD cases) in *DMD*. But, whereas the great majority of DMD-causing deletions and duplications produce frameshifts, the majority of BMD-causing mutations are in-frame alterations (i.e., a multiple of three bases is deleted or duplicated). One would expect that a frameshift, which is likely to produce a premature stop codon (see Chapter 3) and no protein product, would produce more-severe disease than would an in-frame alteration.

The consequences of these different mutations can be observed in the gene product. Although dystrophin is absent in almost all DMD patients, it is usually present in reduced quantity (or as a shortened form of the protein) in

CLINICAL COMMENTARY 4-7
Duchenne Muscular Dystrophy (Continued)

BMD patients. Thus, a dystrophin assay can help to distinguish between the two diseases. This assay also helps to distinguish both diseases from other forms of muscular dystrophy, because several of these forms (e.g., various limb-girdle muscular dystrophies) result from mutations in genes that encode proteins of the dystroglycan-sarcoglycan complex, whereas dystrophin appears to be affected only in BMD and DMD (Figs. 4-23, 4-24, and 4-25).

FIG 4-23   A patient with late-stage Duchenne muscular dystrophy, showing severe muscle loss.

FIG 4-24   Transverse section of gastrocnemius muscle from **(A)** a normal boy and **(B)** a boy with Duchenne muscular dystrophy. Normal muscle fiber is replaced with fat and connective tissue.

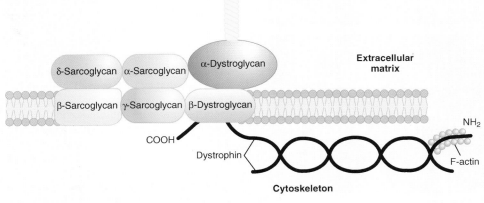

FIG 4-25   The amino terminus of the dystrophin protein binds to F-actin in the cell's cytoskeleton, and its carboxyl terminus binds to elements of the dystroglycan-sarcoglycan complex. The latter complex of glycoproteins spans the cell membrane and binds to proteins in the extracellular matrix, such as laminin.

CLINICAL COMMENTARY 4-7
Duchenne Muscular Dystrophy (Continued)

Genetic testing (see Chapter 10) is now commonly used to help diagnose DMD and BMD; a disease-causing mutation is identified in about 95% of cases. Considerable research has been done on genetically based therapies for muscular dystrophy. For example, small-molecule drugs can cause ribosomes to read through premature stop codons and have shown promise in mouse models. Antisense oligonucleotides (see Chapter 10) can induce the skipping of the altered DMD exon during mRNA translation. These approaches, along with gene therapy in which a normal copy of DMD is inserted into muscle cells, are now being tested in clinical trials.

BOX 4-2   Color Vision: Molecular Biology and Evolution

Human vision depends on a system of retinal photoreceptor cells, about 95% of which are **rod cells.** They contain the light-absorbing protein rhodopsin and allow us to see in conditions of dim light. In addition, the retina contains three classes of **cone cells,** which contain light-absorbing proteins (opsins) that react to light wavelengths corresponding to the three primary colors—red, green, and blue. Color vision depends on the presence of all four of these cell types. Because three major colors are involved, normal color vision is said to be **trichromatic.**

There are many recognized defects of human color vision. The most common of these involve red and green color perception and have been known since 1911 to be inherited in X-linked recessive fashion. Thus, they are much more common in males than in females. Various forms of red-green colorblindness are seen in about 8% of European males, 4% to 5% of Asian males, and 1% to 4% of African and Native American males. Among European males, 2% are **dichromatic:** they are unable to perceive one of the primary colors, usually red or green. The inability to perceive green is termed **deuteranopia,** and the inability to perceive red is termed **protanopia.** About 6% of European males can detect green and red, but with altered perception of the relative shades of these colors. These are respectively termed **deuteranomalous** and **protanomalous** conditions.

It should be apparent that dichromats are not really color blind, because they can still perceive a fairly large array of different colors. True colorblindness (**monochromacy,** the ability to perceive only one color) is much less common, affecting approximately 1 in 100,000 persons. There are two major forms of monochromatic vision. **Rod monochromacy** is an autosomal recessive condition in which all visual function is carried out by rod cells. **Blue cone monochromacy** is an X-linked recessive condition in which both the red and green cone cells are absent.

Cloning of the genes responsible for color perception has revealed a number of interesting facts about both the biology and the evolution of color vision in humans. In the 1980s, Jeremy Nathans and colleagues reasoned that the opsins in all four types of photoreceptor cells might have similar amino acid sequences because they carry out similar functions. Thus, the DNA sequences of the genes encoding these proteins should also be similar. But none of these genes had been located, and the precise nature of the protein products was unknown. How could they locate these genes?

Fortunately, the gene encoding rhodopsin in cattle had been cloned. Even though humans and cattle are separated by millions of years of evolution, their rhodopsin proteins still share about 40% of the same amino acid sequence. Thus, the cattle (bovine) rhodopsin gene could be used as a probe to search for a similar DNA sequence in the human genome. A portion of the bovine rhodopsin gene was converted to single-strand form, radioactively labeled, and hybridized with human DNA (much in the same way that a probe is used in Southern blotting [see Chapter 3]). Low-stringency hybridization conditions were used: Temperature and other conditions were manipulated so that complementary base pairing would occur despite some sequence differences between the two species. In this way, the human rhodopsin gene was identified and mapped to chromosome 3.

The next step was to use the human rhodopsin gene as a probe to identify the cone-cell opsin genes. Each of the conecell opsin amino acid sequences shares 40% to 45% similarity with the human rhodopsin amino acid sequence. By probing with the rhodopsin gene, the gene for blue-sensitive opsin was identified and mapped to

A, Image perceived by a person with normal color vision. **B,** The predicted perception by a person with protanopia, a form of red-green colorblindness. (Copyright George V. Kelvin.)

BOX 4-2   Color Vision: Molecular Biology and Evolution (Continued)

chromosome 7. This gene was expected to map to an autosome because variants in blue sensitivity are inherited in autosomal recessive fashion. The genes for the red and green-sensitive opsins were also identified in this way and, as expected, were found to be on the X chromosome. The red and green genes are highly similar, sharing 98% of their DNA sequence.

Initially, many investigators expected that people with color vision defects would display the usual array of deletions and missense and nonsense mutations seen in other disorders. But further study revealed some surprises. It was found that the red and green opsin genes are located directly adjacent to each other on the distal long arm of the X chromosome and that normal persons have one copy of the red gene but can have one to several copies of the green gene. The multiple green genes are 99.9% identical

in DNA sequence, and the presence of multiple copies of these genes has no effect on color perception because only the red gene and the first green gene are expressed in the retina. However, when there are no green genes, deuteranopia is produced. Persons who lack the single red gene have protanopia.

The unique aspect of these deletions is that they are the result of **unequal crossover** during meiosis. Unlike ordinary crossover, in which equal segments of chromosomes are exchanged (see Chapter 2), unequal crossover results in a loss of chromosome material on one chromosome homolog and a gain of material on the other. Unequal crossover seems to be facilitated by the high similarity in DNA sequence among the red and green genes: It is relatively easy for the cellular machinery to make a mistake in deciding where the crossover should occur. Thus,

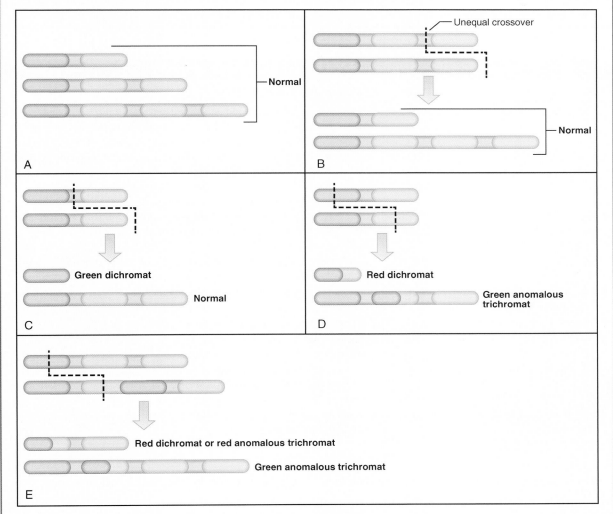

A, Normal individuals have one red gene and one to several green genes. **B,** Unequal crossover causes normal variation in the number of green genes. **C,** Unequal crossover can produce a green dichromat with no green genes (deuteranopia). **D,** Unequal crossover that occurs within the red and green genes can produce a red dichromat (protanopia) or a green anomalous trichromat (deuteranomaly). **E,** Crossovers within the red and green genes can also produce red anomalous trichromats (protanomaly). The degree of red and green color perception depends on where the crossover occurs within the genes. (Based on Nathans J, Merbs SL, Sung C, et al. The genes for color vision. *Sci Am.* 1989;260:42-49.)

BOX 4-2   Color Vision: Molecular Biology and Evolution (Continued)

a female with one red gene and two green genes could produce one gamete containing a red gene with one green gene and another gamete containing a red gene with three green genes. Unequal crossover could also result in gametes with no copies of a gene, producing protanopia or deuteranopia.

Unequal crossover also explains protanomalous and deuteranomalous color vision. Here, crossover takes place within the red or green genes, resulting in new chromosomes with hybrid genes (e.g., a portion of the red gene fused with a portion of the green gene). The relative ratio of red and green components of these **fusion genes** determines the extent and nature of the red-green anomaly.

Because the opsin genes have DNA sequence similarity and perform similar functions, they are members of a gene family, much like the globin genes (see Chapter 3). This suggests that they evolved from a single ancestral gene that, through time, duplicated and diverged to encode different but related proteins. Evidence for this process is provided by comparing these genes in humans and other species. Because the X-linked red and green opsin genes share the greatest degree of DNA sequence similarity, we would expect that these two genes would be the result of the most recent duplication. Indeed, humans share all four of their opsin genes with apes and Old World monkeys, but the less closely related New World monkeys have only a single opsin gene on their X chromosomes. It is therefore likely that the red-green duplication occurred sometime after the split of the New and Old World monkeys, which took place about 30 to 40 million years ago. Similar comparisons date the split of the X-linked and autosomal cone opsin genes to approximately 500 million years ago. And finally, comparisons with the fruit fly, Drosophila melanogaster, indicate that the duplication that produced the rod and cone visual pigment genes may have occurred as much as 1 billion years ago.

TABLE 4-3   Additional Examples of X-Linked Recessive Disorders

NAME	GENE	CLINICAL CHARACTERISTICS
Juvenile retinoschisis	RS1	Progressive visual impairment caused by splitting of the nerve fiber layer of the retina; begins in the first or second decade of life; impairment typically 20/60 to 20/120
Leri-Weill dyschondrosis	SHOX	Madelung deformity of the radius and ulna; mesomelia (shortening of the forearms and lower legs); short stature
ATR-X	ATRX	Mental retardation; genital anomalies; and α-thalassemia without abnormalities of the α-globin gene complex
Hypohydrotic ectodermal hypoplasia	EDA	Diminished sweating and heat intolerance; sparse and light-colored hair, eyelashes, and eyebrows; abnormal and/or missing teeth; recurrent upper airway infections
Vitamin D-resistant rickets	PHEX	Hypophosphatemia due to reduced renal phosphate reabsorption; short stature; bowed legs; poor teeth formation
Aarskog-Scott syndrome (faciogenital dysplasia)	FGD1	Short stature; hypertelorism; genital anomalies
Cleft palate with ankyloglossia	TBX22	Cleft palate with or without ankyloglossia (tongue tie)
Pelizaeus-Merzbacher disease	PLP1	Defect of myelination; typically manifests in infancy or early childhood; characterized by nystagmus, hypotonia, spasticity, early death
Nephrogenic diabetes insipidus	AVPR2	Impaired response to antidiuretic hormone that leads to inability to concentrate urine, polydipsia (excessive thirst), polyuria (excessive urine production)
Otopalatodigital spectrum disorders	FLNA	Skeletal dysplasia ranging from mild to lethal; males more severely affected than females

Thus, as with autosomal recessive traits, the heterozygote will produce about 50% of the normal level of the gene product. Ordinarily this is sufficient for a normal phenotype. The situation is different for males, who are hemizygous for the X chromosome. If a male inherits a recessive disease gene on the X chromosome, he will be affected by the disease because the Y chromosome does not carry a normal allele to compensate for the effects of the disease allele.

An X-linked recessive disease with gene frequency q will be seen in a fraction q of males. This is because a male, having only one X chromosome, will manifest the disease if his X chromosome contains the disease-causing mutation. Females, needing two copies of the mutant allele to express the disease, will have a disease frequency of only q^2, as in autosomal recessive diseases. For example, hemophilia A (see Clinical Commentary 4-6) is seen in about 1 of every 10,000 males in some populations. Thus, in a collection of 10,000 male X chromosomes, one chromosome would, on average, contain the disease-causing mutation ($q = 0.0001$). Affected female homozygotes are almost never seen, because $q^2 = 0.00000001$, or 1 in 100,000,000. This example shows that, in general, males are more frequently affected with X-linked recessive diseases than are females, with this difference becoming more pronounced as the disease becomes rarer.

▶ Because females have two copies of the X chromosome and males have only one (hemizygosity), X-linked recessive diseases are much more common among males than among females.

In addition to their higher prevalence in males than females, X-linked recessive diseases display several patterns of inheritance that distinguish them from autosomal dominant and recessive diseases (Fig. 4-26). Because a father can transmit only a Y chromosome to his son, X-linked genes are not passed from father to son. (In contrast, father-to-son transmission can be observed for autosomal disease alleles.) An X-linked disease allele can be transmitted through a series of phenotypically normal heterozygous females, causing the appearance of skipped generations. The gene is passed from an affected father to all of his daughters, who, as carriers, transmit it to

approximately half of their sons, who are affected.

▶ X-linked recessive inheritance is characterized by an absence of father-to-son transmission, skipped generations when genes are passed through female carriers, and a preponderance of affected males.

The most common mating type involving X-linked recessive genes is the combination of a carrier female and a normal male. The carrier mother will transmit the disease gene to half of her sons and half of her daughters, on average. As Figure 4-27 shows, approximately half of the daughters of such a mating will be carriers, and half will be normal. Half of the sons will be normal, and half, on average, will have the disease.

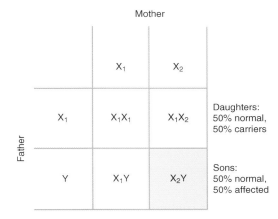

FIG 4-27   Punnett square representation of the mating of a heterozygous female who carries an X-linked recessive disease gene with a normal male. X_1, Chromosome with normal allele; X_2, chromosome with disease allele.

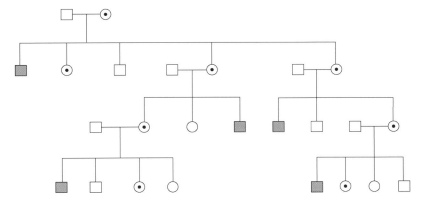

FIG 4-26   A pedigree showing the inheritance of an X-linked recessive trait. *Solid symbols* represent affected individuals, and *dotted symbols* represent heterozygous carriers.

The other common mating type is an affected father and a homozygous unaffected mother (Fig. 4-28). Here, all of the sons must be unaffected, because the father can transmit only his Y chromosome to them. Because all of the daughters must receive the father's X chromosome, they will all be heterozygous carriers. None of the children will manifest the disease, however. Because the father *must* transmit his X chromosome to his daughters and cannot transmit it to his sons, these risks, unlike those in the previous paragraph, are exact figures rather than probability estimates.

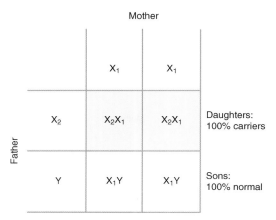

FIG 4-28 Punnett square representation of the mating of a normal female with a male who is affected by an X-linked recessive disease. X_1, Chromosome with normal allele; X_2, chromosome with disease allele.

A much less common mating type is that of an affected father and a carrier mother (Fig. 4-29). Half of the daughters will be heterozygous carriers, and half, on average, will be homozygous for the disease gene and thus affected. Half of the sons will be unaffected, and half will be affected. It may appear that father-to-son transmission of the disease has occurred, but the affected son has actually received the disease allele from his mother.

Recurrence risks for X-linked recessive disorders are more complex than for autosomal disorders. The risk depends on the genotype of each parent and the sex of the offspring.

Occasionally, females who inherit only a single copy of an X-linked recessive disease allele can be affected with the disease. Imagine a female embryo

FIG 4-29 Punnett square representation of the mating of a carrier female with a male affected with an X-linked recessive disease. X_1, Chromosome with normal allele; X_2, chromosome with disease allele.

that has received a normal clotting factor VIII allele from one parent and a mutated clotting factor VIII allele from the other. Ordinarily, X inactivation will result in approximately equal numbers of cells having active paternal and maternal X chromosomes. In this case, the female carrier would produce about 50% of the normal level of factor VIII and would be phenotypically normal. However, because X inactivation is a random process, it sometimes results in a heterozygous female in whom nearly all of the active X chromosomes happen to be the ones carrying the disease-causing mutation. About 5% of female heterozygotes exhibit hemophilia A and are termed **manifesting heterozygotes.** Because they usually maintain at least a small fraction of active normal X chromosomes, manifesting heterozygotes tend to be relatively mildly affected.

Because X inactivation is a random process, some female heterozygotes experience inactivation of most of the normal X chromosomes in their cells. These manifesting heterozygotes are usually mildly affected.

Less commonly, females having only a single X chromosome (Turner syndrome) have been seen with X-linked recessive diseases such as hemophilia A. Females can also be affected with X-linked recessive diseases as a result of translocations or deletions of X chromosome material (see Chapter 6). These events are rare.

X-Linked Dominant Inheritance

X-linked dominant diseases are fewer and less prevalent than are X-linked recessive diseases. An example of an X-linked dominant disease is hypophosphatemic rickets, a disease in which the kidneys are impaired in their ability to reabsorb phosphate. This results in abnormal ossification, with bending and distortion of the bones (rickets). Another example is incontinentia pigmenti type 1, a disorder characterized by abnormal skin pigmentation, conical or missing teeth, and ocular and, in some cases, neurological abnormalities. This disorder is seen only in females. It is thought that hemizygous males are so severely affected that they do not survive to term. Heterozygous females, having one normal X chromosome, tend generally to have milder expression of X-linked dominant traits (just as heterozygotes for most autosomal dominant disease genes are less severely affected than are homozygotes).

X-linked dominant inheritance is also observed in Rett syndrome, a neurodevelopmental disorder seen in 1 in 10,000 females and in a much smaller fraction of males, most of whom do not survive to term. Rett syndrome is characterized by autistic behavior, intellectual disability, seizures, and gait ataxia. The severity of this condition varies substantially among affected females, reflecting the effects of random X inactivation. In mildly affected females, a large percentage of the X chromosomes that bear the disease-causing mutation have been randomly inactivated. About 95% of classic Rett syndrome cases are caused by mutations in the *MECP2* gene, and most of these mutations are *de novo* events that occur in the paternal germline (consistent with a higher mutation rate in male gamete formation, discussed in Chapter 3). The protein product encoded by *MECP2* binds to methylated CG sequences found in the 5′ regions of other genes. After binding to these sequences, the protein helps to recruit other proteins that repress transcription by causing chromatin condensation. Loss-of-function mutations in *MECP2* result in the inappropriate expression of genes thought to be involved in brain development.

Figure 4-30 illustrates a pedigree for X-linked dominant inheritance. As with autosomal dominant diseases, a person need inherit only a single copy of an X-linked dominant disease gene to manifest the disorder. Because females have two X chromosomes, either of which can potentially carry the disease gene, they are about twice as commonly affected as males (unless the disorder is lethal in males, as in incontinentia pigmenti). Affected fathers cannot transmit the trait to their sons. All of their daughters must inherit the disease gene, so all are affected. Affected females are usually heterozygotes and thus have a 50% chance of passing the disease allele to their daughters and sons. The characteristics of X-linked dominant and X-linked recessive inheritance are summarized in Table 4-4. As already mentioned, the distinction between these categories can be blurred by incomplete penetrance in heterozygotes for X-linked dominant mutations and by the presence of disease in heterozygotes for X-linked recessive mutations (manifesting heterozygotes).

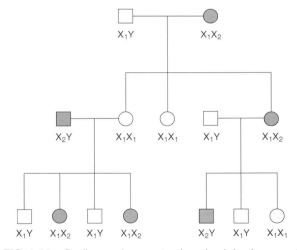

FIG 4-30   Pedigree demonstrating the inheritance of an X-linked dominant trait. X_1, Chromosome with normal allele; X_2, chromosome with disease allele.

X-linked dominant diseases display characteristic patterns of inheritance. They are about twice as common in females as in males, skipped generations are uncommon, and father-to-son transmission is not seen.

TABLE 4-4 **Comparison of the Major Attributes of X-Linked Dominant and X-Linked Recessive Inheritance Patterns**[*]

ATTRIBUTE	X-LINKED DOMINANT	X-LINKED RECESSIVE
Recurrence risk for heterozygous female × normal male mating	50% of sons affected; 50% of daughters affected	50% of sons affected; 50% of daughters heterozygous carriers
Recurrence risk for affected male × normal female mating	0% of sons affected; 100% of daughters affected	0% of sons affected; 100% of daughters heterozygous carriers
Transmission pattern	Vertical; disease phenotype seen in generation after generation	Skipped generations may be seen, representing transmission through carrier females
Sex ratio	Twice as many affected females as affected males (unless disease is lethal in males)	Much greater prevalence of affected males; affected homozygous females are rare
Other	Male-to-male transmission is not seen; expression is less severe in female heterozygotes than in affected males	Male-to-male transmission not seen; manifesting heterozygotes may be seen in females

[*]Compare with the inheritance patterns for autosomal diseases shown in Table 4-1.

Y-Linked Inheritance

Although it consists of approximately 60 Mb of DNA, the Y chromosome contains relatively few genes. Only a few dozen Y-linked, or **holandric,** genes have been identified. These include the gene that initiates differentiation of the embryo into a male (see Chapter 6), several genes that encode testis-specific spermatogenesis factors, a minor histocompatibility antigen (termed HY), and a gene in which mutations can cause hearing loss (*DFNY1*). Several housekeeping genes are located on the Y chromosome, and they all have inactivation-escaping homologs on the X chromosome. Transmission of Y-linked traits is strictly from father to son (Fig. 4-31).

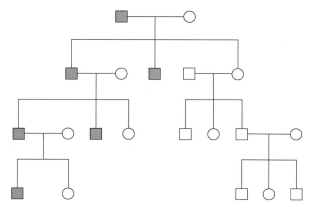

FIG 4-31 Pedigree demonstrating the inheritance of a Y-linked trait. Transmission is exclusively male to male.

SEX-LIMITED AND SEX-INFLUENCED TRAITS

Confusion sometimes exists regarding traits that are sex-linked and those that are **sex-limited** or **sex-influenced**. A **sex-limited trait** occurs in only one of the sexes—due, for instance, to anatomical differences. Inherited uterine or testicular defects would be examples. A good example of a **sex-influenced trait** is male-pattern baldness, which occurs in both males and females but much more commonly in males. This is related in part to sex differences in hormone levels. Contrary to oft-stated belief, male-pattern baldness is not strictly X-linked, although variation in the X-linked androgen receptor gene is associated with baldness. Autosomal genes are also thought to influence male-pattern baldness, helping to explain apparent father-to-son transmission of this trait.

MITOCHONDRIAL INHERITANCE

The great majority of genetic diseases are caused by alterations in the nuclear genome. However, a small but significant number of diseases can be caused by mutations in mitochondrial DNA. Because of the unique properties of the mitochondria, these diseases display characteristic modes of inheritance and a large degree of phenotypic variability.

Each human cell contains several hundred or more mitochondria in its cytoplasm. Through the complex process of oxidative phosphorylation, mitochondria produce adenosine triphosphate (ATP), the energy source essential for cellular metabolism. Mitochondria are thus critically important for cell survival.

The mitochondria have their own DNA molecules, which occur in several copies per mitochondrial body and consist of 16,569 base pairs arranged on a double-stranded circular molecule (Fig. 4-32). The mitochondrial genome encodes two ribosomal RNAs (rRNAs), 22 transfer RNAs (tRNAs), and 13 polypeptides involved in oxidative phosphorylation. (Approximately 1000 nuclear DNA genes also encode polypeptides that are transported into the mitochondria.) Transcription of mitochondrial DNA (mtDNA) takes place in the mitochondrion, independently of the nucleus. Unlike nuclear genes, mtDNA genes contain no introns. Because it is located in the cytoplasm, mtDNA is inherited exclusively through the maternal line (Fig. 4-33). Males do not transmit mtDNA to their offspring because sperm cells contain only a small number of mtDNA molecules, which are not incorporated into the developing embryo. (One isolated case of paternal transmission of a mitochondrial DNA mutation has been reported, but such events appear to be extremely rare.)

The mutation rate of mtDNA is about 10 times higher than that of nuclear DNA. This is caused by a relative lack of DNA repair mechanisms in the mtDNA and also by damage from free oxygen radicals released during the oxidative phosphorylation process.

Because each cell contains a *population* of mtDNA molecules, a single cell can harbor some molecules that have an mtDNA mutation and other molecules that do not. This heterogeneity in DNA composi-

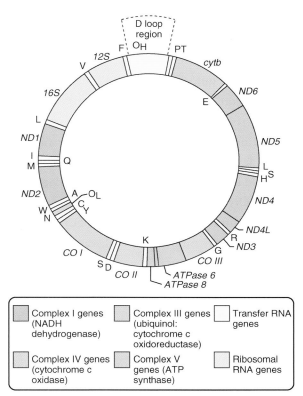

FIG 4-32 The circular mitochondrial DNA genome. Locations of protein-encoding genes (for reduced nicotinamide adenine dinucleotide [NADH] dehydrogenase, cytochrome c oxidase, cytochrome c oxidoreductase, and adenosine triphosphate [ATP] synthase) are shown, as are the locations of the two ribosomal RNA genes and 22 transfer RNA genes (designated by single letters). The replication origins of the heavy (OH) and light (OL) chains and the noncoding D loop (also known as the control region) are shown. (Modified from MITOMAP. A Human Mitochondrial Genome Database. http://www.mitomap.org, 2008.)

FIG 4-33 A pedigree showing the inheritance of a disease caused by a mitochondrial DNA mutation. Only females can transmit the disease mutation to their offspring. Complete penetrance of the disease-causing mutation is shown in this pedigree, but heteroplasmy often results in incomplete penetrance for mitochondrial diseases.

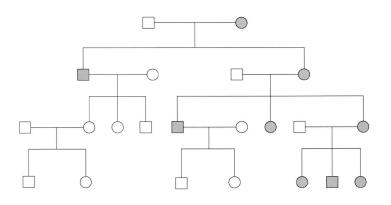

tion, termed **heteroplasmy,** is an important cause of variable expression in mitochondrial diseases. The larger the percentage of mutant mtDNA molecules, the more severe the expression of the disease. As cells divide, changes in the percentage of mutant alleles can occur through chance variation (identical in concept to genetic drift, discussed in Chapter 3) or because of a selective advantage (e.g., deletions produce a shorter mitochondrial DNA molecule that can replicate more quickly than a full-length molecule).

Each tissue type requires a certain amount of ATP for normal function. Although some variation in ATP levels may be tolerated, there is typically a threshold level below which cells begin to degenerate and die. Organ systems with large ATP requirements and high thresholds tend to be the ones most seriously affected by mitochondrial diseases. For example, the central nervous system consumes about 20% of the body's ATP production and therefore is often affected by mtDNA mutations.

Like the globin disorders, mitochondrial disorders can be classified according to the type of mutation that causes them. Missense mutations in protein-coding mtDNA genes cause one of the best-known mtDNA diseases, Leber hereditary optic neuropathy (LHON). This disease, which affects about one in 10,000 persons, is characterized by rapid loss of vision in the central visual field as a result of optic nerve death. Vision loss typically begins in the third decade of life and is usually irreversible. Heteroplasmy is minimal in LHON, so expression tends to be relatively uniform and pedigrees for this disorder usually display a clear pattern of mitochondrial inheritance.

Single-base mutations in a tRNA gene can result in myoclonic epilepsy with ragged-red fiber syndrome (MERRF), a disorder characterized by epilepsy, dementia, ataxia (uncoordinated muscle movement), and myopathy (muscle disease). MERRF is characterized by heteroplasmic mtDNA and is thus highly variable in its expression. Another example of a mitochondrial disease caused by a single-base tRNA mutation is mitochondrial encephalomyopathy and stroke-like episodes (MELAS). Like MERRF, MELAS is heteroplasmic and highly variable in expression.

The final class of mtDNA mutations consists of duplications and deletions. These can produce Kearns-Sayre disease (muscle weakness, cerebellar damage, and heart failure); Pearson syndrome (infantile pancreatic insufficiency, pancytopenia, and lactic acidosis); and chronic progressive external ophthalmoplegia (CPEO). Hundreds of disease-causing mtDNA mutations, including single-base mutations, deletions, and duplications, have been reported.

Mitochondrial mutations are also associated with some common human diseases. A mitochondrial mutation causes a form of late-onset deafness, and the MELAS mutation is seen in 1% to 2% of persons with type 2 diabetes mellitus. Mitochondrial alterations may also be associated with some cases of Alzheimer disease, although it remains unclear whether mitochondrial mutations are a primary cause or a secondary event. It has also been suggested that mtDNA mutations, which accumulate through the life of an individual as a result of free radical formation, could contribute to the aging process.

 The mitochondria, which produce ATP, have their own unique DNA. Mitochondrial DNA is maternally inherited and has a high mutation rate. A number of diseases are known to be caused by mutations in mitochondrial DNA.

GENOMIC IMPRINTING

Mendel's experimental work with garden peas established that the phenotype is the same whether a given allele is inherited from the mother or the father. Indeed, this principle has long been part of the central dogma of genetics. However, research during the past two decades demonstrates that this principle does not always hold. For some human genes, one of the alleles is transcriptionally inactive (no mRNA is produced), depending upon the parent from whom the allele was received. For example, an allele transmitted by the mother would be inactive, and the same allele transmitted by the father would be active. The normal individual would have only one transcriptionally active copy of the gene. This process of gene silencing is known as **genomic imprinting**, and the transcriptionally silenced genes are said to be imprinted. At least 100 human genes are known to be imprinted, and most of these are located in genomic regions that contain clusters of several or more imprinted genes.

Imprinted alleles tend to be heavily methylated (in contrast to the nonimprinted copy of the allele, which typically is not methylated). The attachment of methyl groups to 5′ regions of genes, along with histone hypoacetylation and condensation of chromatin, inhibit the binding of proteins that promote transcription. It should be apparent that this process is similar in many ways to X inactivation, discussed earlier in this chapter.

Prader-Willi and Angelman Syndromes

A striking disease example of imprinting results from a deletion of about 4 Mb of the long arm of chromosome 15. When this deletion is inherited from the father, the child manifests Prader-Willi syndrome (PWS), a disease whose features include short stature, hypotonia (poor muscle tone), small hands and feet, obesity, mild to moderate intellectual disability, and hypogonadism (Fig. 4-34A). When the same deletion is inherited from the mother, the child develops Angelman syndrome (AS), which is characterized by severe intellectual disability, seizures, and an ataxic gait (see Fig. 4-34B). Both diseases are seen in about 1 of every 15,000 persons, and chromosome deletions are responsible for about 70% of cases of both diseases. The deletions that cause PWS and AS are microscopically indistinguishable and affect the same group of genes.

For some time, it was unclear how the same chromosomal deletion could produce such disparate results in different patients. Further analysis showed that the 4-Mb deletion (the critical region) contains several genes that normally are transcribed only on the chromosome inherited from the father. These genes are transcriptionally inactive (imprinted) on the copy of chromosome 15 inherited from the mother. Similarly, other genes in the critical region are active only on the chromosome inherited from the mother and are inactive on the chromosome inherited from the father. Thus, several genes in this region are normally active on only one chromosome (see Fig. 4-34C). If the single active copy of one of these genes is lost through a chromosome deletion, then no gene product is produced at all, and disease results.

Molecular analysis using many of the tools and techniques outlined in Chapter 3 has identified several specific genes in the critical region of chromosome 15. The gene responsible for AS encodes a protein involved in ubiquitin-mediated protein degradation during brain development (consistent with the intellectual disability and ataxia observed in this disorder). In brain tissue, this gene is active only on the chromosome inherited from the mother; thus, a maternally transmitted deletion removes the single active copy of this gene. Several genes in the critical region are involved in PWS, and they are transcribed only on the chromosome transmitted by the father.

Several mechanisms in addition to chromosome deletions can cause PWS and AS. One of these is **uniparental disomy,** in which an individual inherits two copies of a chromosome from one parent and none from the other (see Chapter 6 for further discussion). When two copies of the maternal chromosome 15 are inherited, PWS results because no active paternal genes are present in the critical region. Conversely, disomy of the paternal chromosome 15 produces AS. Point mutations in the maternally transmitted copy of the AS gene produce approximately 10% to 20% of AS cases. Finally, a small percentage of PWS and AS result from defects in the imprinting control center on chromosome 15. This is the DNA sequence that helps to set and reset the imprint itself. The great majority of PWS and AS cases can be diagnosed accurately by analyzing methylation patterns and DNA sequences in the critical region. Box 4-3 presents clinical issues of PWS from the perspective of a patient's family.

FIG 4-34   Illustration of the effect of imprinting on chromosome 15 deletions. **A,** Inheritance of the deletion from the father produces Prader-Willi syndrome (PWS) (note the inverted V-shaped upper lip, small hands, and truncal obesity). **B,** Inheritance of the deletion from the mother produces Angelman syndrome (note the characteristic posture). **C,** Pedigrees illustrating the inheritance pattern of this deletion and the activation status of genes in the critical region.

BOX 4-3   A Mother's Perspective of Prader-Willi Syndrome

We have a 3.5-year-old son, John, who has Prader-Willi syndrome. Months before John was born, we were concerned about his well-being because he wasn't as active in utero as his older siblings had been. At the first sight of John, the doctors suspected that things "weren't quite right." John opened his eyes but made no other movements. He couldn't adequately suck, he required supplemental oxygen, and he was "puffy." He remained hospitalized for nearly 3 weeks. The next 3 years were filled with visits to occupational therapists, physical therapists, home health-care aides, early childhood service providers, and speech therapists.

From the day John was born, we searched diligently for a diagnosis. His father insisted that we need only love and help him. However, I wanted specifics on how to help him and knowledge from other parents who might have traveled a similar path. After extensive testing and three "chromosome checks," John's problem was diagnosed as Prader-Willi syndrome (PWS). We were glad to be provided with some direction and decided that we would deal with further challenges as they came upon us. We used what we learned about PWS to get started helping John reach his potential. We were not going to worry about all the potential problems John could have because of his PWS.

BOX 4-3   A Mother's Perspective of Prader-Willi Syndrome (Continued)

John attends a special education preschool at the local elementary school 4 days a week. The bus ride takes about 5 minutes, but it is long enough for John to very much anticipate it each day. If he is ill, we have to tell him that the bus is broken. He attends a Sunday school class with children of a similar age. He misbehaves by saying "hi" and "bye" very loudly to each participant. He receives speech therapy once a week, and I spend at least 30 minutes each day with John practicing speech, cognitive, and play skills. John has not yet experienced the feeding difficulties commonly observed in children with PWS. However, excessive eating and weight gain are more common in older children with PWS.

Compared with other 3-year-old children, John struggles with speech and motor developmental milestones. Yet, he loves to play with his siblings and their friends and to look at books. In fact, we struggle to keep people from doing too many things for John because they might prevent him from attaining the same goal independently. We feel very privileged to have him in our family.

Our expectations for John are that he achieves everything that is possible for him plus a little bit more. Indeed, some of his care providers are already impressed with his capabilities. I hope that his success is partly a result of the care and support that we have given to him. Moreover, I hope that John continues to overcome the daily challenges that face him.

Beckwith-Wiedemann Syndrome

A second example of imprinting in the human genome is given by Beckwith-Wiedemann syndrome, an overgrowth condition accompanied by an increased predisposition to cancer. Beckwith-Wiedemann syndrome is usually recognizable at birth because of large size for gestational age, neonatal hypoglycemia, a large tongue, creases on the ear lobe, and omphalocele (an abdominal wall defect). Some children with Beckwith-Wiedemann syndrome also develop asymmetrical overgrowth of a limb or one side of the face or trunk (i.e., hemihyperplasia). Children with Beckwith-Wiedemann syndrome have an increased risk for developing Wilms tumor (a kidney cancer) and hepatoblastoma (a liver cancer). Both of these tumors can be treated effectively if they are detected early, so screening at regular intervals is an important part of management (see Chapter 12).

As with Angelman syndrome, a minority of Beckwith-Wiedemann syndrome cases (about 20%-30%) are caused by the inheritance of two copies of a chromosome from the father and no copy of the chromosome from the mother (uniparental disomy, in this case affecting chromosome 11). Several genes on the short arm of chromosome 11 are imprinted on either the paternal or maternal chromosome (Fig. 4-35). These genes are found in two separate, differentially methylated regions (DMRs). In DMR1, the gene that encodes insulin-like growth factor 2 (*IGF2*) is normally inactive on the maternally transmitted chromosome and active on the paternally transmitted chromosome. Normally, then, a person has only one active copy of *IGF2*. When two copies of the paternal chromosome are inherited (i.e., paternal uniparental disomy) or there is loss of imprinting on the maternal copy of *IGF2*, an active *IGF2* gene is present in double dose. This results in increased levels of IGF2 during fetal development, contributing to the overgrowth features of Beckwith-Wiedemann syndrome. (Note that, in contrast to PWS and Angelman syndromes, which are produced by a *missing* gene product, Beckwith-Wiedemann syndrome is caused, at least in part, by *overexpression* of a gene product.)

FIG 4-35 Schematic of the organization of several imprinted genes on chromosome 11p15.5 that are involved in the pathogenesis of Beckwith-Wiedemann syndrome and Silver-Russell syndrome. Beckwith-Wiedemann syndrome can arise from loss of imprinting of the growth promoting gene, *IGF2*, on the maternally transmitted chromosome, two copies of the paternal allele with an active *IGF2* as a consequence of uniparental disomy, or faulty imprinting of the growth-suppressing gene, *CDKN1C*, on the maternally transmitted chromosome. Imprinting defects that lead to downregulation of *IGF2* on the paternal allele cause some cases of Silver-Russell syndrome. *DMR*, Differentially methylated region; *red*, genes that are not methylated and therefore expressed; *green*, genes that are methylated and therefore silenced.

In 50% to 60% of cases, Beckwith-Wiedemann syndrome is caused by a loss of methylation or other alterations of DMR2. This region contains several genes, including *CDKN1C*, an important growth-regulating gene, and *KCNQ1*, a gene that contains a regulatory lncRNA within one of its introns. Altered expression levels of these genes are thought to result in silencing of growth inhibitors and thus overgrowth and increased predisposition to cancer.

Silver-Russell Syndrome

Silver-Russell syndrome is a clinically heterogeneous group of disorders characterized by growth retardation, proportionate short stature, leg length discrepancy, and a small, triangular-shaped face. About half of Silver-Russell syndrome cases are associated with a loss of methylation of DMR1 on chromosome 11p15.5, leading to down-regulation of IGF2 and diminished growth. Thus, whereas up-regulation or extra copies of active IGF2 cause overgrowth in Beckwith-Wiedemann syndrome, down-regulation of IGF2 causes diminished growth in Silver-Russell syndrome.

▶ Some disease genes may be expressed differently when inherited from one sex versus the other. This is genomic imprinting. It is typically associated with methylation of DNA and chromatin condensation, which limit the action of transcription factors and decrease gene expression.

Anticipation and Repeat Expansion

Since the early part of the 20th century, it has been observed that some genetic diseases seem to display an earlier age of onset and/or more severe expression in the more recent generations of a pedigree. This pattern is termed **anticipation**, and it has been the subject of considerable controversy and speculation. Many researchers believed that it was an artifact of better observation and clinical diagnosis in more recent times: a disorder that previously might have remained undiagnosed until age 60 years might

now be diagnosed at age 40 years simply because of better diagnostic tools. Others, however, believed that anticipation could be a real biological phenomenon, although evidence for the actual mechanism remained elusive.

Molecular genetics has now provided good evidence that anticipation does have a biological basis. This evidence has come, in part, from studies of myotonic dystrophy, an autosomal dominant disease that involves progressive muscle deterioration and myotonia (inability to relax muscles after contraction) (Fig. 4-36). Seen in approximately 1 in 8000 persons, myotonic dystrophy is the most common muscular dystrophy that affects adults. This disorder is also typically characterized by cardiac arrhythmias (abnormal heart rhythms), testicular atrophy, insulin resistance, and cataracts. Most cases of myotonic

FIG 4-36 A three-generation family affected with myotonic dystrophy. The degree of severity increases in each generation. The grandmother (*right*) is only slightly affected, but the mother (*left*) has a characteristic narrow face and somewhat limited facial expression. The baby is more severely affected and has the facial features of children with neonatal-onset myotonic dystrophy, including an open, triangle-shaped mouth. The infant has more than 1000 copies of the trinucleotide repeat, whereas the mother and grandmother each have approximately 100 repeats.

dystrophy (termed myotonic dystrophy type 1) are caused by mutations in *DMPK*, a protein kinase gene located on chromosome 19.

Analysis of *DMPK* has shown that the disease-causing mutation is an expanded CTG trinucleotide repeat (see Chapter 3) that lies in the 3′ untranslated portion of the gene (i.e., a region transcribed into mRNA but not translated into protein). The number of these repeats is strongly correlated with severity of the disease. Unaffected persons typically have 5 to 37 copies of the repeat. Those with 50 to 100 copies may be mildly affected or have no symptoms. Those with full-blown myotonic dystrophy have anywhere from 100 to several thousand copies of the repeated sequence. Expansion to large repeat numbers can produce congenital myotonic dystrophy; for reasons that are not well understood, these large expansions are transmitted almost exclusively by females. The number of repeats often increases with succeeding generations: a mildly affected parent with 80 repeats might produce a severely affected offspring who has more than 1000 repeats (Fig. 4-37). As the number of repeats increases through successive generations, the age of onset decreases and severity often increases.

Thus, expansion of this trinucleotide repeat is the primary cause of anticipation in myotonic dystrophy.

How does a mutation in an untranslated portion of *DMPK* produce the many disease features of myotonic dystrophy? The expanded repeat produces an mRNA product that remains in the nucleus of the cell and produces toxic gain-of-function effects. The abnormal mRNA interacts with proteins that normally bind other RNA products to regulate their splicing. As a result, a number of proteins, including several that are expressed in heart and skeletal muscle, are abnormally formed, giving rise to some of the pleiotropic features of the disease phenotype.

A second form of myotonic dystrophy, type 2, is caused by a 4-bp (CCTG) expanded repeat in a gene located on chromosome 3. Again, the repeat is located in an untranslated region of the gene (intron 1), and it results in a toxic mRNA that interferes with the normal function of RNA-binding proteins. The phenotype associated with this mutation is similar to that of myotonic dystrophy type 1, although it sometimes is less severe. Myotonic dystrophy thus illustrates several important genetic principles: anticipation, pleiotropy, and locus heterogeneity.

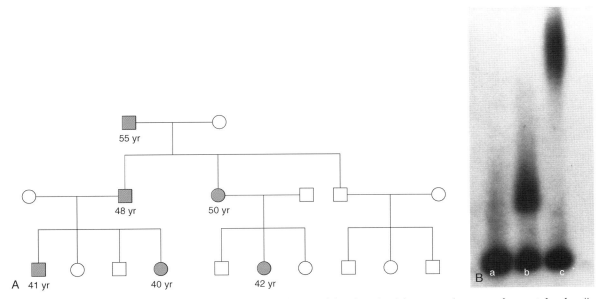

FIG 4-37   A, Myotonic dystrophy pedigree illustrating anticipation. In this case, the age of onset for family members affected with an autosomal dominant disease is lower in more recent generations. **B,** An autoradiogram from a Southern blot analysis of the myotonic dystrophy gene in three individuals. Individual a is homozygous for a 4-to 5-repeat allele and is normal. Individual b has one normal allele and one disease allele of 175 repeats; this individual has myotonic dystrophy. Individual c is also affected with myotonic dystrophy and has one normal allele and a disease-causing allele of approximately 900 repeats. (**B** courtesy Dr. Kenneth Ward and Dr. Elaine Lyon, University of Utah Health Sciences Center.)

Repeat expansions have now been identified as a cause of more than 20 genetic diseases (Table 4-5), which can be assigned to three broad categories. The first includes neurological diseases, such as Huntington disease and most of the spinocerebellar ataxias, that are caused by a CAG or CTG repeat expansion in a protein-coding portion of the gene. The repeats generally expand in number from a normal range of 10 to 35 to a disease-causing range of approximately 50 to 100. Expansions tend to be larger when transmitted through the father than through the mother, and the mutations typically have a gain-of-function effect. The second group consists of phenotypically more diverse diseases in which the expansions are again small in magnitude and are found in exons. The repeat sequence is heterogeneous, however, and anticipation is not a typical feature. The third category includes fragile X syndrome, myotonic dystrophy, two of the spinocerebellar ataxias, juvenile myoclonic epilepsy, and Friedreich ataxia. The repeat expansions are generally much larger than in the first two categories: The normal range is usually 5 to 50 trinucleotides, but the disease-causing range can vary from 100 to several thousand trinucleotides.

TABLE 4-5   Diseases Associated with Repeat Expansions

DISEASE	DESCRIPTION	REPEAT SEQUENCE	NORMAL RANGE; DISEASE RANGE	PARENT IN WHOM EXPANSION USUALLY OCCURS	LOCATION OF EXPANSION
Category 1					
Huntington disease	Loss of motor control, dementia, affective disorder	CAG	6-34; 36-121	More often through father	Exon
Spinal and bulbar muscular atrophy	Adult-onset motor-neuron disease associated with androgen insensitivity	CAG	9-36; 38-62	More often through father	Exon
Spinocerebellar ataxia type 1	Progressive ataxia, dysarthria, dysmetria	CAG	6-39; 40-82	More often through father	Exon
Spinocerebellar ataxia type 2	Progressive ataxia, dysarthria	CAG	15-24; 32-200	—	Exon
Spinocerebellar ataxia type 3 (Machado-Joseph disease)	Dystonia, distal muscular atrophy, ataxia, external ophthalmoplegia	CAG	13-36; 61-84	More often through father	Exon
Spinocerebellar ataxia type 6	Progressive ataxia, dysarthria, nystagmus	CAG	4-19; 20-33	—	Exon
Spinocerebellar ataxia type 7	Progressive ataxia, dysarthria, retinal degeneration	CAG	4-35; 37-306	More often through father	—
Spinocerebellar ataxia type 17	Progressive ataxia, dementia, bradykinesia, dysmetria	CAG	25-42; 47-63	—	Exon
Dentatorubral-pallidoluysian atrophy (Haw River syndrome)	Cerebellar atrophy, ataxia, myoclonic epilepsy, choreoathetosis, dementia	CAG	7-34; 49-88	More often through father	Exon
Huntington disease-like 2	Features very similar to those of Huntington disease	CTG	7-28; 66-78	—	Exon

TABLE 4-5   Diseases Associated with Repeat Expansions (Continued)

DISEASE	DESCRIPTION	REPEAT SEQUENCE	NORMAL RANGE; DISEASE RANGE	PARENT IN WHOM EXPANSION USUALLY OCCURS	LOCATION OF EXPANSION
Category 2					
Pseudoachondroplasia, multiple epiphyseal dysplasia	Short stature, joint laxity, degenerative joint disease	GAC	5; 6-7	—	Exon
Oculopharyngeal muscular dystrophy	Proximal limb weakness, dysphagia, ptosis	GCG	6; 7-13	—	Exon
Cleidocranial dysplasia	Short stature, open skull sutures with bulging calvaria, clavicular hypoplasia, shortened fingers, dental anomalies	GCG, GCT, GCA	17; 27 (expansion observed in one family)	—	Exon
Synpolydactyly	Polydactyly and syndactyly	GCG, GCT, GCA	15; 22-25	—	Exon
Category 3					
Myotonic dystrophy (DM1; chromosome 19)	Muscle loss, cardiac arrhythmia, cataracts, frontal balding	CTG	5-37; 50 to several thousand	Either parent, but expansion to congenital region form through mother	3' untranslated
Myotonic dystrophy (DM2; chromosome 3)	Muscle loss, cardiac arrhythmia, cataracts, frontal balding	CCTG	10-26; 75-11,000	—	3' untranslated region
Friedreich ataxia	Progressive limb ataxia, dysarthria, hypertrophic cardiomyopathy, pyramidal weakness in legs	GAA	6-32; 200-1700	Disorder is autosomal recessive, so disease alleles are inherited from both parents	Intron
Fragile X syndrome (FRAXA)	Intellectual disability, large ears and jaws, macroorchidism in males	CGG	4-39; 200-900	Exclusively through mother	5' untranslated region
Fragile site (FRAXE)	Mild intellectual disability	GCC	6-35; >200	More often through mother	5' untranslated region
Spinocerebellar ataxia type 8	Adult-onset ataxia, dysarthria, nystagmus	CTG	16-34; >74	More often through mother	3' untranslated region
Spinocerebellar ataxia type 10	Ataxia and seizures	ATTCT	10-20; 500-4500	More often through father	Intron
Spinocerebellar ataxia type 12	Ataxia, eye movement disorders; variable age at onset	CAG	7-45; 55-78	—	5' untranslated region
Progressive myoclonic epilepsy type 1	Juvenile-onset convulsions, myoclonus, dementia	12-bp repeat motif	2-3; 30-75	Autosomal recessive inheritance, so transmitted by both parents	5' untranslated region

The repeats are located outside the protein-coding regions of the gene in all of these disorders, and in some cases (e.g., myotonic dystrophy) the mutation produces a harmful RNA product. Repeat expansions are often larger when they are transmitted through the mother. Anticipation is seen in most of the diseases in the first and third categories.

> Anticipation refers to progressively earlier or more severe expression of a disease in more recent generations. Expansion of DNA repeats has been shown to cause anticipation in some genetic diseases. These diseases can be divided into three major categories, depending on the size of the expansion, the location of the repeat, the phenotypic consequences of the expansion, the effect of the mutation, and the parent in whom large expansions typically occur.

The Fragile X Story: Molecular Genetics Explains a Puzzling Pattern of Inheritance

Since the 19th century, it has been observed that there is an approximate 25% excess of males among persons with intellectual disability. This excess is partly explained by X-linked conditions that cause cognitive impairment, of which the fragile X syndrome is the most common. In addition to intellectual disability, fragile X syndrome is characterized by a distinctive facial appearance, with large ears and long face (Fig. 4-38), hypermobile joints, and macroorchidism (increased testicular volume) in postpubertal males. The degree of intellectual disability tends to be milder and more variable in females than in males. The syndrome is termed "fragile X" because the X chromosomes of affected persons, when cultured in a medium that is deficient in folic acid, sometimes exhibit breaks and gaps near the tip of the long arm (Fig. 4-39).

Although the presence of a single fragile X mutation is sufficient to cause disease in either males or females, the prevalence of this condition is higher in males (1/4000) than in females (1/8000). The lower degree of penetrance in females, as well as variability in expression, reflects variation in patterns of X inactivation (i.e., the percentage of active X chromosomes that carry the disease-causing mutation). Males who have affected descendants but are not affected themselves are termed *normal transmitting males*. In the mid-1980s, studies of fragile X syndrome pedigrees revealed a perplexing pattern: the mothers of transmitting males had a much lower percentage of affected sons than did the daughters of these males (Fig. 4-40). Because the mothers and daughters of normal transmitting males are both obligate carriers of the X-linked mutation, they should have equal risks of producing affected sons. Daughters

FIG 4-38 Boys with fragile X syndrome. Note the long faces, prominent jaws, and large ears and the similar characteristics of children from different ethnic groups: European **(A)**, Asian **(B)**, and Latin American **(C)**.

FIG 4-39 An X chromosome from a male with fragile X syndrome, showing an elongated, condensed region near the tip of the long arm. (From Stein CK. Applications of cytogenetics in modern pathology. In: McPherson RA, Pincus MR, eds. *Henrys Clinical Diagnosis and Management by Laboratory Methods.* 21st ed. Philadelphia: Saunders; 2006.)

FIG 4-40 A pedigree showing the inheritance of the fragile X syndrome. Females who carry a premutation (50 to 200 CGG repeats) are shown by *dotted symbols*. Affected individuals are represented by *solid symbols*. A normal transmitting male, who carries a premutation of 70 to 90 repeat units, is designated NTM. Note that the number of repeats increases each time the mutation is passed through another female. Also, only 5% of the NTM's sisters are affected, and only 9% of his brothers are affected, but 40% of his grandsons and 16% of his granddaughters are affected. This is the Sherman paradox.

of normal transmitting males were never affected with the disorder, but these women's sons could be affected. This pattern, dubbed the *Sherman paradox*, appeared to be inconsistent with the rules of X-linked inheritance.

Many mechanisms were proposed to explain this pattern, including autosomal and mitochondrial modifier loci. Resolution of the Sherman paradox came only with the identification of the disease-causing gene, labeled *FMR1*. DNA sequence analysis showed that the 5′ untranslated region of the gene contains a CGG repeat unit that is present in 6 to 50 copies in unaffected persons. Those with fragile X syndrome have 200 to 1000 or more CGG repeats (a full mutation). An intermediate number of repeats, ranging approximately from 50 to 200 copies, is seen in normal transmitting males and their female offspring and is termed a **premutation**. When these female offspring transmit the gene to their offspring, there is sometimes an expansion from the premutation of 50 to 200 repeats to the full mutation of more than 200 repeats. These expansions do not occur in male transmission. Furthermore, premutations tend to become larger in successive generations, and larger premutations are more likely to expand to a full mutation. These findings explain the Sherman paradox. Males with the premutation do not have daughters with fragile X syndrome because expansion to the full mutation occurs only in female transmission. Grandsons and great-grandsons of transmitting

males are more likely to be affected by the disorder than are brothers of transmitting males because of progressive repeat expansion through successive generations of female premutation carriers.

Measurement of mRNA transcribed from *FMR1* has shown that the highest mRNA expression levels are in the brain, as would be expected. Persons with normal and premutation *FMR1* genes both produce mRNA. In fact, mRNA production is elevated in those with premutations, and it has been shown that this mRNA accumulates in the nucleus and has toxic effects, as do mutated mRNAs in myotonic dystrophy. Consequently, about more than half of males with premutations develop a neurological disease characterized by ataxia and tremors by age 70 (the risk for female carriers is less than 20%). Approximately 25% of females with *FMR1* premutations experience premature ovarian failure (amenorrhea before age 40 years), again because of toxic mRNA effects. In contrast, those with full mutations have no *FMR1* mRNA in their cells, indicating no transcription of the gene. The CGG repeat is heavily methylated in those with the full mutation, as is a series of CG sequences 5′ of the gene. The degree of methylation, which is likely to influence transcription of *FMR1*, is correlated with severity of expression of the disorder. A small percentage of persons with fragile X syndrome (<5%) do not have an expansion of the CGG repeat but instead have other loss-of-function mutations in *FMR1*.

The protein product of *FMR1*, FMRP, binds to RNA and is capable of shuttling back and forth between the nucleus and the cytoplasm. It appears that FMRP is involved in transporting mRNA from the nucleus to the cytoplasm, and it is thought to be involved in regulating the translation of mRNA.

Identification of the *FMR1* gene and the nature of its repeat expansion have already explained a great deal about the inheritance and expression of the fragile X syndrome. These advances have also improved diagnostic accuracy for the condition, because cytogenetic analysis of chromosomes often fails to identify fragile X heterozygotes. In contrast, DNA diagnosis, which consists of measurement of the length of the CGG repeat sequence and the degree of methylation of *FMR1*, is much more accurate.

SUMMARY

Single-gene disorders are caused by mutations in one gene, and they follow mendelian inheritance patterns. Mendel's contributions with respect to inheritance are the theoretical foundation for our understanding of single-gene disorders. Pedigree analyses of large families can be used to determine whether a disease-associated gene is located on an autosome or on a sex chromosome and whether the related disease phenotype is dominant or recessive.

Autosomal dominant single-gene diseases occur in individuals who have a single mutant copy of the disease-associated gene. The risk of occurrence is 50%. Autosomal recessive single-gene diseases occur only in individuals with two mutant alleles of the disease-associated gene. The risk of occurrence is usually 25%. Single-gene diseases that involve genes on the sex chromosomes have somewhat different inheritance patterns than those that involve genes on autosomes. Because females have two copies of the X chromosome and males have one, X-linked recessive diseases are much more common among males than among females. The risk of occurrence depends on the genotype of each parent and the sex of the offspring. X-linked dominant diseases are approximately twice as common in females as in males. Y-linked single-gene diseases are always passed from affected fathers to their sons. A Y-linked disease-associated phenotype is always revealed, regardless of whether the mutation is dominant or recessive.

A number of diseases are known to be caused by mutations in mitochondrial DNA. Because mitochondrial DNA is maternally inherited and has a high mutation rate, diseases caused by abnormal mitochondrial genes are almost always transmitted by the mother. The composition of mitochondrial DNA varies from cell to cell throughout the body. This heterogeneity is an important cause of variable expression in mitochondrial diseases. However, some mitochondrial disorders are caused by genes in the cell nucleus that affect mitochondria.

Some factors, such as new mutations, germline mosaicism, penetrance, expressivity, pleiotropy, heterogeneity, consanguinity, genomic imprinting, and anticipation, complicate the patterns of inheritance of diseases in families. Attention should be paid to these factors in estimating the risk of occurrence of a genetic disorder in a family.

IMPORTANT TERMINOLOGY

principle of segregation　分离定律
principle of independent assortment　自由组合定律
genotype　基因型
phenotype　表现型
proband　先证者
consanguinity　近亲结婚

penetrance 外显率
heterogeneity 异质性
pleiotropy 基因多效性
coefficient of relationship 近婚系数
dosage compensation 剂量补偿
hemizygous 半合子

Barr body 巴氏小体
heterozygote 杂合子
sex-limited trait 限性性状
sex-influenced trait 从性性状
genomic imprinting 基因组印记
anticipation 遗传早现

REVIEW QUESTIONS

1. A man who has achondroplasia marries a phenotypically normal woman. If they have four children, what is the probability that none of their children will be affected with this disorder? What is the probability that *all* of them will be affected?

2. The estimated penetrance for familial retinoblastoma is approximately 90%. If a man has had familial retinoblastoma and mates with a woman who does not have a retinoblastoma mutation, what is the risk that their offspring will develop retinoblastoma?

3. Two mating individuals, labeled A and B in Figure 4-41, share a single great-grandparent. What is their coefficient of relationship? Suppose that one member of this couple is a heterozygous carrier for PKU. What is the probability that this couple will produce a child affected with PKU?

FIG 4-41 Diagram for study question 3.

4. A man implicated in a paternity suit has had his DNA tested to establish whether or not he is the father of the baby. Four STR loci were tested for him, the mother, and the baby. The baby's alleles and the man's alleles match for all four loci. The frequencies of these alleles in the general population are 0.05, 0.01, 0.01, and 0.02. What is the probability that someone else in the general population could be the father of the baby?

5. Females have been observed with five X chromosomes in each somatic cell. How many Barr bodies would such females have?

6. Explain why 8% to 10% of female carriers of the *DMD* gene have muscle weakness.

7. Figure 4-42 shows the inheritance of hemophilia A in a family. What is the risk that the male in generation IV is affected with hemophilia A? What is the risk that the female in generation IV is a heterozygous carrier? What is the risk that she is affected by the disorder?

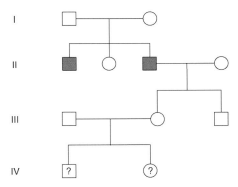

FIG 4-42 Pedigree for study question 7

8. Pedigrees for autosomal dominant and X-linked dominant diseases are sometimes difficult to distinguish. Name as many features as you can that would help to tell them apart.

9. How would you distinguish mitochondrial inheritance from other modes of inheritance?

10. A boy and his brother both have hemophilia A. If there is no family history of hemophilia A in previous generations, what is the probability that the boys' aunt (the mother's sister) is a heterozygous carrier of the disease gene?

SUGGESTED READINGS AND WEBSITES

1. Barrett PM, Alagely A, Topol EJ. Cystic fibrosis in an era of genomically guided therapy. *Hum Mol Genet.* 2012; 21: R66-R71.

2. Biesecker LG, Spinner NB. A genomic view of mosaicism and human disease. *Nat Rev Genet.* 2013; 14: 307-320.

3. Bolar N, Van Laer L, Loeys BL. Marfan syndrome: from gene to therapy. *Curr Opin Pediatr.* 2012; 24: 498-504.

4. Deeb SS. The molecular basis of variation in human color vision. *Clin Genet.* 2005; 67: 369-377.

5. Dimaras H, Kimani K, Dimba EAO, et al. Retinoblastoma. *Lancet.* 2012; 379: 1436-1446.

6. Graw J, Brackmann HH, Oldenburg J, et al. Haemophilia A: from mutation analysis to new therapies. *Nat Rev Genet.* 2005; 6: 488-501.

7. High KA. The gene therapy journey for hemophilia: are we there yet? *Blood.* 2012; 120: 4482-4487.

8. Horsthemke B. In brief: genomic imprinting and imprinting diseases. *J Pathol.* 2014; 232: 485-487.

9. Jorde LB. Inbreeding in human populations. In: Dulbecco R, ed. *Encyclopedia of Human Biology.* Vol. 5. New York: Academic Press; 1997: 1-13.

10. Koopman WJH, Willems PHGM, Smeitink JAM. Monogenic mitochondrial disorders. *N Engl J Med.* 2012; 366: 1132-1141.

11. Lee JT, Bartolomei MS. X-inactivation, imprinting, and long noncoding RNAs in health and disease. *Cell.* 2013; 152: 1308-1323.

12. Mercuri E, Muntoni F. Muscular dystrophy: new challenges and review of the current clinical trials. *Curr Opin Pediatr.* 2013; 25: 701-707.

13. Modell B, Darr A. Science and society: genetic counselling and customary consanguineous marriage. *Nat Rev Genet.* 2002; 3: 225-229.

14. Nelson DL, Orr HT, Warren ST. The unstable repeats—three evolving faces of neurological disease. *Neuron.* 2013; 77: 825-843.

15. Pasmant E, Vidaud M, Vidaud D, Wolkenstein P. Neurofibromatosis type 1: from genotype to phenotype. *J Med Genet.* 2012; 49: 483-489.

16. Peters J. The role of genomic imprinting in biology and disease: an expanding view. *Nat Rev Genet.* 2014; 15: 517-530.

17. Potter A, Phillips JA, Rimoin DL. Genetic disorders of the pituitary gland. In: Rimoin DL, Connor JM, Pyeritz RE, Korf BR, eds. *Emery and Rimoin's Principles and Practice of Medical Genetics.* Vol. 2. Philadelphia: Churchill Livingstone; 2007: 1889-1931.

18. Ross CA, Tabrizi SJ. Huntington's disease: from molecular pathogenesis to clinical treatment. *Lancet Neurol.* 2011; 10: 83-98.

19. Wutz A, Gribnau J. X inactivation Xplained. *Curr Opin Genet Dev.* 2007; 17: 387-393.

20. Cystic Fibrosis Mutation Database (also contains links to other useful cystic fibrosis websites): http://www.genet.sickkids.on.ca/cftr/

21. Eye Cancer Network: Retinoblastoma (descriptions, photographs, and useful links): http://www.eyecancer.com/Patient/Condition.aspx?nID=53&Category=Retinal+Tumors&Condition=Retinoblastoma

22. MITOMAP (extensive information about the mitochondrial genome and its role in disease): http://www.mitomap.org/

23. Muscular Dystrophy Association (information about various types of muscular dystrophy with links to other websites): http://www.mdausa.org/

24. National Center for Biotechnology Information: Genes and Disease (brief summaries of many of the genetic diseases discussed in this text): http://www.ncbi.nlm.nih.gov/ books/bv.fcgi?call=bv.View..ShowTOC&rid=gnd.TOC&depth=2

25. National Hemophilia Foundation (information about hemophilia and links to other websites): http://www.hemophilia.org/home.htm

26. National Institute of Neurological Diseases and Stroke: Huntington Disease Information Page: http://www.ninds.nih.gov/disorders/huntington/huntington.htm

27. National Marfan Foundation (basic information about Marfan syndrome, with links to other sites): http://www.marfan.org/

28. National Neurofibromatosis Foundation (many useful links to online resources): http://www.ctf.org/

(Li Li)

Chapter 5

Multifactorial Inheritance and Common Diseases

The focus of previous chapters has been on diseases that are caused primarily by mutations in single genes. Much progress has been made in identifying specific mutations that cause these diseases, leading to better risk estimates and in some cases more effective treatment. However, these conditions form only a small portion of the total burden of human genetic disease. A much larger component of our disease burden is composed of congenital malformations and common adult diseases, such as cancer, heart disease, and diabetes. Although they are usually not the result of single-gene mutations or chromosome abnormalities, these diseases have significant genetic components. They are the result of a complex interplay of multiple genetic and environmental factors. Because of the significance of common diseases in health care, it is vital to understand the ways in which genes contribute to causing them.

PRINCIPLES OF MULTIFACTORIAL INHERITANCE

The Multifactorial Model

Traits in which variation is thought to be caused by the combined effects of multiple genes are called **polygenic** ("many genes"). When environmental factors are also believed to cause variation in the trait, which is usually the case, the term **multifactorial** is used. Many **quantitative traits** (those, such as blood pressure, that are measured on a continuous numerical scale) are multifactorial. Because they are caused by the additive effects of many genetic and environmental factors, these traits tend to follow a normal, or bell-shaped, distribution in populations.

Let us use an example to illustrate this concept. To begin with the simplest case, suppose (unrealistically) that height is determined by a single gene with two alleles, A and a. Allele A tends to make people tall, and allele a tends to make them short. If there is no dominance at this locus, then the three possible genotypes, AA, Aa, and aa, will produce three phenotypes: tall, intermediate, and short. Assume that the allele frequencies of A and a are each 0.50. If we assemble a population of individuals, we will observe the height distribution depicted in Figure 5-1A.

Now suppose, a bit more realistically, that height is determined by two loci instead of one. The second locus also has two alleles, B (tall) and b (short), and they affect height in exactly the same way as alleles A and a do. There are now nine possible genotypes in our population: aabb, aaBb, aaBB, Aabb, AaBb, AaBB, AAbb, AABb, and AABB. Because an individual might have zero, one, two, three, or four "tall" alleles, there are now five distinct phenotypes (see Fig. 5-1B).Although the height distribution in our population is not yet normal, it approaches a normal distribution more closely than in the single-gene case.

We now extend our example so that many genes and environmental factors influence height, each having a small effect. Then there are many possible phenotypes, each differing slightly, and the height distribution approaches the bell-shaped curve shown in Figure 5-1C. Genome-wide association studies have identified more than 200 loci associated with human height, affirming that this is indeed a polygenic, multifactorial trait. The loci underlying variation in a quantitative trait such as height are termed **quantitative trait loci.**

FIG 5-1 A, The distribution of height in a population, assuming that height is controlled by a single locus with genotypes *AA*, *Aa*, and *aa*. **B**, The distribution of height, assuming that height is controlled by two loci. There are now five distinct phenotypes instead of three, and the distribution begins to look more like the normal distribution. **C**, Distribution of height, assuming that multiple factors, each with a small effect, contribute to the trait (the multifactorial model).

It should be emphasized that the individual genes underlying a multifactorial trait such as height follow the mendelian principles of segregation and independent assortment, just like any other genes. The only difference is that many of them act together to influence the trait.

Blood pressure is another example of a multifactorial trait. There is a correlation between parents' blood pressures (systolic and diastolic) and those of their children, and there is good evidence that this

correlation is due in part to genes. But blood pressure is also influenced by environmental factors, such as diet and stress. One of the goals of genetic research is identification of the genes responsible for multifactorial traits such as blood pressure and of the interactions of those genes with environmental factors.

 Many traits are thought to be influenced by multiple genes as well as by environmental factors. These traits are said to be multifactorial. When they can be measured on a continuous scale, they often follow a normal distribution.

The Threshold Model

A number of diseases do not follow the bell-shaped distribution. Instead, they appear to be either present or absent in individuals. Yet they do not follow the patterns expected of single-gene diseases. A commonly used explanation is that there is an underlying **liability distribution** for these diseases in a population (Fig. 5-2). Persons who are on the low end of the distribution have little chance of developing the disease in question (i.e., they have few of the alleles or environmental factors that would cause the disease). Those who are closer to the high end of the distribution have more of the disease causing alleles and environmental factors and are more likely to develop the disease. For multifactorial diseases that are either present or absent, a **threshold of liability** must be crossed before the disease is expressed. Below the threshold, the person appears unaffected; above it, he or she is affected by the disease.

A disease that is thought to correspond to this threshold model is pyloric stenosis, a disorder that manifests shortly after birth and is caused by a narrowing or obstruction of the pylorus, the area between the stomach and intestine. Chronic vomiting, constipation, weight loss, and electrolyte imbalance result from the condition, which can be corrected by surgery or sometimes resolves spontaneously. The prevalence of pyloric stenosis among whites is about 3/1000 live births. It is much more common in males than in females, affecting 1/200

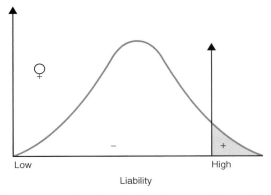

FIG 5-2 A liability distribution for a multifactorial disease in a population. To be affected with the disease, a person must exceed the threshold on the liability distribution. This figure shows two thresholds, a lower one for males and a higher one for females (as in pyloric stenosis).

	MALE PROBANDS		FEMALE PROBANDS	
RELATIVES	LONDON	BELFAST	LONDON	BELFAST
Brothers	3.8	9.6	9.2	12.5
Sisters	2.7	3.0	3.8	3.8

TABLE 5-1   Receurrence Risks (%) for Pyloric Stenosis, Subdivided by Gender of Affected Probands and Relatives*

Adapted from Carter Co. Genetics of common single malformation. *Br Med Bull.* 1976, 32: 21-26.
*Note that the risks differ somewhat between the two populations

males and 1/1000 females. It is thought that this difference in prevalence reflects two thresholds in the liability distribution; a lower one in males and a higher one in females (see Fig. 5-2). A lower male threshold implies that fewer disease-causing factors are required to generate the disorder in males.

The liability threshold concept can explain the pattern of sibling recurrence risks for pyloric stenosis, shown in Table 5-1. Notice that males, having a lower threshold, always have a higher risk than females. However, the recurrence risk also depends on the sex of the proband. It is higher when the proband is female than when the proband is male. This reflects the concept that females, having a higher liability threshold, must be exposed to more disease-causing factors than males in order to develop the disease. Thus, a family with an affected female must have more genetic and environmental risk factors, producing a higher recurrence risk for pyloric steno-

sis in future offspring. In such a situation, we would expect that the highest risk category would be *male* relatives of *female* probands; Table 5-1 shows that this is indeed the case.

A number of other congenital malformations are thought to correspond to this model. They include isolated (In this context, the term "isolated" means that this is the only observed disease feature, i.e., the feature is not part of a large constellation of findings, as in cleft lip/palate secondary to trisomy 13.) cleft lip and/or cleft palate, neural tube defects (anencephaly and spina bifida), club foot (talipes), and some forms of congenital heart disease.

 The threshold model applies to many multifactorial diseases. It assumes that there is an underlying liability distribution in a population and that a threshold on this distribution must be passed before a disease is expressed.

Recurrence Risks and Transmission Patterns

Whereas recurrence risks can be given with confidence for single-gene diseases (50% for a completely penetrant autosomal dominant disease, 25% for autosomal recessive diseases, and so on), risk estimation is more complex for multifactorial diseases. This is because the number of genes contributing to the disease is usually not known, the precise allelic constitution of the parents is not known, and the extent of environmental effects can vary substantially. For most multifactorial diseases, **empirical risks** (i.e., risks based on direct observation of data) have been derived. To estimate empirical risks, a large series of families is examined in which one child (the proband) has developed the disease. The relatives of each proband are surveyed in order to calculate the percentage who have also developed the disease. For example, in North America neural tube defects are seen in about 2% to 3% of the siblings of probands with this condition (Clinical Commentary 5-1). Thus, the recurrence risk for parents who have had one child with a neural tube defect is 2% to 3%. For conditions that are not lethal or severely debilitating, such as cleft lip and cleft palate, recurrence risks can also be estimated for the offspring of affected parents. Because risk factors vary among diseases, empirical recurrence risks are specific for each multifactorial disease.

In contrast to most single-gene diseases, recurrence risks for multifactorial diseases can change substantially from one population to another (notice the differences between the London and Belfast populations in Table 5-1). This is because allele frequencies as well as environmental factors can differ among populations.

 Empirical recurrence risks for multifactorial diseases are based on studies of large collections of families. These risks are specific to a given population.

It is sometimes difficult to differentiate polygenic or multifactorial diseases from single-gene diseases that have reduced penetrance or variable expression. Large data sets and good family history data are necessary to make the distinction. Several criteria are usually used to define multifactorial inheritance.

- *The recurrence risk is higher if more than one family member is affected.* For example, the sibling recurrence risk for a ventricular septal defect (VSD, a type of congenital heart defect) is 3% if one sibling has had a VSD but increases to approximately 10% if two siblings have had VSDs. In contrast, the recurrence risk for single-gene diseases remains the same regardless of the number of affected siblings. This increase does not mean that the family's risk has actually changed.

Rather, it means that we now have more information about the family's true risk: because they have had two affected children, they are probably located higher on the liability distribution than a family with only one affected child. In other words, they have more risk factors (genetic and/ or environmental) and are more likely to produce an affected child.

- *If the expression of the disease in the proband is more severe, the recurrence risk is higher.* This is again consistent with the liability model, because a more-severe expression indicates that the affected person is at the extreme tail of the liability distribution (see Fig. 5-2). His or her relatives are thus at a higher risk to inherit disease-causing genes. For example, the occurrence of a bilateral (both sides) cleft lip/palate confers a higher recurrence risk on family members than does the occurrence of a unilateral (one side) cleft.

- *The recurrence risk is higher if the proband is of the less commonly affected sex* (see, for example, the previous discussion of pyloric stenosis). This is because an affected individual of the less susceptible sex is usually at a more extreme position on the liability distribution.

- *The recurrence risk for the disease usually decreases rapidly in more remotely related relatives* (Table 5-2). Although the recurrence risk for single-gene diseases decreases by 50% with each degree of relationship (e.g., an autosomal dominant disease has a 50% recurrence risk for offspring of affected persons, 25% for nieces or nephews, 12.5% for first cousins, and so on), it decreases much more quickly for multifactorial diseases. This reflects the fact that many genetic and environmental factors must combine to produce a trait. All of the necessary risk factors are unlikely to be present in less closely related family members.

- *If the prevalence of the disease in a population is f (which varies between zero and one), the risk for offspring and siblings of probands is approximately* $\sqrt{f}$. This does not hold true for single-gene traits, because their recurrence risks are independent of population prevalence. It is not an absolute rule

CLINICAL COMMENTARY 5-1

Neural Tube Defects

Neural tube defects (NTDs) include anencephaly, spina bifida, and encephalocele, as well as several other less-common forms (Fig. 5-3). They are one of the most important classes of birth defects, with a newborn prevalence of approximately 1 per 1000. There is considerable variation in the prevalence of NTDs among populations, with an especially high rate among some northern Chinese populations (as high as 6 per 1000 births). The prevalence of NTDs has been decreasing in many parts of the United States and Europe during the past three decades.

Normally the neural tube closes at about the fourth week of gestation. A defect in closure or a subsequent reopening of the neural tube results in an NTD. Spina bifida is the most commonly observed NTD and consists of a protrusion of spinal tissue through the vertebral column (the tissue usually includes meninges, spinal cord, and nerve roots). About 75% of spina bifida patients have secondary hydrocephalus, which sometimes in turn produces intellectual disability. Paralysis or muscle weakness, lack of sphincter control, and club feet are often observed. A study conducted in British Columbia showed that survival rates for spina bifida patients have improved dramatically over the past several decades. Less than 30% of such children born between 1952 and 1969 survived to 10 years of age, but 65% of those born between 1970 and 1986 survived to this age.

Anencephaly is characterized by partial or complete absence of the cranial vault and calvarium and partial or complete absence of the cerebral hemispheres. At least two thirds of anencephalics are stillborn; term deliveries do not survive more than a few hours or days. Encephalocele consists of a protrusion of the brain into an enclosed sac. It is seldom compatible with survival.

NTDs are thought to arise from a combination of genetic and environmental factors. In most populations surveyed thus far, empirical recurrence risks for siblings of affected individuals range from 2% to 5%. Consistent with a multifactorial model, the recurrence risk increases with additional affected siblings. A Hungarian study showed that the overall prevalence of NTDs in that country was 1/300 births and that the sibling recurrence risks were 3%, 12%, and 25% after one, two, and three affected offspring, respectively. Recurrence risks tend to be slightly lower in populations with lower NTD prevalence rates, as predicted by the multifactorial model. Recurrence risk data support the idea that the major forms of NTDs are caused by shared or similar factors. An anencephalic conception increases the recurrence risk for subsequent spina bifida conceptions, and vice versa.

NTDs can usually be diagnosed prenatally, sometimes by ultrasound and usually by an elevation in **α-fetoprotein (AFP)** in the maternal serum or amniotic fluid. A spina bifida lesion can be either open or closed (i.e., covered with a layer of skin). Open spina bifida is more likely to be detected by an AFP assay. A major epidemiological finding is that mothers who supplement their diet with folic acid at the time of conception are less likely to produce children with NTDs. This result has been replicated in several different populations and is thus well confirmed. It has been

FIG 5-3 The major neural tube defects. **A,** An infant with an open spina bifida (meningomyelocele). **B,** A fetus with anencephaly. Note the abnormalities of the orbits of the eye and the cranial defect. **C,** An occipital encephalocele. (A and B from Jones KL. *Smith's Recognizable Patterns of Human Malformation.* 6th ed. Philadelphia: Saunders; 2006:705.)

CLINICAL COMMENTARY 5-1
Neural Tube Defects (Continued)

estimated that approximately 50% to 70% of NTDs can be avoided simply by dietary folic acid supplementation. (Traditional prenatal vitamin supplements would not have an effect because administration does not usually begin until well after the time that the neural tube closes.) Since mothers would be likely to ingest similar amounts of folic acid from one pregnancy to the next, folic acid deficiency could well account for at least part of the elevated sibling recurrence risk for NTDs.

Dietary folic acid is an important example of a nongenetic factor that contributes to familial clustering of a dis-

ease. However, it is likely that there is genetic variation in response to folic acid, which helps to explain why most mothers with folic acid deficiency do not bear children with NTDs and why some who ingest adequate amounts of folic acid nonetheless bear children with NTDs. To address this issue, researchers are testing for associations between NTDs and variants in several genes whose products (e.g., methylene tetrahydrofolate reductase) are involved in folic acid metabolism (see Clinical Commentary 12-6 for further information on dietary folic acid supplementation and NTD prevention).

TABLE 5-2   Recurrence Risks for First-, Second-, and Third-Degree Relatives of Probands

DISEASE	PREVALENCE IN GENERAL POPULATION	DEGREE OF RELATION		
		FIRST DEGREE	SECOND DEGREE	THIRD DEGREE
Cleft lip/palate	0.001	0.04	0.007	0.003
Club foot	0.001	0.025	0.005	0.002
Congenital hip dislocation	0.002	0.005	0.006	0.004

---

for multifactorial traits either, but many such diseases do tend to conform to this prediction. Examination of the risks given in Table 5-2 shows that these three diseases follow the prediction fairly well.

> Risks for multifactorial diseases usually increase if more family members are affected, if the disease has more severe expression, and if the affected proband is a member of the less commonly affected sex. Recurrence risks decrease rapidly with more-remote degrees of relationship. In general, the sibling recurrence risk is approximately equal to the square root of the prevalence of the disease in the population.

Multifactorial versus Single-Gene Inheritance

It is important to clarify the difference between a multifactorial disease and a single-gene disease in which there is locus heterogeneity. In the former case, a disease is caused by the simultaneous influence of multiple genetic and environmental factors, each of which has a relatively small effect. In contrast, a disease with locus heterogeneity, such as osteogenesis

imperfecta, requires only a single mutation to cause it. Because of locus heterogeneity, a single mutation at either of two or more loci can cause disease; some affected persons have one mutation while others have the other mutation.

In some cases, a trait may be influenced by the combination of both a single gene with large effects and a multifactorial background in which additional genes and environmental factors have small individual effects (Fig. 5-4). Imagine that variation in height, for example, is caused by a single locus (termed a **major gene**) and a multifactorial component. Individuals with the *AA* genotype tend to be taller, those with the *aa* genotype tend to be shorter, and those with *Aa* tend to be intermediate. But additional variation is caused by other factors (the multifactorial component). Thus, those with the *aa* genotype vary in height from 130 cm to about 170 cm, those with the *Aa* genotype vary from 150 cm to 190 cm, and those with the *AA* genotype vary from 170 to 210 cm. There is substantial overlap among the three major genotypes because of the influence of the multifactorial background. The total distribution of height, which is bell-shaped, is caused by the superposition of the three distributions about each genotype.

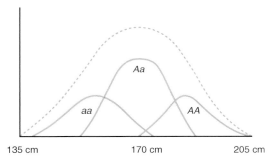

FIG 5-4   The distribution of height, assuming the presence of a major gene (genotypes *AA*, *Aa*, and *aa*) combined with a multifactorial background. The multifactorial background causes variation in height among individuals of each genotype. If the distributions of each of the three genotypes were superimposed, then the overall distribution of height would be approximately normal, as shown by the dotte line.

Many of the diseases to be discussed later can be caused by a major gene and/or multifactorial inheritance. That is, there are subsets of the population in which diseases such as colon cancer, breast cancer, or heart disease are inherited as single-gene disorders (with additional variation in disease susceptibility contributed by other genetic and environmental factors). These subsets usually account for only a small percentage of the total number of disease cases. It is nevertheless important to identify the responsible major genes, because their function can provide important clues to the pathophysiology and treatment of the disease.

 Multifactorial diseases can be distinguished from single-gene disorders caused by mutations at different loci (locus heterogeneity). Sometimes a disease has both single-gene and multifactorial components.

NATURE AND NURTURE: DISENTANGLING THE EFFECTS OF GENES AND ENVIRONMENT

Family members share genes and a common environment. Family resemblance in traits such as blood pressure therefore reflects both genetic and environmental commonality ("nature" and "nurture,"

respectively). For centuries, people have debated the relative importance of these two types of factors. It is a mistake, of course, to view them as mutually exclusive. Few traits are influenced only by genes or only by environment. Most are influenced by both.

Determining the relative influence of genetic and environmental factors can lead to a better understanding of disease etiology. It can also help in the planning of public health strategies. A disease in which hereditary influence is relatively small, such as lung cancer, may be prevented most effectively through emphasis on lifestyle changes (avoidance of tobacco). When a disease has a relatively larger hereditary component, as in breast cancer, examination of family history should be emphasized in addition to lifestyle modification.

In the following sections, we review two research strategies that are often used to estimate the relative influence of genes and environment: twin studies and adoption studies. We then discuss methods that aim to delineate the individual genes responsible for multifactorial diseases.

Twin Studies

Twins occur with a frequency of about 1/100 births in populations of European ancestry. They are slightly more common among Africans and a bit less common among Asians. **Monozygotic** (MZ, or identical) twins originate when the developing embryo divides to form two separate but genetically identical embryos. Because they are genetically identical, MZ twins are an example of natural clones. Their physical appearances can be strikingly similar (Fig. 5-5). **Dizygotic** (DZ, or fraternal) twins are the result of a double ovulation followed by the fertilization of each egg by a different sperm (While MZ twinning rates are quite constant across populations, DZ twinning rates vary somewhat. DZ twinning increases with maternal age until about age 40 years, after which the rate declines. The frequency of DZ twinning has increased dramatically in developed countries during the past several decades because of the use of ovulation-inducing drugs). Thus, DZ twins are genetically no more similar than siblings. Because two different

FIG 5-5 Monozygotic twins, showing a striking similarity in physical appearance. Both twins developed myopia as Teenagers.

sperm cells are required to fertilize the two eggs, it is possible for each DZ twin to have a different father.

Because MZ twins are genetically identical, any differences between them should be due only to environmental effects. MZ twins should thus resemble each other very closely for traits that are strongly influenced by genes. DZ twins provide a convenient comparison: their environmental differences should be similar to those of MZ twins, but their genetic differences are as great as those between siblings. Twin studies thus usually consist of comparisons between MZ and DZ twins. If both members of a twin pair share a trait (e.g., cleft lip), they are said to be **concordant**. If they do not share the trait, they are **discordant**. For a trait determined completely by genes, MZ twins should always be concordant, and DZ twins should be concordant less often. Like siblings, DZ twins share only 50% of their DNA because each parent transmits half of his or her DNA to each offspring. Concordance rates can differ between opposite-sex DZ twin pairs and same-sex DZ pairs for some traits, such as those that have different frequencies in males and females. For such traits, only same-sex DZ twin pairs should be used when comparing MZ and DZ concordance rates.

A concordance estimate would not be appropriate for quantitative traits, such as blood pressure or height. Here the **intraclass correlation coefficient** is used. This statistic varies between −1.0 and +1.0 and measures the degree of homogeneity of a trait in a sample of individuals. For example, we may wish to assess the degree of similarity between twins for a trait such as height. The measurements are made in a collection of twins, and correlation coefficients are estimated separately for the MZ sample and the DZ sample. If a trait were determined entirely by genes, we would expect the correlation coefficient for MZ pairs to be 1.0 (i.e., each pair of twins would have exactly the same height). A correlation coefficient of 0.0 would mean that the similarity between MZ twins for the trait in question is no greater than chance. Because DZ twins share half of their DNA, we would expect a DZ correlation coefficient of 0.50 for a trait determined entirely by genes.

 Monozygotic (identical) twins are the result of an early cleavage of the embryo, whereas dizygotic (fraternal) twins are caused by the fertilization of two eggs by two sperm cells. Comparisons of concordance rates and correlations in MZ and DZ twins help to estimate the extent to which a trait is influenced by genes.

Concordance rates and correlation coefficients for a number of traits are given in Table 5-3. The concordance rates for contagious diseases like measles are quite similar in MZ and DZ twins. This is expected, because most contagious diseases are unlikely to be influenced markedly by genes. On the other hand, the concordance rates for schizophrenia are quite dissimilar between MZ and DZ twins, indicating a sizable genetic component for this disease. The MZ correlation for dermatoglyphics (fingerprints), a series of traits determined almost entirely by genes, is close to 1.0.

Correlations and concordance rates in MZ and DZ twins can be used to measure the **heritability** of multifactorial traits. Essentially, heritability is the percentage of population variation in a trait that is due to genes (statistically, it is the proportion of the total **variance** of a trait that is caused by genes). A simple formula for estimating heritability (h) from twin correlations or concordance rates is as follows:

$$h = \frac{C_{MZ} - C_{DZ}}{1 - C_{DZ}}$$

where C_{MZ} is the concordance rate (or intraclass correlation) for MZ twins and C_{DZ} is the concordance rate (or intraclass correlation) for DZ twins. As this formula illustrates, traits that are largely determined by genes result in a heritability estimate that approaches 1.0 (i.e., C_{MZ} approaches 1.0, and C_{DZ} approaches 0.5). As the difference between MZ and DZ concordance rates becomes smaller, heritability approaches zero. Correlations and concordance rates in other types of relatives (e.g., between parents and offspring) can also be used to measure heritability.

Like recurrence risks, heritability values are specific for the population in which they are estimated. However, there is usually agreement from one population to another regarding the general range of heritability estimates of most traits (e.g., the heritability of height is almost always high, and the heritability of contagious diseases is almost always low). The same is true of empirical recurrence risks.

 Comparisons of correlations and concordance rates in MZ and DZ twins allow the estimation of heritability, a measure of the percentage of population variation in a disease that can be attributed to genes.

TABLE 5-3	Concordance Rates in Twins for Selected Traits and Diseases[*]		
	CONCORDANCE RATE		
TRAIT OR DISEASE	**MZ TWINS**	**DZ TWINS**	**HERITABILITY**
Affective disorder (bipolar)	0.79	0.24	>1.0[‡]
Affective disorder (unipolar)	0.54	0.19	0.70
Alcoholism	>0.60	<0.30	0.60
Autism	0.58	0.23	0.70
Blood pressure (diastolic)[†]	0.58	0.27	0.62
Blood pressure (systolic)[†]	0.55	0.25	0.60
Body fat percentage[†]	0.73	0.22	>1.0
Body mass index[†]	0.95	0.53	0.84
Cleft lip/palate	0.38	0.08	0.60
Club foot	0.32	0.03	0.58
Dermatoglyphics (finger ridge count)[†]	0.95	0.49	0.92
Diabetes mellitus	0.45-0.96	0.03-0.37	>1.0
Diabetes mellitus (type 1)	0.35-0.50	0.05-0.10	0.60-0.80
Diabetes mellitus (type 2)	0.70-0.90	0.25-0.40	0.90-1.0
Epilepsy (idiopathic)	0.69	0.14	>1.0
Height[†]	0.94	0.44	1.0
IQ[†]	0.76	0.51	0.50
Measles	0.95	0.87	0.16
Multiple sclerosis	0.28	0.03	0.50
Myocardial infarction (males)	0.39	0.26	0.26
Myocardial infarction (females)	0.44	0.14	0.60
Schizophrenia	0.47	0.12	0.70
Spina bifida	0.72	0.33	0.78

DZ, Dizygotic; *IQ*, intelligence quotient; *MZ*, monozygotic.
[*]These figures were compiled from a large variety of sources and represent primarily European and U.S. populations. Heritability is estimated here using the formula 2 ($C_{MZ}-C_{DZ}$).
[†]Because these are quantitative traits, correlation coefficients are given rather than concordance rates.
[‡]Several heritability estimates exceed 1.0. Because it is impossible for >100% of the variance of a trait to be genetically determined, these values indicate that other factors, such as shared environmental factors, must be operating.

At one time, twins were thought to provide a perfect "natural laboratory" in which to determine the relative influences of genetics and environment. But several difficulties arise. One of the most important is the assumption that the environments of MZ and DZ twins are equally similar. MZ twins are often treated more similarly than DZ twins. A greater similarity in environment can make MZ twins more concordant for a trait, inflating the apparent influence of genes. In addition, MZ twins may be more likely to seek the same type of environment, further reinforcing environmental similarity. On the other hand, it has been suggested that some MZ twins tend to develop personality differences in an attempt to assert their individuality.

Another difficulty is that the uterine environments of different pairs of MZ twins can be more or less similar, depending on whether there are two amnions and two chorions, two amnions and one shared chorion, or one shared amnion and one shared chorion. In addition, somatic mutations can occur during mitotic divisions of the cells of MZ twin embryos after cleavage occurs. Thus, the MZ twins might not be quite "identical," especially if a mutation occurred early in the development of one of the twins. Finally, methylation patterns, which can influence the transcription of specific genes, become more dissimilar in MZ twin pairs as they age. This dissimilarity is greater when the twins adopt markedly different habits and lifestyles (e.g., when one twin smokes cigarettes and the other does not).

Of the various problems with the twin method, the greater degree of environmental sharing among MZ twins is perhaps the most serious. One way to circumvent this problem, at least in part, is to study MZ twins who were raised in separate environments. Concordance among these twin pairs should be caused by genetic, rather than environmental, similarities. As one might expect, it is not easy to find such twin pairs. A major effort to do so has been undertaken by researchers at the University of Minnesota, whose studies have shown a remarkable congruence among MZ twins reared apart, even for many behavioral traits. However, these studies must

be viewed with caution, because the sample sizes are relatively small and because many of the twin pairs had at least some contact with each other before they were studied.

 Although twin studies provide valuable information, they are also affected by certain biases. The most serious is greater environmental similarity between MZ twins than between DZ twins. Other biases include somatic mutations that might affect only one MZ twin and differences in the uterine environments of twins.

Adoption Studies

Studies of adopted children are also used to estimate the genetic contribution to a multifactorial trait. Offspring who were born to parents who have a disease but who were adopted by parents lacking the disease can be studied to find out whether the offspring develop the disease. In some cases, these adopted persons develop the disease more often than do children in a comparative control population (i.e., adopted children who were born to parents who do not have the disease). This provides evidence that genes may be involved in causing the disease, because the adopted children do not share an environment with their affected natural parents. For example, schizophrenia is seen in 8% to 10% of adopted children whose natural parent had schizophrenia, whereas it is seen in only 1% of adopted children of unaffected parents.

As with twin studies, several precautions must be exercised in interpreting the results of adoption studies. First, prenatal environmental influences could have long-lasting effects on an adopted child. Second, children are sometimes adopted after they are several years old, ensuring that some nongenetic influences have been imparted by the natural parents. Finally, adoption agencies sometimes try to match the adoptive parents with the natural parents in terms of attributes such as socioeconomic status. All of these factors could exaggerate the apparent influence of biological inheritance.

 Adoption studies provide a second means of estimating the influence of genes on multifactorial diseases. They consist of comparing disease rates among the adopted offspring of affected parents with the rates among adopted offspring of unaffected parents. As with the twin method, several biases can influence these studies.

These reservations, as well as those summarized for twin studies, underscore the need for caution in basing conclusions on twin and adoption studies. These approaches do not provide definitive measure of the role of genes in multifactorial disease, nor can they identify specific genes responsible for disease. Instead, they provide a preliminary indication of the extent to which a multifactorial disease may be influenced by genetic factors. Methods for the direct detection of genes underlying multifactorial traits are summarized in Box 5-1.

Box 5-1 Finding Genes That Contribute to Multifactorial Disease

As mentioned in the text, twin and adoption studies are not designed to reveal specific genes that cause multifactorial diseases. The identification of specific causative genes is an important goal, because only then can we begin to understand the underlying biology of the disease and undertake to correct the defect. For complex multifactorial traits, this is a formidable task because of locus heterogeneity, the interactions of multiple genes, decreased penetrance, age-dependent onset, and **phenocopies** (persons who have a phenotype, such as breast cancer, but who do not carry a known disease-causing mutation, such as a *BRCA1* alteration). Fortunately, recent technological advances promise to make this goal more attainable. Here, we discuss several approaches that are used to identify the genes underlying multifactorial traits.

One way to search for these genes is to use conventional linkage analysis. Disease families are collected, a single-gene mode of inheritance is assumed, and linkage analysis is undertaken with a large series of marker polymorphisms that span the genome (this is termed a **genome scan**). If a sufficiently large LOD score is obtained with a polymorphism, it is assumed that the region around this polymorphism might contain a disease-causing gene. This approach is sometimes successful, especially when there are subsets of families in which a single-gene mode of inheritance is seen (e.g., autosomal dominant, autosomal recessive). This was the case, for example, with familial breast cancer and familial Alzheimer disease, where some families presented a clear autosomal dominant mode of inheritance.

With many multifactorial disorders, however, such subsets are not readily apparent. Because of obstacles such as heterogeneity and phenocopies, traditional linkage analyses are often impractical. One alternative to traditional linkage analysis is the **affected sib-pair method**. The logic of this approach is simple: if two siblings are both affected by a genetic disease, we would expect to see increased sharing of marker alleles in the genomic region that contains a susceptibility gene. To conduct an analysis using this approach, we begin by collecting DNA samples from a large number of sib pairs in which both members of the pair are affected by the disease. Then a genome scan is undertaken, and the proportion of affected-sib pairs who share the same allele is estimated for each polymorphism. Because siblings share with half their DNA (see Chapter 4), we would expect this proportion to be 50% for marker polymorphisms that are not linked to a disease-susceptibility locus. However, if we find that siblings share the same allele for a marker polymorphism more than half the time (say, 75% of the time), this would be evidence that the marker is linked to a susceptibility locus. This approach was used, for example, to show that the genes in the HLA region contribute to susceptibility for type 1 diabetes.

The affected sib-pair method has the advantage that one does not have to assume a specific mode of inheritance. In addition, the method is unaffected by reduced penetrance, because both members of the sib pair must be affected to be included in the analysis. It is especially useful for disorders with late age of onset (e.g., prostate cancer), for which it would be difficult to assemble multigenerational families from whom DNA samples could be taken. Affected sib-pair analyses are sometimes made more powerful by selecting subjects with extreme values of a trait (e.g., sib pairs with very high blood pressure) to enrich the sample for genes likely to contribute to the trait. A variation on this approach is to sample sib pairs that are highly discordant for a trait (e.g., one with very high blood pressure and one with very low blood pressure) and then to look for markers in which there is less allele sharing than the expected 50%.

During the past decade or so, genome-wide association studies (GWAS) have become common in searches for genes that cause complex diseases. GWAS became more practical after the Human Genome Project developed dense sets of SNPs that span the human genome. It is now common to use microarrays that can assay millions of SNPs or high-throughput DNA sequencing strategies in a collection of cases and controls. GWAS are carried out using both SNPs as well as larger CNVs (which can contain multiple genes). Because the differences in the frequencies of disease causing variants can be quite small, thousands or even tens of thousands of cases and controls are often tested in these studies. A major challenge with GWAS is that the variants detected by this technique typically have only a small effect on disease risk (5%-20%), and their biologic significance is usually difficult to inter-

Box 5-1   Finding Genes That Contribute to Multifactorial Disease (Continued)

pret. Confidence in the plausibility of disease associated genes increases if an appreciable number of the genes encode products in the same disease-associated pathway (e.g., the folate metabolism pathway for neural tube defects or the dopaminergic pathway for schizophrenia).

As the cost of exome and whole-genome sequencing has decreased, it has become increasingly common to compare DNA sequences in affected cases and matched controls. This approach has the advantage that it can detect all variants, including rare alleles, that differ in the two groups. Because these alleles are rare, large sample sizes must be used to detect their effects. This problem can be overcome somewhat by adding the effects of all disease associated alleles at a given locus together (this is termed a **burden test**). In addition, there has been a resurgence of interest in sequencing families, in which even a rare allele is likely to be observed in multiple cases. This

approach has been successful, for example, in identifying new genes associated with late-onset Alzheimer disease.

In addition to searching for variants in protein-coding DNA there is now considerable interest in identifying non-coding regulatory variants that may contribute to complex diseases. Indeed, about 80% of the SNPs associated with complex diseases in GWAS are found in non-coding DNA. This motivates whole-genome sequencing studies. Our understanding of variation in regulatory sequences such as enhancers and promoters is limited, however, but initial results (e.g., the association between enhancer elements and prostate cancer, discussed in the text) suggest that much will be learned by analyzing noncoding variation in the genome. Studies of epigenetic regulation (e.g., methylation and chromatin modification patterns) are also likely to yield new insights.

THE GENETICS OF COMMON DISEASES

Having discussed the principles of multifactorial inheritance, we turn next to a discussion of the common **multifactorial disorder**s themselves. Some of these disorders, the congenital malformations, are by definition present at birth. Others, including heart disease, cancer, diabetes, and most psychiatric disorders, are seen primarily in adolescents and adults. Because of their complexity, unraveling the genetics of these disorders is a daunting task. Nonetheless, significant progress is now being made.

Congenital Malformations

Approximately 2% of newborns present with a **congenital malformation** (i.e., one that is present at birth); most of these conditions are considered to be multifactorial in etiology. Some of the more common congenital malformations are listed in Table 5-4. In general, sibling recurrence risks for most of these disorders range from 1% to 5%.

Some congenital malformations, such as cleft lip/palate and pyloric stenosis, are relatively easy to repair and thus do not cause lasting problems. Others, such as neural tube defects, usually have more severe consequences. Although some cases of congenital malformations can occur in the absence of any other problems, it is quite common for them to be associated with other disorders. For example, cleft

lip/palate is often seen in babies with trisomy 13, and congenital heart defects are seen in many syndromes, including trisomy of chromosomes 13, 18, and 21.

Considerable progress is now being made in isolating single genes including the HOX, PAX, and TBX families of genes, that can cause congenital malformations. Another example is the RET proto-oncogene, which is responsible for some cases of Hirschsprung disease. However, the causes of many cases of this disorder remain undiscovered. Indeed, most of the genetic factors that contribute to important congenital malformations (e.g., neural tube defects, common congenital heart defects, cleft lip/palate) are as yet unidentified.

Environmental factors have also been shown to cause some congenital malformations. An example is thalidomide, a sedative used during pregnancy in the

TABLE 5-4 Prevalence Rates of Common Congenital Malformations in Persons of European Descent	
DISORDER	APPROXIMATE PREVALENCE PER 1000 BIRTHS
Cleft lip/palate	1.0
Club foot	1.0
Congenital heart defects	4.0-8.0
Hydrocephaly	0.5-2.5
Isolated cleft palate	0.4
Neural tube defects	1.0-3.0
Pyloric stenosis	3.0

early 1960s (and recently reintroduced for the treatment of dermatological conditions such as leprosy). When ingested during early pregnancy, this drug often can cause phocomelia (severely shortened limbs) in babies. Maternal exposure to retinoic acid, which is used to treat acne, can cause congenital defects of the heart, ear, and central nervous system. Maternal rubella infection can cause congenital heart defects. Other environmental factors that can cause congenital malformations are discussed in Chapter 12.

▶ Congenital malformations are seen in roughly 1 of every 50 live births. Most of them are considered to be multifactorial disorders. Specific genes and environmental causes have been detected for some congenital malformations, but the causes of most congenital malformations remain largely unknown.

Multifactorial Disorders in the Adult Population

Until recently, very little was known about specific genes responsible for common adult diseases. With more powerful laboratory and analytical techniques, this situation is changing. We next review recent progress in understanding the genetics of the major common adult diseases.

Cardiovascular Disorders

Heart disease. Heart disease is the leading cause of death worldwide, and it accounts for approximately 25% of all deaths in the United States. The most common underlying cause of heart disease is **coronary artery disease** (CAD), which is caused by atherosclerosis (a narrowing of the coronary arteries resulting from the formation of lipid-laden lesions). This narrowing impedes blood flow to the heart and can eventually result in a myocardial infarction (death of heart tissue caused by an inadequate supply of oxygen). When atherosclerosis occurs in arteries that supply blood to the brain, a stroke can result. A number of risk factors for CAD have been identified, including obesity, cigarette smoking, hypertension, elevated cholesterol

level, and positive family history (usually defined as having one or more affected first degree relatives). Many studies have examined the role of family history in CAD, and they show that a person with a positive family history is at least twice as likely to suffer from CAD than is a person with no family history. Generally, these studies also show that the risk is higher if there are more affected relatives, if the affected relative is female (the less commonly affected sex) rather than male, and if the age of onset in the affected relative is early (before 55 years of age). For example, one study showed that men between the ages of 20 and 39 years had a threefold increase in CAD risk if they had one affected first-degree relative. This risk increased to 13-fold if there were two first-degree relatives affected with CAD before 55 years of age.

What part do genes play in the familial clustering of CAD? Because of the key role of lipids in atherosclerosis, many studies have focused on the genetic determination of variation in circulating lipoprotein levels. An important advance was the identification of the gene that encodes the low-density lipoprotein (LDL) receptor. Heterozygosity for a mutation in this gene roughly doubles LDL cholesterol levels and is seen in approximately 1 in 500 persons. (This condition, known as familial hypercholesterolemia, is described further in Clinical Commentary 5-2.) Mutations in the gene encoding apolipoprotein B, which are seen in about 1 in 1000 persons, are another genetic cause of elevated LDL cholesterol. These mutations occur in the portion of the gene that is responsible for binding of apolipoprotein B to the LDL receptor, and they increase circulating LDL cholesterol levels by 50% to 100%. Dozens of other genes involved in lipid metabolism and transport have been identified, including those genes that encode various apolipoproteins (these are the protein components of lipoproteins) (Table 5-5). In addition, several genes whose protein products contribute to inflammation have been associated with CAD, reflecting the critical role of inflammation in generating atherosclerotic plaques. Functional analysis of these genes is leading to increased understanding and more effective treatment of CAD.

Clinical Commentary 5-2
Familial Hypercholesterolemia

Autosomal dominant familial hypercholesterolemia (FH) is an important cause of heart disease, accounting for approximately 5% of myocardial infarctions (MIs) in persons younger than 60 years. FH is one of the most common autosomal dominant disorders: in most populations surveyed to date, about 1 in 500 persons is a heterozygote. Plasma cholesterol levels are approximately twice as high as normal (i.e., about 300-400 mg/dl), resulting in substantially accelerated atherosclerosis and the occurrence of distinctive cholesterol deposits in skin and tendons, called xanthomas (Fig. 5-6). Data compiled from multiple studies showed that approximately 75% of men with FH developed coronary artery disease, and 50% had a fatal MI, by age 60 years. The corresponding percentages for women were lower (45% and 15%, respectively), because women generally develop heart disease at a later age than men.

FIG 5-6   Xanthomas, seen here on the knuckles, are often seen in patients with familial hypercholesterolemia.

Consistent with Hardy-Weinberg predictions, about 1/1,000,000 births is homozygous for the FH gene. Homozygotes are severely affected, with cholesterol levels ranging from 600 to 1200 mg/dl. Most homozygotes experience MIs before 20 years of age, and an MI at 18 months of age has been reported. Without treatment, most FH homozygotes die before the age of 30 years.

All cells require cholesterol as a component of their plasma membrane. They can either synthesize their own cholesterol, or preferentially they obtain it from the extracellular environment, where it is carried primarily by low-density lipoprotein (LDL). In a process known as **endocytosis**, LDL-bound cholesterol is taken into the cell via LDL receptors on the cell's surface. FH is caused by a reduction in the number of functional LDL receptors on cell surfaces. Cellular cholesterol uptake is reduced, and circulating cholesterol levels increase.

Much of what we know about endocytosis has been learned through the study of LDL receptors. The process of endocytosis and the processing of LDL in the cell is described in detail in Figure 5-7. These processes result in

a fine-tuned regulation of cholesterol levels within cells, and they influence the level of circulating cholesterol as well.

The identification of the LDL receptor gene (*LDLR*) in 1984 was a critical step in understanding exactly how LDL receptor defects cause FH. More than a thousand different mutations, two thirds of which are missense and nonsense substitutions, have been identified. Most of the remaining mutations are insertions and deletions, many of which arise from unequal crossovers (see Chapters 4 and 6) that occur between *Alu* repeat sequences (see Chapter 2) scattered throughout the gene. The *LDLR* mutations can be grouped into five broad classes, according to their effects on the activity of the receptor:

- Class I mutations in *LDLR* result in no detectable protein product. Thus, heterozygotes would produce only half the normal number of LDL receptors.
- Class II mutations result in production of the LDL receptor, but it is altered to the extent that it cannot leave the endoplasmic reticulum. It is eventually degraded.
- Class III mutations produce an LDL receptor that is capable of migrating to the cell surface but is incapable of normal binding to LDL.
- Class IV mutations, which are comparatively rare, produce receptors that are normal except that they do not migrate specifically to coated pits and thus cannot carry LDL into the cell.
- Class V mutations produce an LDL receptor that cannot disassociate from the LDL particle after entry into the cell.

The receptor cannot return to the cell surface and is degraded. Each class of mutations reduces the number of effective LDL receptors, resulting in decreased LDL uptake and hence elevated levels of circulating cholesterol. The number of effective receptors is reduced by about half in FH heterozygotes, and homozygotes have virtually no functional LDL receptors.

Understanding the defects that lead to FH has helped in the development of effective therapies for the disorder. Dietary reduction of cholesterol (primarily through the reduced intake of saturated fats) has only modest effects on cholesterol levels in FH heterozygotes. Because cholesterol is reabsorbed into the gut and then recycled through the liver (where most cholesterol synthesis takes place), serum cholesterol levels can be reduced by the administration of bile acid absorbing resins, such as cholestyramine. The absorbed cholesterol is excreted. It is interesting that reduced recirculation from the gut causes the liver cells to form additional LDL receptors, lowering circulating cholesterol levels. However, the decrease in intracellular cholesterol also stimulates cholesterol synthesis by liver cells, so the overall reduction in plasma LDL is only about 15% to 20%. This treatment is much more effective when combined with one of the statin drugs (e.g., lovastatin, pravastatin), which reduce cholesterol synthesis by inhibiting 3-hydroxy-3-methylglutaryl coenzyme A (HMG-CoA) reductase. Decreased synthesis leads to further production of LDL receptors. When these therapies are used in combination, serum cholesterol levels in FH heterozygotes can often be reduced to approximately normal levels.

Clinical Commentary 5-2
Familial Hypercholesterolemia (Continued)

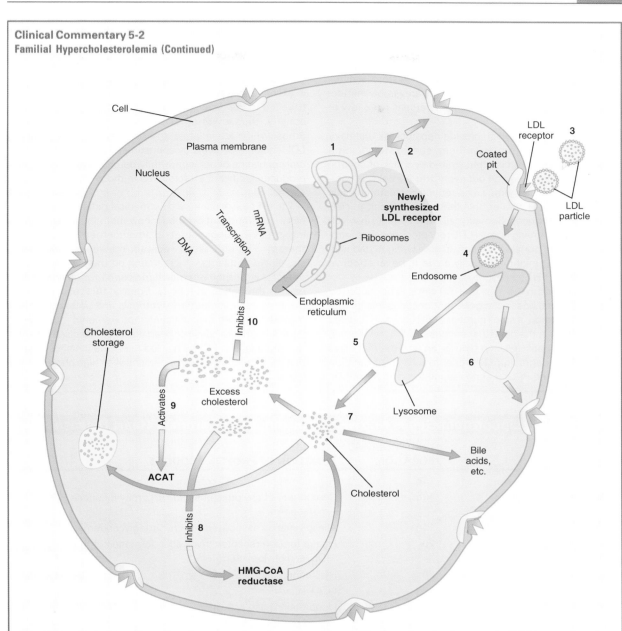

FIG 5-7   The process of receptor-mediated endocytosis. *1,* The low-density lipoprotein (LDL) receptors, which are glycoproteins, are synthesized in the endoplasmic reticulum of the cell. *2,* They pass through the Golgi apparatus to the cell surface, where part of the receptor protrudes outside the cell. *3,* The circulating LDL particle is bound by the LDL receptor and localized in cell-surface depressions called coated pits (so named because they are coated with a protein called clathrin). *4,* The coated pit invaginates, bringing the LDL particle inside the cell. *5,* Once inside the cell, the LDL particle is separated from the receptor, taken into a lysosome, and broken down into its constituents by lysosomal enzymes. *6,* The LDL receptor is recirculated to the cell surface to bind another LDL particle. Each LDL receptor goes through this cycle approximately once every 10 minutes, even if it is not occupied by an LDL particle. *7,* Free cholesterol is released from the lysosome for incorporation into cell membranes or metabolism into bile acids or steroids. Excess cholesterol can be stored in the cell as a cholesterol ester or removed from the cell by association with high-density lipoprotein (HDL). *8,* As cholesterol levels in the cell rise, cellular cholesterol synthesis is reduced by inhibition of the rate-limiting enzyme, HMG-CoA reductase. *9,* Rising cholesterol levels also increase the activity of acyl-coenzyme A: cholesterol acyltransferase (ACAT), an enzyme that modifies cholesterol for storage as cholesterol esters. *10,* In addition, the number of LDL receptors is decreased by lowering the transcription rate of the LDL receptor gene itself. This decreases cholesterol uptake.

Clinical Commentary 5-2
Familial Hypercholesterolemia (Continued)

The picture is less encouraging for FH homozygotes. The therapies mentioned can enhance cholesterol elimination and reduce its synthesis, but they are largely ineffective in homozygotes because these persons have few or no LDL receptors.

Liver transplants, which provide hepatocytes that have normal LDL receptors, have been successful in some cases, but this option is often limited by a lack of donors. Plasma exchange, carried out every 1 to 2 weeks, in combination with drug therapy, can reduce cholesterol levels by about 50%. However, this therapy is difficult to continue for long periods. Somatic cell gene therapy, in which hepatocytes carrying normal LDL receptor genes are introduced into the portal circulation, is now being tested (see Chapter 10). It might eventually prove to be an effective treatment for FH homozygotes.

As discussed in the main text, FH can also be caused by inherited mutations in the gene that encodes apolipoprotein B. In addition, a small number of FH cases are caused by mutations in the gene that encodes PCSK9 (proprotein convertase subtilisin/kexin type 9), an enzyme that plays a key role in degrading LDL receptors. Gain-of-function mutations in the PCSK9 gene reduce the number of LDL receptors, causing FH. Loss-of-function mutations in this gene can increase the number of LDL receptors, resulting in exceptionally low circulating LDL levels. These findings have led to the development of drugs that inhibit PCSK9 activity, thus lowering LDL cholesterol levels. These drugs, which are in late-stage clinical trials, can reduce LDL cholesterol levels by approximately 50% in the general population of persons with hypercholesterolemia and produce significant effects even in those who are using statin drugs.

The FH story illustrates how medical genetics research has made important contributions to both the understanding of basic cell biology and advancements in clinical therapy. The process of receptor-mediated endocytosis, elucidated largely by research on the LDL receptor defects, is of fundamental significance for cellular processes throughout the body. Equally, this research, by clarifying how cholesterol synthesis and uptake can be modified, has led to significant improvements in therapy for this important cause of heart disease. The discovery of rare mutations in PCSK9 has led to PCSK9 inhibitor drugs that may benefit millions of persons with high cholesterol levels.

TABLE 5-5 Lipoprotein Genes Known to Contribute to Coronary Heart Disease Risk

GENE	CHROMOSOME LOCATION	FUNCTION OF PROTEIN PRODUCT
Apolipoprotein A-I	11q	HDL component; LCAT cofactor
Apolipoprotein A-IV	11q	Component of chylomicrons and HDL; may influence HDL metabolism
Apolipoprotein C-III	11q	Allelic variation associated with hypertriglyceridemia
Apolipoprotein B	2p	Ligand for LDL receptor; involved in formation of VLDL, LDL, IDL, and chylomicrons
Apolipoprotein D	2p	HDL component
Apolipoprotein C-I	19q	LCAT activation
Apolipoprotein C-II	19q	Lipoprotein lipase activation
Apolipoprotein E	19q	Ligand for LDL receptor
Apolipoprotein A-II	1p	HDL component
LDL receptor	19p	Uptake of circulating LDL particles
Lipoprotein(a)	6q	Cholesterol transport
Lipoprotein lipase	8p	Hydrolysis of lipoprotein lipids
Hepatic triglyceride lipase	15q	Hydrolysis of lipoprotein lipids
LCAT	16q	Cholesterol esterification
Cholesterol ester transfer protein	16q	Facilitates transfer of cholesterol esters and phospholipids between lipoproteins

Adapted in part from King RA, Rotter JI, eds. *The Genetic Basis of Common Diseases*. 2nd ed. New York: Oxford University Press; 2002. *HDL*, High-density lipoprotein; *IDL*, Intermediate-density lipoprotein; *LCAT*, lecithin cholesterol acyltransferase; *LDL*, low-density lipoprotein; *VLDL*, very-low-density lipoprotein.

Environmental factors, many of which are easily modified, are also important causes of CAD. There is abundant epidemiological evidence that cigarette smoking and obesity increase the risk of CAD, whereas exercise and a diet low in saturated fats decrease the risk. Indeed, the approximate 60% reduction in age-adjusted mortality due to CAD and stroke in the United States since 1950 is usually attributed to a decrease in the percentage of adults who smoke cigarettes, decreased consumption of saturated fats, improved medical care, and increased emphasis on healthy lifestyle factors such as exercise.

Another form of heart disease is cardiomyopathy, an abnormality of the heart muscle that leads to inadequate cardiac function. Cardiomyopathy is a common cause of heart failure, resulting in approximately 10,000 deaths annually in the United States. Nearly 100 different genes have been linked to cardiomyopathy. Hypertrophic cardiomyopathy, one major form of the disease, is characterized by thickening (hypertrophy) of portions of the left ventricle and is seen in as many as 1 in 500 adults. About half of hypertrophic cardiomyopathy cases are familial and are caused by autosomal dominant mutations in any of the multiple genes that encode various components of the cardiac sarcomere. The most commonly mutated genes are those that encode the β-myosin heavy chain (35% of familial cases), myosin-binding protein C (20% of cases), and troponin T (15% of cases).

In contrast to the hypertrophic form of cardiomyopathy, dilated cardiomyopathy, which is seen in about 1 in 2500 persons, consists of increased size and impaired contraction of the ventricles. The end result is impaired pumping of the heart. This disease is familial in about one third of affected persons; although autosomal dominant mutations are most common, mutations can also be X-linked or mitochondrial. The most commonly mutated gene encodes titin, a cytoskeletal protein. Other genes that can cause dilated cardiomyopathy encode other cytoskeletal proteins, including actin, cardiac roponin T, desmin, and components of the dystroglycan-sarcoglycan complex. (Recall from Chapter 4 that abnormalities of the latter proteins can also cause muscular dystrophies.)

Mutations have also been identified in more than a dozen genes that cause the long QT (LQT) syndrome. LQT, which is seen in approximately 1 in 2000 persons, describes the characteristically elongated QT interval in the electrocardiogram of affected individuals, indicative of delayed cardiac repolarization. This disorder, which can be caused either by inherited mutations or by exposure to drugs that block potassium channels, predisposes affected persons to potentially fatal cardiac arrhythmia. An autosomal dominant form, known as Romano-Ward syndrome, can be caused by loss-of-function mutations in genes that encode potassium channels (such as *KCNQ1*, *KCNH2*, *KCNE1*, *KCNE2*, or *KCNJ2*). These mutations delay cardiac repolarization. Gain-of-function mutations in several of these same genes have been shown to produce a shortened QT interval, as might be expected. Romano-Ward syndrome can also be caused by gain-of-function mutations in sodium or calcium channel genes (*SCN5A* and *CACNA1C*, respectively), which result in a prolonged depolarizing current. (Other examples of mutations that can cause LQT are given in Table 5-6.)

An autosomal recessive form of LQT syndrome, known as Jervell-Lange-Nielsen syndrome, is less common than the Romano-Ward syndrome but is associated with a longer QT interval, a higher incidence of sudden cardiac death, and sensorineural deafness. This syndrome is caused by mutations in either *KCNQ1* or *KCNE1*. Because LQT syndrome can be difficult to diagnose clinically, genetic testing enables more accurate diagnosis of affected persons. In addition, the identification of disease-causing genes and their protein products is now guiding the development of drug therapy to activate the encoded ion channels. Because cardiac arrhythmias account for most of the 300,000 sudden cardiac deaths that occur annually in the United States, a better understanding of the genetic defects underlying arrhythmia is of considerable public health significance.

▶ Heart disease aggregates in families. This aggregation is especially strong if there is early age of onset and if there are several affected relatives. Specific genes have been identified for some subsets of families with heart disease, and lifestyle changes (exercise, diet avoidance of tobacco) can modify heart disease risks appreciably.

TABLE 5-6 Examples of Mendelian Subtypes of Complex Disorders*

MENDELIAN SUBTYPE	PROTEIN (GENE)	CONSEQUENCE OF MUTATION
Heart Disease		
Familial hypercholesterolemia	LDL receptor *(LDLR)*	Elevated LDL level
	Apolipoprotein B *(APOB)*	Elevated LDL level
	Proprotein convertase subtilisin/kexin type 9 *(PCSK9)*	Gain-of-function mutations elevate LDL; loss-of-function mutations reduce LDL
Tangier disease	ATP-binding cassette 1 *(ABC1)*	Reduced HDL level
Familial dilated cardiomyopathy	Cardiac troponin T *(TNNT2)*	Reduced force generation by sarcomere
	Titin *(TTN)*	Destabilized sarcomere
	Cardiac β-myosin heavy chain *(MYH7)*	Reduced force generation by sarcomere
	β-Sarcoglycan *(SGCB)*	Destabilized sarcolemma and signal transduction
	δ-Sarcoglycan *(SGCD)*	Destabilized sarcolemma and signal transduction
	Dystrophin	Destabilized sarcolemma in cardiac myocytes
Familial hypertrophic cardiomyopathy	Cardiac β-myosin heavy chain *(MYH7)*	Reduced force generation by sarcomere
	Cardiac troponin T *(TNNT2)*	Reduced force generation by sarcomere
	Myosin-binding protein C *(MYBPC)*	Sarcomere damage
Long QT syndrome	Cardiac potassium channel α subunit *(LQT1, KCNQ1)*	Prolonged QT interval on electrocardiogram, arrhythmia
	Cardiac potassium channel α subunit *(LQT2, KCNH2)*	Prolonged QT interval on electrocardiogram, arrhythmia
	Cardiac sodium channel *(LQT3, SCN5A)*	Prolonged QT interval on electrocardiogram, arrhythmia
	Ankyrin B anchoring protein *(LQT4, ANK2)*	Prolonged QT interval on electrocardiogram, arrhythmia
	Cardiac potassium channel β subunit *(LQT5, KCNE1)*	Prolonged QT interval on electrocardiogram, arrhythmia
	Cardiac potassium channel subunit *(LQT6, KCNE2)*	Prolonged QT interval on electrocardiogram, arrhythmia
Hypertension		
Liddle syndrome	Renal epithelial sodium channel subunits *(SCNN1B, SCNN1G)*	Severe hypertension, low renin and suppressed aldosterone
Gordon syndrome	*WNK1* or *WNK4* kinase genes	High serum potassium level and increased renal salt reabsorption
Glucocorticoid-remediable aldosteronism	Fusion of genes that encode aldosterone synthase and steroid 11β-hydroxylase	Early-onset hypertension with suppressed plasma renin and normal or elevated aldosterone levels
Syndrome of apparent mineralocorticoid excess	11β-Hydroxysteroid dehydrogenase *(11β-HSD2)*	Early-onset hypertension, low potassium and renin levels, low aldosterone
Diabetes		
MODY1	Hepatocyte nuclear factor-4α *(HNF4A)*	Decreased insulin secretion
MODY2	Glucokinase *(GCK)*	Impaired glucose metabolism, leading to mild nonprogressive hyperglycemia
MODY3	Hepatocyte nuclear factor-1α *(HNF1α)*	Decreased insulin secretion
MODY4	Insulin promoter factor-1 *(IPF1)*	Decreased transcription of insulin gene
MODY5	Hepatocyte nuclear factor-1β *(HNF1β)*	β-cell dysfunction leads to decreased insulin secretion
MODY6	NeuroD transcription factor *(NEUROD1)*	Decreased insulin secretion
Alzheimer Disease		
Familial Alzheimer disease	Amyloid-β precursor protein *(APP)*	Alteration of cleavage sites in amyloid-β precursor protein, producing longer amyloid fragments
	Presenilin 1 *(PS1)*	Altered cleavage of amyloid-β precursor protein, producing larger proportion of long amyloid fragments
	Presenilin 2 *(PS2)*	Altered cleavage of amyloid-β precursor protein, producing larger proportion of long amyloid fragments

TABLE 5-6 Examples of Mendelian Subtypes of Complex Disorders* (Continued)

MENDELIAN SUBTYPE	PROTEIN (GENE)	CONSEQUENCE OF MUTATION
Parkinson Disease		
Familial Parkinson disease (autosomal dominant)	α-Synuclein *(PARK1, SNCA)*	Formation of α-synuclein aggregates
Familial Parkinson disease (autosomal recessive)	Parkin: E3 ubiquityl ligase, thought to ubiquinate α-synuclein *(PARK2)*	Compromised degradation of α-synuclein
Familial Parkinson disease (autosomal dominant)	Ubiquitin C-hydrolase-L1 *(PARK5)*	Accumulation of α-synuclein
Amyotrophic Lateral Sclerosis		
Familial amyotrophic lateral sclerosis	Superoxide dismutase 1 *(SOD1)*	Neurotoxic gain of function
Familial amyotrophic lateral sclerosis	*C9ORF72*	Expanded repeat mutation
Juvenile amyotrophic lateral sclerosis (autosomal recessive)	Alsin *(ALS2)*	Presumed loss of function
Epilepsy		
Benign neonatal epilepsy, types 1 and 2	Voltage-gated potassium channels *(KCNQ2* and *KCNQ3,* respectively)	Reduced M current increases neuronal excitability
Generalized epilepsy with febrile seizures plus type 1	Sodium channel β1 subunit *(SCN1B)*	Sodium current persistence leading to neuronal hyperexcitability
Autosomal dominant nocturnal frontal lobe epilepsy	Neuronal nicotinic acetylcholine receptor subunits *(CHRNA4* and *CHRNB2)*	Increased neuronal excitability in response to cholinergic stimulation
Generalized epilepsy with febrile seizures plus type 3	GABA$_A$ receptor *(GABRG2)*	Loss of synaptic inhibition leading to neuronal excitability

HDL, High-density lipoprotein; *LDL,* low-density lipoprotein; *MODY,* maturity-onset diabetes of the young.
*This table is not meant to provide an exhaustive list of genes; additional genes are discussed in the review papers cited at the end of Chapter 5.

Stroke. Stroke, which refers to brain damage caused by a sudden and sustained loss of blood flow to the brain, can result from arterial obstruction (ischemic stroke, which accounts for 80% of stroke cases) or breakage (hemorrhagic stroke). This disease is the fourth leading cause of mortality in the United States, accounting for approximately 140,000 deaths per year. As with heart disease, strokes cluster in families: One's risk of having a stroke increases by two- to three-fold if a parent has had a stroke. The largest twin study conducted to date showed that concordance rates for stroke death in MZ and DZ twins were 10% and 5%, respectively. These figures imply that genes might influence one's susceptibility to this disease.

Stroke can be caused by any of more than a dozen single-gene disorders, including sickle cell disease (see Chapter 3), MELAS (*m*itochondrial myopathy, *e*ncephalopathy, *l*actic *a*cidosis, and *s*troke, a mitochondrial disorder discussed in Chapter 4), and cerebral autosomal dominant arteriopathy with subcortical infarcts and leukoencephalopathy (CADASIL, a condition characterized by recurrent strokes and dementia and caused by mutations in the *NOTCH3* gene). Because blood clots are a common cause of stroke, it is expected that mutations in genes that encode coagulation factors might affect stroke susceptibility. For example, inherited deficiencies of protein C and protein S, both of which are coagulation inhibitors a associated with an increased risk of stroke, especially in children. A specific mutation in clotting factor V, the factor V Leiden allele, causes resistance to activated protein C and thus produces an increased susceptibility to clotting. Heterozygosity for this allele, which is seen in approximately 5% of whites, produces a sevenfold increase in the risk of venous thrombosis (clots). In homozygotes, the risk increases to 100-fold. However, the evidence for an association between the factor V Leiden allele and stroke is inconsistent.

In addition to family history and specific genes, several factors are known to increase the risk of stroke. These include hypertension, obesity, atherosclerosis, diabetes, and smoking.

▶ Stroke, which clusters in families, is associated with several single-gene disorders and with some inherited coagulation disorders.

Hypertension. Systemic hypertension is a key risk factor for heart disease, stroke, and kidney disease. It is estimated that hypertension is responsible for approximately half of all cardiovascular mortality. Studies of blood pressure correlations within families yield heritability estimates of approximately 30% to 50% for both systolic and diastolic blood pressure. Heritability estimates based on twin studies tend to be higher (about 60%) and may be inflated because of greater similarities in the environments of MZ compared with DZ twins. The fact that the heritability estimates are substantially less than 100% indicates that environmental factors must also be sig-

nificant causes of blood pressure variation. The most important environmental risk factors for hypertension are increased sodium intake, decreased physical activity, psychosocial stress, and obesity (as discussed later, the latter factor is itself influenced both by genes and environment).

Blood pressure regulation is a highly complex process that is influenced by many physiological systems, including various aspects of kidney function, cellular ion transport, vascular tone, and heart function. Because of this complexity, much research is now focused on specific components that might influence blood pressure variation, such as the renin-angiotensin system (Fig. 5-8) (involved in sodium reabsorption and vasoconstriction); vasodilators such as nitric oxide and the kallikrein-kinin system; and ion transport systems such as adducin and sodium-lithium countertransport. These individual factors are more likely to be under the control of smaller numbers of genes than is blood pressure itself, simplifying the task of identifying these genes and their role in regulating blood pressure. For example, linkage and association studies have implicated several genes involved in the renin-angiotensin system (e.g.,

FIG 5-8   The renin-angiotensin-aldosterone system. ↑, Increased; ↓, decreased; *AT_1*, angiotensin type II receptor 1. (Modified from King RA, Rotter JI, Motulsky AG, eds. *The Genetic Basis of Common Diseases*. New York: Oxford University Press; 1992.)

the genes that encode angiotensinogen, angiotensin-converting enzyme type 1, and angiotensin II type 1 receptor) in causing hypertension.

A small percentage of hypertension cases are the result of rare single-gene disorders, such as Liddle syndrome (low plasma aldosterone and hypertension caused by mutations that alter the ENaC epithelial sodium channel) and Gordon syndrome (hypertension, high serum potassium level, and increased renal salt reabsorption caused by mutations in the *WNK1* or *WNK4* kinase genes); see Table 5-6 for additional examples. More than 20 genes have been identified that can lead to rare inherited forms of hypertension, and many of them affect the reabsorption of water and salt by the kidney, which in turn affects blood volume and blood pressure. It is hoped that isolation and study of these genes, and the pathways in which they act, will lead to the identification of genetic factors underlying essential hypertension.

Large-scale genome scans, undertaken in more than 100,000 humans and in experimental animals such as mice and rats, have sought to identify additional loci (see Box 5-1) that might underlie essential hypertension. These studies have identified dozens of genes that influence susceptibility to hypertension. Although the individual effects of each of these genes is small (as expected for a multifactorial trait), they collectively explain a significant proportion of the genetic risk for hypertension.

Heritability estimates for systolic and diastolic blood pressure range from 30% to 50%. A number of genes responsible for rare hypertension syndromes have been identified, and genome scans have implicated regions that might contain genes that underlie susceptibility to essential hypertension. Other risk factors for hypertension include increased sodium intake, lack of exercise, psychosocial stress, and obesity.

Cancer

Cancer is the second leading cause of death in the United States, although it is estimated that it might soon surpass heart disease as the leading cause of death. It is well established that many major types of cancer (e.g., breast, colon, prostate, ovarian) cluster strongly in families. This is due both to shared genes and shared environmental factors. Although numerous cancer genes have been isolated, environmental factors also play an important role in causing cancer by inducing somatic mutations. In particular, tobacco use is estimated to account for one third of all cancer cases in developed countries, making it the most important known cause of cancer. Diet (i.e., carcinogenic substances and the lack of "anticancer" components such as fiber, fruits, and vegetables) is another leading cause of cancer and may also account for as much as one third of cancer cases. It is estimated that approximately 15% of worldwide cancer cases are caused primarily by infectious agents (e.g., human papilloma virus for cervical cancer, hepatitis B and C for liver cancer). Because cancer genetics was the subject of Chapter 8, we confine our attention here to **genetic** and **environmental factors** that influence susceptibility to some of the most common cancers.

Breast cancer. Breast cancer is the second most commonly diagnosed cancer (after skin cancer) among women, affecting approximately 12% of American women who live to age 85 years or older. Invasive breast cancer was diagnosed in approximately 230,000 American women in 2014.

Although the breast cancer mortality rate has been declining for 25 years, about 40,000 women in the United States die from this disease each year. Breast cancer was formerly the leading cause of cancer death among women, but it has been surpassed by lung cancer. Breast cancer can also occur in men, with a lifetime prevalence that is roughly 100 times lower than that of women (2400 cases diagnosed in 2014). The familial aggregation of breast cancer has been recognized for centuries, having been described by physicians in ancient Rome. If a woman has one affected first-degree relative, her risk of developing breast cancer doubles. The risk increases further with additional affected relatives, and it increases if those relatives developed cancer at a relatively early age (before 50 years of age).

Several genes are now known to predispose women to developing hereditary breast cancer. Most important among these are **BRCA1** and **BRCA2**, two genes involved in DNA repair (see Chapter 8). Germline mutations in the *TP53* and *CHK2* genes can cause Li-Fraumeni syndrome, which also predisposes to breast cancer. Cowden disease, a rare autosomal dominant condition that includes multiple hamartomas and breast cancer, is caused by mutations in the *PTEN* tumor suppressor gene (see Chapter 8). Ataxia-telangiectasia, an autosomal recessive disorder caused by defective DNA repair, includes breast cancer in its presentation. Mutations in the *MSH2* and *MLH1* DNA repair genes, which lead to hereditary nonpolyposis colorectal cancer (HNPCC), also confer an increased risk of breast cancer. Despite the significance of these genes, it should be emphasized that more than 90% of breast cancer cases are not inherited as mendelian diseases.

A number of environmental factors are known to increase the risk of developing breast cancer. These include nulliparity (never bearing children), bearing the first child after 30 years of age, a high-fat diet, alcohol use, and estrogen replacement therapy.

Colorectal cancer. It is estimated that 1 in 20 Americans will develop colorectal cancer, and roughly one third of those with this cancer will die from it. With approximately 135,000 new cases and 50,000 deaths in the United States each year, colorectal cancer is second only to lung cancer in the total number of annual cancer deaths. Like breast cancer, it clusters in families; familial clustering of this form of cancer was reported in the medical literature as early as 1881. The risk of colorectal cancer in people with one affected first-degree relative is two to three times higher than that of the general population.

As discussed in Chapter 8, familial colorectal cancer can be the result of mutations in the **APC** tumor suppressor gene or in one of several DNA mismatch-repair genes (HNPCC). Another, less common, inherited cause of colorectal cancer is the autosomal dominant Peutz-Jeghers syndrome. About half of Peutz-Jeghers cases are caused by mutations in the *STK11* tumor suppressor gene, which encodes a protein kinase. Juvenile intestinal polyposis, an autosomal dominant disease defined by the presence of 10 or more polyps before adult-hood, can be caused by mutations in *SMAD4* (see Chapter 8), in *BMPRA1* (a receptor serine-threonine kinase gene), or, in rare cases, in *PTEN*.

As with breast cancer, most colorectal cancer cases (>90%) are not inherited as mendelian conditions and are likely to be caused by a complex interaction of inherited and somatic genetic alterations and environmental factors. The latter risk factors include a lack of physical activity and a high-fat, low-fiber diet.

Prostate cancer. Prostate cancer is the second most commonly diagnosed cancer in men (after skin cancer), with approximately 220,000 new cases annually in the United States. Prostate cancer is second only to lung cancer as a cause of cancer death in men, causing more than 27,000 deaths each year. Having an affected first-degree relative increases the risk of developing prostate cancer by a factor of two to three, and the heritability of prostate cancer is estimated to be approximately 40%.

The relatively late age of onset of most prostate cancer cases (median age, 72 years) makes genetic analysis especially difficult. However, **loss of heterozygosity** (see Chapter 8) has been observed in a number of genomic regions in prostate tumor cells, possibly indicating the presence of genetic alterations in these regions. In addition, genome scans (GWAS) have identified several dozen polymorphisms associated with prostate cancer risk. Several of these are located in chromosome 8q24, which contains polymorphisms associated with several other cancers as well (colon, pancreas, and esophagus). Although the 8q24 region contains no protein-coding genes, it contains enhancer elements that affect expression of the *MYC* oncogene, located about 250 kb from 8q24.

Nongenetic risk factors for prostate cancer may include a high-fat diet. Because prostate cancer usually progresses slowly and because it can be detected by digital examination and by the prostate-specific antigen (PSA) test, fatal metastasis can usually be prevented.

Most common cancers have genetic components. Recurrence risks tend to be higher if there are several affected relatives and if those relatives developed cancer at an early age. Specific genes have been discovered that cause inherited colon, breast, and prostate cancer in some families.

Diabetes Mellitus

Like the other disorders discussed in this chapter, the etiology of diabetes mellitus is complex and not fully understood. Nevertheless, progress is being made in understanding the genetic basis of this disorder, which is the leading cause of adult blindness, kidney failure, and lower-limb amputation and a major cause of heart disease and stroke. An important advance has been the recognition that diabetes mellitus is actually a heterogeneous group of disorders, all characterized by elevated blood sugar. We focus here on the three major types of diabetes, type 1 (formerly termed insulin-dependent diabetes mellitus, or IDDM), type 2 (formerly termed non-insulin-dependent diabetes mellitus, or NIDDM), and maturity-onset diabetes of the young (MODY).

Type 1 diabetes. Type 1 diabetes, which is characterized by T-cell infiltration of the pancreas and destruction of the insulin-producing beta cells, usually (though not always) manifests before 40 years of age. Patients with type 1 diabetes must receive exogenous insulin to survive. In addition to T-cell infiltration of the pancreas, autoantibodies are formed against pancreatic cells, insulin, and enzymes such as glutamic acid decarboxylase; these autoantibodies can be observed long before clinical symptoms occur. These findings, along with a strong association between type 1 diabetes and the presence of several human leukocyte antigen (HLA) class II alleles, indicate that this is an autoimmune disease. Over the past few decades, the incidence of type 1 diabetes has increased substantially.

Siblings of persons with type 1 diabetes face a substantial elevation in risk: approximately 6%, as opposed to a risk of about 0.3% to 0.5% in the general population. The recurrence risk is also elevated when there is a diabetic parent, although this risk varies with the sex of the affected parent. The risk for offspring of diabetic mothers is only 1% to 3%, but it is 4% to 6% for the offspring of diabetic fathers. (Because type 1 diabetes affects males and females in roughly equal proportions in the general population, this risk difference is inconsistent with the sex-specific threshold model for multifactorial traits.) Twin studies show that the empirical risk for MZ twins of type 1 diabetes patients ranges from 30% to 50%. In contrast, the concordance rate for DZ twins is 5% to 10%. The fact that type 1 diabetes is not 100% concordant among identical twins indicates that genetic factors are not solely responsible for the disorder. There is evidence that specific viral infections contribute to the cause of type 1 diabetes in at least some persons, possibly by activating an autoimmune response.

The association of specific HLA class II alleles and type 1 diabetes has been studied extensively, and it is estimated that the HLA loci account for about 40% to 50% of the genetic susceptibility to type 1 diabetes. Approximately 95% of whites with type 1 diabetes have the *HLA DR3* and/or *DR4* alleles, whereas only about 50% of the general white population has either of these alleles. If an affected proband and a sibling are both heterozygous for the *DR3* and *DR4* alleles, the sibling's risk of developing type 1 diabetes is nearly 20% (i.e., about 40 times higher than the risk in the general population). This association may in part reflect linkage disequilibrium between alleles of the *DR* locus and those of the *HLA-DQ* locus. The absence of aspartic acid at position 57 of the *DQ* polypeptide is strongly associated with susceptibility to type 1 diabetes; in fact, those who do not have this amino acid at position 57 (and instead are homozygous for a different amino acid) are 100 times more likely to develop type 1 diabetes. The aspartic acid substitution alters the shape of the HLA class II molecule and thus its ability to bind and present peptides to T cells (see Chapter 9). Altered T-cell recognition might help to protect persons with the aspartic acid substitution from an autoimmune episode.

The insulin gene, which is located on the short arm of chromosome 11, is another logical candidate for type 1 diabetes susceptibility. Polymorphisms within and near this gene have been tested for association with type 1 diabetes. Intriguingly, a strong risk association is seen with allelic variation in a VNTR polymorphism (see Chapter 3) located just 5′ of the **insulin gene**. Differences in the number of VNTR repeat units might affect transcription of the insulin gene (possibly by altering chromatin structure), which would result in variation in susceptibility. It is estimated that inherited genetic variation in the insulin region accounts for approximately 10% of the familial clustering of type 1 diabetes.

Affected sib-pair and genome-wide association analyses have been used extensively to map additional genes that can cause type 1 diabetes. In addition, an animal model, the nonobese diabetic (NOD) mouse, has been used to identify diabetes susceptibility genes that could have similar roles in humans (see Box 5-1). These studies have identified dozens of additional genes associated with type 1 diabetes susceptibility. One of these is the *CTLA4* (cytotoxic lymphocyte associated-4) gene, which encodes an inhibitory T-cell receptor. Several studies have demonstrated that alleles of *CTLA4* are associated with an increased risk of type 1 diabetes. There is growing evidence that variation in *CTLA4* is also associated with other autoimmune diseases, such as rheumatoid arthritis and celiac disease. Another gene associated with type 1 diabetes susceptibility, *PTPN22*, is involved in T-cell regulation and is also associated with other autoimmune disorders, including rheumatoid arthritis and systemic lupus erythematosus.

Type 2 diabetes. Type 2 diabetes accounts for more than 90% of all diabetes cases, and its incidence is rising rapidly in populations with access to high-calorie diets. It currently affects approximately 10% to 20% of the adult populations of many developed countries. One study estimates that because of the rapid rate of increase of this disease, one third of Americans born in 2000 will eventually develop type 2 diabetes.

A number of features distinguish type 2 diabetes from type 1 diabetes. Persons with type 2 diabetes usually have some degree of endogenous insulin production, at least in earlier stages of the disease, and they can sometimes be treated successfully with dietary modification, oral drugs, or both. In contrast to those with type 1 diabetes, patients with type 2 diabetes have **insulin resistance** (i.e., their cells have difficulty using insulin) and are more likely to be obese. This form of diabetes has traditionally been seen primarily in patients older than 40 years, but because of increasing obesity among adolescents and young adults, it is now increasing rapidly in this segment of the population. Neither HLA associations nor autoantibodies are seen commonly in this form of diabetes. MZ twin concordance rates are substantially higher than in type 1 diabetes, often exceeding 90% (because of age dependence, the concordance rate increases if older subjects are studied). The empirical recurrence risks for first-degree relatives of patients with type 2 diabetes are higher than those for type 1 patients, generally ranging from 15% to 40%. The differences between type 1 and type 2 diabetes are summarized in Table 5-7.

The two most important risk factors for type 2 diabetes are a positive family history and obesity; the latter increases insulin resistance. The disease tends to rise in prevalence when populations adopt a diet and exercise pattern typical of United States and European populations. Increases have been seen, for example, among Japanese immigrants to the United States and among some native populations of the South Pacific, Australia, and the Americas. Several studies, conducted on both male and female subjects,

TABLE 5-7 Comparison of the Major Features of Type 1 and Type 2 Diabetes Mellitus		
FEATURE	**TYPE 1 DIABETES**	**TYPE 2 DIABETES**
Age of onset	Usually <40 yr	Usually >40 yr
Insulin production	None	Partial
Insulin resistance	No	Yes
Autoimmunity	Yes	No
Obesity	Not common	Common
MZ twin concordance	0.35-0.50	0.90
Sibling recurrence risk	1%-6%	15%-40%

MZ, Monozygotic

have shown that regular exercise can substantially lower one's risk of developing type 2 diabetes, even among persons with a family history of the disease. This is partly because exercise reduces obesity. However, even in the absence of weight loss, exercise increases insulin sensitivity and improves glucose tolerance.

Extensive linkage and genome-wide association analyses have identified more than 70 genes that contribute to type 2 diabetes susceptibility. The most significant gene identified thus far is *TCF7L2*, which encodes a transcription factor involved in secreting insulin. A variant of *TCF7L2* is associated with a 50% increased risk of developing type 2 diabetes. A significant association has also been observed between type 2 diabetes and a common allele of the gene that encodes peroxisome proliferator-activated receptor-γ (PPAR-γ), a nuclear receptor that is involved in adipocyte differentiation and glucose metabolism. This receptor is the target of thiazolidinediones [TZDs], a class of drugs commonly used to increase insulin sensitivity in those with type 2 diabetes. Although the common *PPARG* allele confers only a 25% increase in the risk of developing type 2 diabetes, it is found in more than 75% of persons of European descent and thus helps to account for a significant fraction of type 2 diabetes cases. Variation in *KCNJ11*, which encodes a potassium channel necessary for glucose-stimulated insulin secretion, confers an additional 20% increase in type 2 diabetes susceptibility. The associations between diabetes susceptibility and each of these genes have been widely replicated in numerous populations. Many rare susceptibility alleles in each of these diabetes-associated genes are now being discovered through high-throughput DNA sequencing studies.

Maturity-onset diabetes of the young. MODY, which accounts for 1% to 5% of all diabetes cases, typically occurs before 25 years of age and follows an autosomal dominant mode of inheritance. In contrast to type 2 diabetes, it is not associated with obesity. Studies of MODY pedigrees have shown that about 50% of cases are caused by mutations in the gene that encodes glucokinase, a rate-limiting enzyme in the conversion of glucose to glucose-6-phosphate in the

pancreas. Another 40% of MODY cases are caused by mutations in any of five genes that encode transcription factors involved in pancreatic development or insulin regulation: hepatocyte nuclear factor-1α (*HNF1α*), hepatocyte nuclear factor-1β (*HNF1β*), hepatocyte nuclear factor-4α (*HNF4α*), insulin promoter factor-1 (*IPF1*), and neurogenic differentiation 1 (*NEUROD1*). Mutations in these genes, all of which are expressed in pancreatic beta cells, lead to beta cell abnormalities and thus to diabetes.

 Type 1 (insulin-dependent) and type 2 (non-insulindependent) diabetes both cluster in families, with stronger familial clustering observed for type 2 diabetes. Type 1 has an earlier average age of onset, is HLA-associated, and is an autoimmune disease. Type 2 is not an autoimmune disorder and is more likely to be seen in obese persons. Several genes have been identified that increase susceptibility to type 1 or type 2 diabetes. Most cases of autosomal dominant MODY are caused by mutations in any of six specific genes.

Obesity

The worldwide prevalence of obesity is increasing rapidly among adults and children. Approximately 70% of American adults and 60% of British adults are overweight (body mass index [BMI] >25), and about half of these overweight persons are obese (BMI >30). Although obesity itself is not a disease, it is an important risk factor for several common diseases, including heart disease, stroke, type 2 diabetes, and cancers of the prostate, breast, and colon.

As one might expect, there is a strong correlation between obesity in parents and obesity in their children. This could easily be ascribed to common environmental effects: parents and children usually share similar diet and exercise habits. However, there is good evidence for genetic components as well. Four adoption studies each showed that the body weights of adopted persons correlated significantly with their natural parents' body weights but not with those of their adoptive parents. Twin studies also provide evidence for a genetic effect on body weight, with most studies yielding heritability estimates between 0.60 and 0.80. The heritability of "fatness" (measured, for example, by skinfold thickness) is approximately 0.50.

Research, aided substantially by mouse models, has shown that several genes likely play a role in human obesity. Important among these are the genes that encode **leptin** (Greek, "thin") and its receptor. The leptin hormone is secreted by adipocytes (fat storage cells) and binds to receptors in the hypothalamus, the site of the body's appetite control center. Increased fat stores lead to an elevated leptin level, which produces satiety and a loss of appetite. Lower leptin levels lead to increased appetite. Mice with loss-of-function mutations in the leptin gene have uncontrolled appetites and become obese. When injected with leptin, these mice lose weight Mice with mutations in the leptin receptor gene cannot respond to increased leptin levels and also develop obesity.

Identification of the leptin gene and its receptor in mice led to their identification in humans, which in turn prompted optimistic predictions that leptin could be a key to weight loss in humans (without the perceived unpleasantness of dieting and exercise). However, most obese humans have *high* levels of leptin, indicating that the leptin gene is functioning normally. Leptin receptor defects were then suspected, but these are also uncommon in humans. Although mutations in the human leptin gene and its receptor have now been identified in a few humans with severe obesity (BMI >40), they both appear to be extremely rare. Unfortunately, studying these genes will not solve the problem of human obesity. However, clinical trials using recombinant leptin have demonstrated moderate weight loss in a subset of obese individuals.

In addition, leptin participates in important interactions with other components of appetite control, such as neuropeptide Y, as well as α-melanocyte-stimulating hormone and its receptor, the melanocortin-4 receptor (MC4R). Mutations in the gene that encodes MC4R have been found in 3% to 5% of severely obese individuals. Several genome-wide association studies have demonstrated an association between an intronic variant in the brain-expressed *FTO* gene and obesity in whites. Homozygosity for this variant, which is seen in about 16% of whites, confers increased risks of overweight and obesity of 40% and 70%, respectively. Recent evidence shows that the *FTO* variant is part of an enhancer that binds to the *IRX* gene, which is located 2 Mb away from *FTO* and is involved in regulation of fat mass. Identification of these and other obesity-predisposing genes is leading to a better understanding of appetite control in humans and could eventually lead to effective treatments for some cases of obesity.

 Adoption and twin studies indicate that at least half of the population variation in obesity may be caused by genes. Specific genes and gene products involved in appetite control and susceptibility to obesity, including leptin and its receptor, MC4R, and FTO, are now being studied.

Alzheimer Disease

Alzheimer disease (AD), which is responsible for 60% to 70% of cases of **progressive cognitive impairment** among the elderly, affects approximately 10% of the population older than 65 years and 40% of the population older than 85 years. Because of the aging of the population, the number of Americans with AD, which is currently about 5 million, continues to increase. Alzheimer disease is characterized by progressive dementia and memory loss and by the formation of amyloid plaques and neurofibrillary tangles in the brain, particularly in the cerebral cortex and hippocampus. The plaques and tangles lead to progressive neuronal loss, and death usually occurs within 7 to 10 years after the first appearance of symptoms.

The risk of developing AD doubles in persons who have an affected first-degree relative. Although most cases do not appear to be caused by single genes, approximately 10% follow an autosomal dominant mode of transmission. About 3% to 5% of AD cases occur before age 65 years and are considered early onset; these are much more likely to be inherited in autosomal dominant fashion.

Alzheimer disease is a genetically **heterogeneous disorder**. Approximately half of early-onset cases can be attributed to mutations in any of three genes, all of which affect amyloid-β deposition. Two of the genes, presenilin 1 (*PS1*) and presenilin 2 (*PS2*), are very similar to each other, and their protein products are involved in cleavage of the amyloid-β precursor protein (APP) by γ-secretase (posttranslational modification; see Chapter 2). Gain-of-function mutations in *PS1* or *PS2* affect the cleavage of APP such that amyloid-producing forms of it accumulate excessively and are deposited in the brain (Fig. 5-9). This is thought to be a primary cause of AD. Mutations in *PS1* typically result in especially early onset of AD, with the first occurrence of symptoms in the fifth decade of life.

A small percentage of cases of early-onset AD are caused by mutations of the gene (*APP*) that encodes APP itself, which is located on chromosome 21. These mutations disrupt normal secretase cleavage sites in APP (see Fig. 5-9), again leading to the accumulation of the longer protein product. It is interesting that this gene is present in three copies in persons with trisomy 21, where the extra gene copy leads to amyloid deposition and the frequent occurrence of early-onset AD in Down syndrome patients (see Chapter 6). High-throughput DNA sequencing stud-

ies have revealed an allele in *APP* that is protective against Alzheimer disease and may help to prevent cognitive decline.

An important risk factor for the more common late-onset form of AD is allelic variation in the **apolipoprotein E** (*APOE*) locus, which has three major alleles: ε2, ε3, and ε4. Studies conducted in diverse populations have shown that persons who have one copy of the ε4 allele are 2 to 5 times more likely to develop AD, and those with two copies of this allele are 5 to 10 times more likely to develop AD. The risk varies some what by population, with higher ε4-associated risks in whites and Japanese and relatively lower risks in Latin Americans and African Americans. Despite the strong association between ε4 and AD, approximately half of persons who develop late-onset AD do not have a copy of the ε4 allele, and many who are homozygous for ε4 remain free of AD even at advanced age. The apolipoprotein E protein product is not involved in cleavage of APP but instead appears to be associated with learance of amyloid from the brain.

Genome-wide association studies, based on microarrays and high-throughput sequencing, indicate that there are many additional genes associated with late-onset AD. Disease-associated variants that are relatively common in populations tend to

FIG 5-9 **A**, Cleavage of the amyloid-β precursor protein (APP) by α-secretase disrupts the amyloid-β protein and prevents the formation of amyloid plaques. **B**, An alternate cleavage pathway involves cleavage of APP by β-secretase at the N terminus and γ-secretase at the C terminus, producing a protein product of 40 to 42 amino acids. Gain-of-function mutations in the presenilin genes result in increased cleavage activity via this pathway. This yields an excessive amount of the 42-amino acid form of APP, which leads to formation of amyloid plaques. Mutations in the *APP* gene can also alter the α-secretase cleavage sites such that excess amounts of the longer form of APP are produced.

confer only a modest increase in risk, as is the case with most multifactorial conditions. Less common disease-associated variants, revealed by high-throughput sequencing, confer a higher relative risk of AD but are generally rare in populations.

AD has several features that have made it somewhat refractory to genetic analysis. Its genetic heterogeneity has already been described. In addition, because a definitive diagnosis can be obtained only by a brain autopsy, it is often difficult to diagnose AD in living family members (although clinical features and brain imaging studies can provide strong evidence that a person is affected with AD). Finally, because onset of the disease can occur very late in life, persons carrying an AD-predisposing mutation could die from another cause before developing the disease. They would then be misidentified as noncarriers. These types of difficulties arise not only with AD but with many other common adult diseases as well. Despite these obstacles, multiple AD-associated genes have now been identified, leading to a better understanding of the disorder and to the possibility of more effective AD treatment.

▶ Approximately 10% of AD cases are caused by autosomal dominant genes. Early-onset cases cluster more strongly in families and are more likely to follow an autosomal dominant inheritance pattern. This disease is genetically heterogeneous, and many AD susceptibility genes have been identified. Three genes (encoding presenilin 1, presenilin 2, and amyloid-β precursor protein) cause early-onset AD and affect the cleavage and processing of the amyloid precursor protein. The most significant gene associated with late-age onset AD encodes the apolipoprotein E protein.

Psychiatric Disorders

The major psychiatric diseases, including schizophrenia and autism spectrum disorder, have been the subjects of numerous genetic studies. Twin, adoption, and family studies have shown that these disorders aggregate in families. Moreover, schizophrenia, and autism tend to occur together in the same families. In part, this reflects the fact that some of the same genes influence susceptibility to each of these conditions.

Schizophrenia. Schizophrenia is a severe emotional disorder characterized by delusions, hallucinations, retreat from reality, and bizarre, withdrawn, or inappropriate behavior (contrary to popular belief, schizophrenia is not a "split personality" disorder). The lifetime recurrence risk for schizophrenia among the offspring of one affected parent is approximately 8% to 10%, which is about 10 times higher than the risk in the general population. The empirical risks increase when more relatives are affected. For example, a person with an affected sibling and an affected parent has a risk of about 15% to 20%, and a person with two affected parents has a risk of 40% to 50%. The risks decrease when the affected family member is a second- or third-degree relative. Details are given in Table 5-8. On inspection of this table, it may seem puzzling that the proportion of schizophrenic probands who have a schizophrenic parent is only about 5%, which is substantially lower than the risk for other first-degree relatives (e.g., siblings, affected parents, and their offspring). This can be explained by the fact that schizophrenics are less likely to marry and produce children than are other persons. There is thus substantial selection against schizophrenia in the population.

TABLE 5-8 **Recurrence Risks for Relatives of Schizophrenic Probands, Based on Multiple Studies of Western European Populations**	
RELATIONSHIP TO PROBAND	RECURRENCE RISK (%)
Monozygotic twin	44.3
Dizygotic twin	12.1
Offspring	9.4
Sibling	7.3
Niece or nephew	2.7
Grandchild	2.8
First cousin	1.6
Spouse	1.0

Adapted from McGue M, Gottesman II, Rao DC. The analysis of schizophrenia family data. *Behav Genet.* 1986;16:75-87.

Twin and adoption studies indicate that genetic factors are likely to be involved in schizophrenia. Data pooled from multiple twin studies show a 47% concordance rate for MZ twins, compared with only 12% for DZ twins. The concordance rate for MZ twins reared apart, 46%, is about the same as the rate for MZ twins reared together. The risk of developing the disease for offspring of a schizophrenic parent who are adopted by normal parents is about 10%, approximately the same as the risk when the offspring are raised by a schizophrenic biological parent.

Dozens of genome scans have been performed in an effort to locate schizophrenia genes. The techniques have identified significant associations between schizophrenia and polymorphisms in more than 100 genomic regions. A number of the genes in these regions encode components of the glutamatergic and dopaminergic neuronal signaling pathways. These findings are biologically plausible because the major drugs used to treat schizophrenia block dopamine receptors.

Bipolar disorder. Bipolar disorder, also known as manic depressive disorder, is characterized by extreme mood swings and emotional instability. The prevalence of the disorder in the general population is approximately 0.5% to 1%, but it rises to 5% to 10% among those with an affected first-degree relative. A study based on the Danish twin registry yielded concordance rates of 79% and 24% for MZ and DZ twins, respectively, yielding a heritability estimate of approximately 72% (other studies have yielded even higher heritability estimates—up to 90%). The corresponding concordance rates for major **depressive disorder** (sometimes termed unipolar depression) were 54% and 19%. Thus, it appears that bipolar disorder is more strongly influenced by genetic factors than is major depressive disorder.

As with schizophrenia, many linkage and genome-wide association studies have been carried out to identify genes contributing to bipolar disorder. These studies have implicated many chromosome regions in multiple population samples. Some of the best-replicated results are for genes that encode voltage-gated calcium channels. Ion-channel modu-

lating drugs are frequently used as mood stabilizers, giving these results functional plausibility. Many of the genes associated with bipolar disorder are also associated with schizophrenia.

Autism spectrum disorder. Autism spectrum disorder (ASD) is characterized by **impairments** in social interaction and communication, as well as restricted, repetitive, and stereotyped behaviors and activities. The definition of ASD has been broadened considerably in the past decade or so (e.g., it now includes Asperger syndrome), resulting in a much higher current prevalence estimate (approximately 1% worldwide). ASD is 3-4 times more common in males than in females and is usually diagnosed during the first three years of life. As predicted by the multifactorial threshold model, the empirical recurrence risk is substantially higher in the siblings of females with ASD. Genetic factors play a large role in the etiology of ASD, with twin studies suggesting a heritability of approximately 70%. Many large, well-controlled studies have investigated the relationship between ASD and vaccination (in particular for measles, mumps, and rubella), and no relationship has been found.

Approximately 10% of ASD cases have a known mendelian condition or genetic syndrome, most of which have been discussed in previous chapters. These include Fragile X syndrome (1%-2% of cases), Rett syndrome (0.5%), tuberous sclerosis (1%), and neurofibromatosis type 1 (<1%). The most frequent cytogenetic abnormality seen in persons with ASD (1%-3%) is a maternally transmitted duplication of chromosome 15q11-q13, the region that is deleted in Prader-Willi and Angelman syndromes (see Chapter 4). A 600 kb duplication or deletion of 16p11.2 is seen in about 1% of ASD cases.

Numerous GWAS and sequencing studies have been carried out to identify additional loci associated with ASD, and more than 100 susceptibility loci (each with small effect) have been identified. An increased number of de novo mutations are seen in children with ASD, most of which are inherited paternally (these are detected by comparing the DNA sequences of affected cases with those of their unaffected parents). This may help to explain the increased risk of autism among the offspring of older fathers. In addition, an increase in the number of copy number variants (CNVs) is seen in persons with autism.

Psychiatric disorders, such as schizophrenia, bipolar disorder, and ASD, present a number of challenges for genetic analysis. These diseases are undoubtedly heterogeneous, reflecting the influence of numerous genetic and environmental factors (the same is true of other psychiatric diseases, such as attention hyperactivity deficit disorder, which are not discussed here). This genetic heterogeneity is to be expected, in part because at least one-third of human genes are expressed in the brain. Also, the definition of a psychiatric phenotype is not always straightforward, and it can change through time. Several measures are being taken to improve the likelihood of finding genes underlying these conditions. Phenotypes are being defined in standardized and rigorous fashion. Larger sample sizes of affected persons (often tens of thousands), with more rigorous phenotype definition, are being collected in efforts to increase the power to detect linkage and association. Heterogeneity can be decreased by studying clinically defined subtypes of these diseases and by carrying out studies in genetically homogeneous populations.

▶ Marked familial aggregation, as well as familial co-occurrence, has been observed for schizophrenia and autism spectrum disorder. Case-control and family studies have revealed evidence that these conditions are caused by brain-expressed genes that encode neurotransmitters, receptors, ion channels, and neurotransmitter-related enzymes.

Other Complex Disorders

The disorders discussed in this chapter represent some of the most common multifactorial disorders and those for which significant progress has been made in identifying genes. Many other multifactorial disorders are being studied as well, and in some cases specific susceptibility genes have been identified. These include, for example, Parkinson disease, hear-

ing loss, multiple sclerosis, amyotrophic lateral sclerosis, epilepsy, asthma, inflammatory bowel disease, and some forms of blindness (see Table 5-6).

SOME GENERAL PRINCIPLES AND CONCLUSIONS

Some general principles can be deduced from the results obtained thus far regarding the genetics of complex disorders. First, the more strongly inherited forms of complex disorders generally have an earlier age of onset (examples include breast cancer, Alzheimer disease, and heart disease). Often, these include subsets of cases in which there is single-gene inheritance. Second, when there is laterality, bilateral forms sometimes cluster more strongly in families (e.g., cleft lip/palate or breast cancer). Third, while the sex-specific threshold model fits some of the complex disorders (e.g., pyloric stenosis, cleft lip/palate, autism, heart disease), it fails to fit others (e.g., type 1 diabetes).

There is a tendency, particularly among the lay public, to assume that the presence of a genetic component means that the course of a disease cannot be altered ("If it's genetic, you can't change it"). This is incorrect. Most of the diseases discussed in this chapter have both genetic and environmental components. Thus, environmental modification (e.g., diet, exercise, stress reduction) can often reduce risk significantly. Such modifications may be especially important for persons who have a family history of a disease, because they are likely to develop the disease earlier in life. Those with a family history of heart disease, for example, can often add many years of productive living with relatively minor lifestyle alterations. By targeting those who can benefit most from intervention, genetics helps to serve the goal of preventive medicine.

In addition, the identification of a specific genetic alteration can lead to more effective prevention and treatment of the disease. Identification of mutations causing familial colorectal cancer can allow early screening and prevention of metastasis. Pinpointing a gene responsible for a neurotransmitter defect in a psychiatric disorder such as schizophrenia could lead to the development of more effective drug treatments. In some cases, such as familial hypercholesterolemia, gene therapy may be useful. It is important for health-care practitioners to make their patients aware of these facts. Although the genetics of common disorders is complex and sometimes confusing, the public health impact of these diseases and the evidence for hereditary factors in their etiology demand that genetic studies be pursued. Substantial progress is already being made. The next decade will undoubtedly witness many advancements in our understanding and treatment of these disorders.

SUMMARY

Multifactorial traits are determined by a combination of many genes and the environment. Multifactorial traits reflect the cumulative effect of genetic variation at several loci, each with a relatively small contribution to the phenotype. Polygenic traits are continuous, also called quantitative traits. The phenotypic distribution of a polygenic trait in a population has bell shaped or normal distribution pattern. Polygenic diseases are caused by an interplay of multiple genes with multiple environment factors. Thus, the relatives of an affected individual are more likely to experience the same gene-gene and gene-environment interactions that lead to the disease in the proband compared to individuals who are unrelated to the proband. The threshold model applies to many multifactorial diseases. It assumes that there is an underlying liability distribution in a population and that a threshold must be reached before a disease is expressed. Heritability measures the genetic contribution to the variability of a multifactorial trait in a population. Heritability estimates are specific to a particular population at a particular time. The risk of multifactorial diseases usually increases if more

family members are affected, if the disease is more severely expressed, and if the proband is a member of the less commonly affected sex. The risk of occurrence decreases rapidly with more remote degrees of relationship. In some cases, the risk of occurrence in siblings is approximately equal to the square root of the prevalence of the disease in the population. Multifactorial diseases can be distinguished from single-gene disorders caused by mutations at different loci (locus heterogeneity). Sometimes a disease has both single-gene and multifactorial components. Many disorders, such as cardiovascular disorders, cancer, diabetes mellitus, and Alzheimer disease, were discussed in this chapter. Many other multifactorial disorders are being studied, and in some cases specific susceptibility genes have been identified. These include genes associated with Parkinson disease, hearing loss, amyotrophic lateral sclerosis, some forms of blindness, and other diseases. The identification of a specific genetic alteration can lead to more effective prevention and treatment of a disease.

IMPORTANT TERMINOLOGY

polygenic   多基因的
multifactorial   多因子的
quantitative traits   数量性状
liability   易患性
threshold   阈值
major gene   主基因
heritability   遗传率
cardiovascular disorder   心血管疾病
heart disease   心脏病
hypertension   高血压
cancer   癌症
diabetes mellitus   糖尿病
obesity   肥胖
Alzheimer disease   阿尔茨海默病
psychiatric disorder   精神疾病

REVIEW QUESTIONS

1. Consider a multifactorial trait that is twice as common in females as in males. Indicate which

type of mating is at higher risk for producing affected children (affected father and normal mother versus normal father and affected mother). Is the recurrence risk higher for their sons or their daughters?

2. Consider a disease that is known to have a 5% sibling recurrence risk. This recurrence risk could be the result of either multifactorial inheritance or a single autosomal dominant gene with 10% penetrance. How would you test which of these possibilities is correct?

3. One member of a pair of monozygotic twins is affected by an autosomal dominant disease, and the other is not. List two different ways this could happen.

4. Suppose that the heritability of body fat percentage is 0.80 when correlations between siblings are studied but only 0.50 when correlations between parents and offspring are studied. Suppose also that a significant positive correlation is observed in the body fat percentages of spouses. How would you interpret these results?

SUGGESTED READINGS AND WEBSITES

1. Behere SP, Shubkin CD, Weindling SN. Recent advances in the understanding and management of long QT syndrome. *Curr Opin Pediatr.* 2014; 26(6): 727-733.

2. Bonnefond A, Froguel P. Rare and common genetic events in type 2 diabetes: what should biologists know? *Cell Metab.* 2015; 21(3): 357-368.

3. Chouraki V, Seshadri S. Genetics of Alzheimer's disease. *Adv Genet.* 2014; 87: 245-294.

4. Copp AJ, Stanier P, Greene NDE. Neural tube defects: recent advances, unsolved questions, and controversies. *Lancet Neurol.* 2013; 12: 799-810.

5. Craddock N, Sklar P. Genetics of bipolar disorder. *Lancet.* 2013; 381: 1654-1662.

6. Lai M-C, Lombardo MV, Baron-Cohen S. Autism. *Lancet.* 2014; 383: 896-910.

7. Lambert G, Sjouke B, Choque B, et al. The PCSK9 decade. *J Lipid Res.* 2012; 53: 2515-2524.

8. McNally EM, Barefield DY, Puckelwartz MJ. The genetic landscape of cardiomyopathy and its role in heart failure. *Cell Metab.* 2015; 21: 174-182.

9. Munroe PB, Barnes MR, Caulfield MJ. Advances in blood pressure genomics. *Circ Res.* 2013; 112: 1365-1379.

10. O'Donnell CJ, Nabel EG. Genomics of cardiovascular disease. *N Engl J Med.* 2011; 365: 2098-2109.

11. Pomerantz MM, Freedman ML. The genetics of cancer risk. *Cancer J.* 2011; 17: 416-422.

12. Pugh TJ, Kelly MA, Gowrisankar S, et al. The landscape of genetic variation in dilated cardiomyopathy as surveyed by clinical DNA sequencing. *Genet Med.* 2014; 16(8): 601-608.

13. Roberts R. A genetic basis for coronary artery disease. *Trends Cardiovasc Med.* 2014; 64(23): 2525-2540.

14. Schizophrenia Working Group. Biological insights from 108 schizophrenia-associated genetic loci. *Nature.* 2014; 511: 421-427.

15. Stankov K, Benc D, Draskovic D. Genetic and epigenetic factors in etiology of diabetes mellitus type 1. *Pediatrics.* 2013; 132(6): 1112-1122.

16. van Dongen J, Slagboom PE, Draisma HH, et al. The continuing value of twin studies in the omics era. *Nat Rev Genet.* 2012; 13: 640-653.

17. Visscher PM, Brown MA, McCarthy MI, Yang J. Five years of GWAS discovery. *Am J Hum Genet.* 2012; 90(1): 7-24.

18. Waalen J. The genetics of human obesity. *Transl Res.* 2014; 164: 293-301.

19. Willsey JA, State MW. Autism spectrum disorders: from genes to neurobiology. *Curr Opin Neurobiol.* 2015; 30C: 92-99.

20. Willyard C. Heritability: the family roots of obesity. *Nature.* 2014; 508: S58-S60.

21. Human Genome Epidemiology Network Reviews (contains links to review articles on genetics of mendelian and common diseases): http://www.cdc.gov/genomics/hugenet/reviews/

22. International Clearinghouse for Birth Defects Web Guide: http:// www.icbdsr.org/page.asp?n=WebGuide

(Jinbo Zhang, Cuiying Peng)

Chapter 6

Clinical Cytogenetics: The Chromosomal Basis of Human Disease

The previous chapter has dealt with single-gene diseases. We turn now to diseases caused by alterations in the number or structure of chromosomes. The study of chromosomes and their abnormalities is called **cytogenetics**.

Chromosome abnormalities are responsible for a significant fraction of genetic diseases, occurring in approximately 1 of every 150 live births. They are the leading known cause of intellectual disability and pregnancy loss. Chromosome abnormalities are seen in 50% of first-trimester and 20% of second-trimester spontaneous abortions. Thus, they are an important cause of morbidity and mortality.

As in other areas of medical genetics, advances in molecular genetics have contributed many new insights in the field of cytogenetics. For example, molecular techniques have permitted the identification of chromosome abnormalities, such as deletions, that affect very small regions. In many cases, specific genes that contribute to the phenotypes of cytogenetic syndromes are being pinpointed. In addition, the ability to identify DNA polymorphisms in parents and offspring has enabled researchers to specify whether an altered chromosome is derived from the mother or from the father. This has increased our understanding of the biological basis of meiotic errors and chromosome abnormalities.

In this chapter we discuss abnormalities of chromosome number and structure. The genetic basis of sex determination is reviewed. Emphasis is given to the recent contributions of molecular genetics to cytogenetics.

CYTOGENETIC TECHNOLOGY

Although it was possible to visualize chromosomes under microscopes as early as the mid-1800s, it was quite difficult to observe individual chromosomes and thus to count the number of chromosomes in a cell or to examine structural abnormalities. Beginning in the 1950s, several techniques were developed that improved our ability to observe chromosomes. These included the use of spindle poisons, such as **colchicine** and **colcemid**, that arrest dividing somatic cells in metaphase, when chromosomes are maximally condensed and easiest to see; the use of a hypotonic (low-salt) solution, which causes swelling of cells, rupture of the nucleus, and better separation of individual chromosomes; and the use of staining materials that are absorbed differently by different parts of chromosomes, producing the characteristic light and dark bands that help to identify individual chromosomes.

▶ Our ability to study chromosomes has been improved by the visualization of chromosomes in metaphase, by hypotonic solutions that cause nuclear swelling, and by staining techniques that label chromosome bands.

Karyotype

Chromosomes are typically analyzed by collecting a living tissue (usually blood), culturing the tissue for the appropriate amount of time (usually 48 to 72 hours for peripheral lymphocytes), adding colcemid to produce metaphase arrest, harvesting the cells, placing the cell sediment on a slide, rupturing the cell nucleus with a hypotonic saline solution, staining with a designated nuclear stain, and photographing the metaphase spreads of chromosomes on the slide.

FIG 6-1   A banded karyogram (karyotype) of a normal male. The banded metaphase chromosomes are arranged from largest to smallest.

The images of the 22 pairs of autosomes are arranged according to length, with the sex chromosomes in the right-hand corner. This ordered display of chromosomes is termed a **karyogram** or **karyotype** (Fig. 6-1). (The term *karyotype* refers to the number and type of chromosomes present in an individual, and *karyogram* is now often used to designate the printed display of chromosomes.) Currently, computerized image analyzers are usually used to display chromosomes.

After sorting by size, chromosomes are further classified according to the position of the centromere. If the centromere occurs near the middle of the chromosome, the chromosome is said to be **metacentric** (Fig. 6-2). An **acrocentric** chromosome

has its centromere near the tip, and **submetacentric** chromosomes have centromeres somewhere between the middle and the tip. The tip of each chromosome is the telomere. The short arm of a chromosome is labeled *p* (for "petite"), and the long arm is labeled *q*. In metacentric chromosomes, where the arms are of roughly equal length, the p and q arms are designated by convention.

> A karyotype, or karyogram, is a display of chromosomes ordered according to length. Depending on the position of the centromere, a chromosome may be acrocentric, submetacentric, or metacentric.

A normal female karyotype is designated 46,XX; a normal male karyotype is designated 46,XY. The nomenclature for various chromosome abnormalities is summarized in Table 6-1 and is indicated for each condition discussed in this chapter.

Chromosome Banding

Early karyotypes were useful in counting the number of chromosomes, but structural abnormalities, such as balanced rearrangements or small chromosomal deletions, were often undetectable. Staining

FIG 6-2   Metacentric, submetacentric, and acrocentric chromosomes. Note the stalks and satellites present on the short arms of the acrocentric chromosomes.

TABLE 6-1 Standard Nomenclature for Chromosome Karyotypes

KARYOTYPE	DESCRIPTION
46,XY	Normal male chromosome constitution
47,XX,+21	Female with trisomy 21, Down syndrome
47,XY,+21[10]/46,XY[10]	Male who is a mosaic of trisomy 21 cells and normal cells (10 cells scored for each karyotype)
46,XY,del(4)(p14)	Male with distal and terminal deletion of the short arm of chromosome 4 from band p14 to terminus
46,XX,dup(5)(p14p15.3)	Female with a duplication within the short arm of chromosome 5 from bands p14 to p15.3
45,XY,der(13;14)(q10;q10)	A male with a balanced Robertsonian translocation of chromosomes 13 and 14; karyotype shows that one normal 13 and one normal 14 are missing and replaced with a derivative chromosome composed of the long arms of chromosomes 13 and 14
46,XY,t(11;22)(q23;q22)	A male with a balanced reciprocal translocation between chromosomes 11 and 22; the breakpoints are at 11q23 and 22q22
46,XX,inv(3)(p21q13)	An inversion on chromosome 3 that extends from p21 to q13; because it includes the centromere, this is a pericentric inversion
46,X,r(X)(p22.3q28)	A female with one normal X chromosome and one ring X chromosome formed by breakage at bands p22.3 and q28 with subsequent fusion
46,X,i(Xq)	A female with one normal X chromosome and an isochromosome of the long arm of the X chromosome

techniques were developed in the 1970s to produce the chromosome bands characteristic of modern karyotypes. **Chromosome banding** helps greatly in the detection of deletions, duplications, and other structural abnormalities, and it facilitates the correct identification of individual chromosomes. The major bands on each chromosome are systematically numbered (Fig. 6-3). For example, 14q32 refers to the second band in the third region of the long arm of chromosome 14. Sub-bands are designated by decimal points following the band number (e.g., 14q32.3 is the third sub-band of band 2).

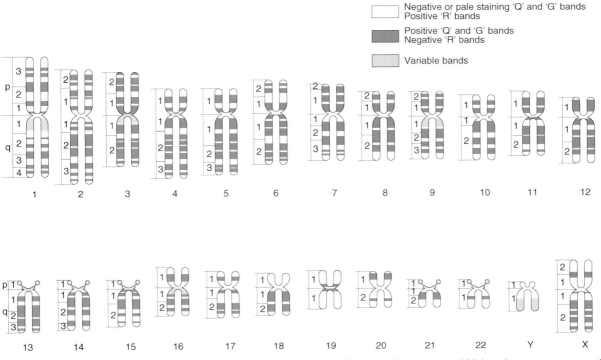

FIG 6-3 A schematic representation of the banding pattern of a G-banded karyotype; 300 bands are represented in this ideogram. The short and long arms of the chromosomes are designated, and the segments are numbered according to the standard nomenclature adopted at the Paris conference in 1971. In this illustration, both sister chromatids are shown for each chromosome.

Several chromosome-banding techniques are used in cytogenetics laboratories. **Quinacrine banding** (Q-banding) was the first staining method used to produce specific banding patterns. This method requires a fluorescence microscope and is no longer as widely used as **Giemsa banding** (G-banding). To produce G-bands, a Giemsa stain is applied after the chromosomal proteins are partially digested by trypsin. **Reverse banding** (R-banding) requires heat treatment and reverses the usual white and black pattern that is seen in G-bands and Q-bands. This method is particularly helpful for staining the distal ends of chromosomes. Other staining techniques include **C-banding** and nucleolar organizing region stains (NOR stains). These latter methods specifically stain certain portions of the chromosome. C-banding stains the **constitutive heterochromatin**, which usually lies near the centromere, and NOR staining highlights the satellites and stalks of acrocentric chromosomes (see Fig. 6-2).

High-resolution banding involves staining chromosomes during prophase or early metaphase (prometaphase), before they reach maximal condensation. Because prophase and prometaphase chromosomes are more extended than metaphase chromosomes, the number of bands observable for all chromosomes increases from about 300 to 450 (as in Fig. 6-3) to as many as 800. This allows the detection of less obvious abnormalities usually not seen with conventional banding.

> ▶ Chromosome bands help to identify individual chromosomes and structural abnormalities in chromosomes. Banding techniques include quinacrine, Giemsa, reverse, C, and NOR banding. High-resolution banding, using prophase or prometaphase chromosomes, increases the number of observable bands.

Fluorescence in Situ Hybridization

In the widely used **fluorescence in situ hybridization** (**FISH**) technique, a labeled single-stranded DNA segment (probe) is exposed to denatured metaphase, prophase, or interphase chromosomes from a patient. The probe undergoes complementary base pairing (hybridization) only with the complementary DNA sequence at a specific location on one of the denatured chromosomes. Because the probe is labeled with a fluorescent dye, the location at which it hybridizes with the patient's chromosomes can be visualized under a fluorescence microscope. A common use of FISH is to determine whether a portion of a chromosome is deleted in a patient. In an unaffected person, a probe hybridizes in two places, reflecting the presence of two homologous chromosomes in a somatic cell nucleus. If a probe from the chromosome segment in question hybridizes to only one of the patient's chromosomes, then the patient probably has the deletion on the copy of the chromosome to which the probe fails to hybridize. FISH provides considerably better resolution than high-resolution banding approaches and can typically detect deletions as small as 1 million base pairs (1 Mb) in size. It is widely used to detect common deletion syndromes such as Prader-Willi syndrome (microdeletion of 15q11.2) and Williams syndrome (microdeletion of 7q11.2) (discussed later).

Extra copies of a chromosome region can also be detected using FISH. In this case, the probe hybridizes in three or more places instead of two. Combinations of FISH probes can also be used to detect chromosome rearrangements such as translocations (see later discussion).

Figure 6-4A illustrates a FISH result for a child who is missing a small piece of the short arm of chromosome 17. Although a centromere probe (used as a control) hybridizes to both copies of chromosome 17, a probe corresponding to a specific region of 17p hybridizes to only one chromosome. This demonstrates the deletion that causes the Smith-Magenis syndrome (see Fig. 6-4B; also see Table 6-3).

Because FISH detection of missing or extra chromosomes can be carried out with interphase chromosomes, it is not necessary to stimulate cells to divide in order to obtain metaphase chromosomes (a time-consuming procedure required for traditional microscopic approaches). This allows analyses

FIG 6-4   **A**, A fluorescence in situ hybridization (FISH) result. The *thinner arrows* point to a centromere-hybridizing probe for chromosome 17, and the *thicker arrow* points to a probe that hybridizes to 17p. The latter probe reveals only one spot in this individual, who has a deletion of 17p, producing the Smith-Magenis syndrome. (Courtesy Dr. Arthur Brothman, University of Utah Health Sciences Center.) **B**, Face of an infant girl with Smith-Magenis syndrome. Note the broad forehead and relatively flat face. (Courtesy Dr. Marilyn C. Jones, Children's Hospital, San Diego.)

and diagnoses to be completed more rapidly. FISH analysis of interphase chromosomes is commonly used in the prenatal detection of fetal chromosome abnormalities and in the analysis of chromosome rearrangements in tumor cells.

The FISH technique has been extended by using multiple probes, each labeled with a different color, so that several of the most common numerical abnormalities (e.g., those of chromosomes 13, 18, 21, X, and Y) can be tested simultaneously in the same cell. In addition, techniques such as **spectral karyotyping** use varying combinations of five different fluorescent probes in conjunction with special cameras and image-processing software so that each chromosome is uniquely colored (painted along its entire length with a series of same-colored probes) for ready identification. Such images can be especially useful for identifying small chromosome rearrangements (Fig. 6-5).

FIG 6-5   Spectral karyotype. An application of spectral karyotyping is demonstrated by the identification of a rearrangement between chromosomes 2 and 22. Note that a portion of chromosome 2 (*purple*) has exchanged places with a portion of chromosome 22 (*yellow*). (Courtesy Dr. Arthur Brothman, University of Utah Health Sciences Center.)

With the increasing use of techniques such as comparative genomic hybridization (see below), spectral karyotyping is now less used in clinical practice.

▶ FISH is a technique in which a labeled probe is hybridized to metaphase, prophase, or interphase chromosomes. FISH can be used to test for missing or additional chromosomal material as well as chromosome rearrangements. The FISH technique can be extended with multiple colors to detect several possible alterations of chromosome number simultaneously. Multiple probes can be used to paint each chromosome with a unique color, facilitating the detection of structural rearrangements.

Comparative Genomic Hybridization

Losses or duplications of whole chromosomes or specific chromosome regions can be detected by a widely used technique known as **comparative genomic hybridization** (**CGH**) (Fig. 6-6). DNA is extracted from a test source, such as cells from a tumor or whole-blood cells from a patient. The DNA is then labeled with a substance that exhibits one color (e.g., red) under a fluorescence microscope; DNA taken from normal control cells is labeled with a second color (e.g., green). In the earliest version of CGH, both sets of DNA are then hybridized to normal metaphase chromosomes on a slide. If any chromosome region is duplicated in the tumor cell, then the corresponding region of the metaphase chromosome will hybridize with excess quantities of the red-labeled DNA. This region will appear red under

FIG 6-6 The comparative genomic hybridization (CGH) technique. **A**, Red-labeled test DNA (from a tumor sample in this case) and green-labeled reference DNA (from normal cells) are both denatured and hybridized to normal chromosomes. The ratio of green to red signal on the hybridized chromosomes indicates the location of duplications (*red signal*) or deletions (*green signal*) in the tumor chromosomes. **B**, Array CGH: Test and normal DNA are hybridized to probes embedded in a microarray. Duplications are indicated by hybridization of more red-labeled DNA to a probe containing a DNA sequence that is complementary to the duplicated region. Conversely, hybridization of only green-labeled DNA (reference DNA) indicates a deletion of the corresponding region. **C**, In a patient with DiGeorge sequence, an aCGH test was performed in which the patient's DNA was labeled green and the control DNA was labeled red. The figure demonstrates a lack of green signal and excess red signal, signifying a deletion of chromosome 22q11.

the microscope. Conversely, if a region is deleted in the tumor cell, then the corresponding region of the metaphase chromosome will hybridize only with green-labeled control DNA, and the region will appear green under the microscope. CGH is especially useful in scanning for deletions and duplications of chromosome material in cancer cells, where detection of such alterations can help to predict the type and/or severity of the cancer.

A serious limitation of CGH when used with metaphase chromosomes is that deletions or duplications smaller than 5 to 10 Mb cannot be detected microscopically. Higher resolution is offered by **array CGH (aCGH)**, in which test and control DNA is hybridized with a microarray (see Chapter 3) that contains hundreds of thousands to millions of oligonucleotide probes (see Chapter 3) whose DNA sequences correspond to specific regions of the genome. These microarrays provide resolution to 50 to 100 kb or even less, allowing the detection of duplications and deletions that may affect only a single gene.

Array CGH offers a number of other advantages over traditional karyotype analysis. The process is highly automated, requiring less time from laboratory personnel. There is no need for dividing cells (in contrast to the analysis of metaphase chromosomes), and less than a microgram of DNA is sufficient for analysis of the entire genome. For these reasons, aCGH has become one of the most commonly used techniques in cytogenetics laboratories. The primary disadvantage of aCGH is that it cannot detect balanced rearrangements of chromosomes (i.e., reciprocal translocations or inversions) because the quantity of chromosome material remains unchanged.

▶ The CGH technique, in which differentially labeled DNA from test and control sources is hybridized to probes in microarrays, allows the detection of chromosome duplications and deletions but not balanced rearrangements. Array CGH can detect deletions and duplications shorter than 100 kb and requires only small amounts of DNA.

ABNORMALITIES OF CHROMOSOME NUMBER

Polyploidy

A cell that contains a multiple of 23 chromosomes in its nucleus is said to be **euploid** (Greek, *eu* = "good," *ploid* ="set"). Thus, haploid gametes and diploid somatic cells are euploid. **Polyploidy**, the presence of a complete set of extra chromosomes in a cell, is seen commonly in plants and often improves their agricultural value. Polyploidy also occurs in humans, although much less frequently. The polyploid conditions that have been observed in humans are **triploidy** (69 chromosomes in the nucleus of each cell) and **tetraploidy** (92 chromosomes in each cell nucleus). The karyotypes for these two conditions are designated 69,XXX and 92,XXXX, respectively (assuming that all of the sex chromosomes were X; other combinations of the X and Y chromosomes may be seen). Because the number of chromosomes present in each of these conditions is a multiple of 23, the cells are euploid in each case. However, the additional chromosomes encode a large amount of surplus gene product, causing multiple anomalies such as defects of the heart and central nervous system.

Triploidy is seen in about 1 in 10,000 live births, but it accounts for an estimated 15% of the chromosome abnormalities occurring at conception. Thus, the vast majority of triploid conceptions are spontaneously aborted, and this condition is one of the most common causes of fetal loss in the first two trimesters of pregnancy. Triploid fetuses that survive to term typically die shortly after birth. The most common cause of triploidy is the fertilization of an egg by two sperm (**dispermy**). The resulting zygote receives 23 chromosomes from the egg and 23 chromosomes from each of the two sperm cells. Triploidy can also be caused by the fusion of an ovum and a polar body, each containing 23 chromosomes, and subsequent fertilization by a sperm cell. **Meiotic failure**, in which a diploid sperm or egg cell is produced, can also produce a triploid zygote.

Tetraploidy is much rarer than triploidy, both at

conception and among live births. It has been recorded in only a few live births, and those infants survived for only a short period. Tetraploidy can be caused by a mitotic failure in the early embryo: all of the duplicated chromosomes migrate to one of the two daughter cells. It can also result from the fusion of two diploid zygotes.

▶ Cells that have a multiple of 23 chromosomes are said to be euploid. Triploidy (69 chromosomes) and tetraploidy (92 chromosomes) are polyploid conditions found in humans. Most polyploid conceptions are spontaneously aborted, and all are incompatible with long term survival.

Autosomal Aneuploidy

Cells that contain missing or additional individual chromosomes are termed **aneuploid** (not a multiple of 23 chromosomes). Usually only one chromosome is affected, but it is possible for more than one chromosome to be missing or duplicated. Aneuploidies of the autosomes are among the most clinically important of the chromosome abnormalities. They consist primarily of **monosomy** (the presence of only

one copy of a chromosome in an otherwise diploid cell) and **trisomy** (three copies of a chromosome). Autosomal monosomies are nearly always incompatible with survival to term, so only a small number of them have been observed among live-born individuals. In contrast, some trisomies are seen with appreciable frequencies among live births. The fact that trisomies produce less-severe consequences than monosomies illustrates an important principle: *the body can tolerate excess genetic material more readily than it can tolerate a deficit of genetic material.*

The most common cause of aneuploidy is **nondisjunction**, the failure of chromosomes to disjoin normally during meiosis (Fig. 6-7). Nondisjunction can occur during meiosis I or meiosis II (see Chapter 2). The resulting gamete either lacks a chromosome or has two copies of it, producing a monosomic or trisomic zygote, respectively.

▶ Aneuploid conditions consist primarily of monosomies and trisomies. They are usually caused by nondisjunction. Autosomal monosomies are almost always lethal, but some autosomal trisomies are compatible with survival.

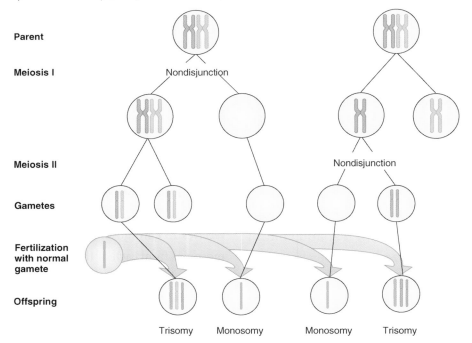

FIG 6-7   In meiotic nondisjunction, two chromosome homologs migrate to the same daughter cell instead of disjoining normally and migrating to different daughter cells. This produces monosomic and trisomic offspring.

Trisomy 21

Trisomy 21 (karyotype 47,XY,+21 or 47,XX,+21) (For brevity, the remainder of the karyotype designations for abnormalities not involving the sex chromosomes will indicate an affected male.) is seen in approximately 1 of every 700 to 1000 live births, making it the most common autosomal aneuploid condition compatible with survival to term. This trisomy is the most common cause of Down syndrome, a phenotype originally described by John Langdon Down in 1866. Almost 100 years elapsed between Down's description of this syndrome and the discovery (in 1959) that it is caused by the presence of an extra copy of chromosome 21.

Although there is considerable variation in the appearance of persons with Down syndrome, they present with a constellation of features that help the clinician to make a clinical diagnosis. The facial features include a depressed nasal root, upslanting palpebral fissures, measurably small and sometimes overfolded ears, and a flattened maxillary and malar region, giving the face a characteristic appearance (Fig. 6-8). Some of these features led to the use of the term "mongolism" in earlier literature, but this term is inappropriate and is no longer used. The cheeks are round, and the corners of the mouth are sometimes downturned. The neck is short, and the skin is redundant at the nape of the neck, especially in newborns. The occiput is flat, and the hands and feet tend to be rather broad and short. Approximately 50% of persons with Down syndrome have a single flexion crease across their palms (single palmar crease, formerly termed a "simian crease," though this term is also now considered inappropriate). Decreased muscle tone (hypotonia) is a highly consistent feature that is also helpful in making a diagnosis. None of these features are diagnostic per se as all are observed in the general population of infants; it is the clustering together that suggests the diagnosis.

Several medically significant problems occur with increased frequency among infants and children with Down syndrome. About 3% of these infants develop an obstruction of the duodenum or atresia (closure or absence) of the esophagus, duodenum, or anus.

Respiratory infections are quite common, and the risk of developing leukemia is 15 to 20 times higher in patients with Down syndrome than in the general population. The most significant medical problem is that approximately 40% of these persons are born with structural heart defects. The most common of these is an atrioventricular (AV) canal, a defect in which the interatrial and interventricular septa fail to fuse normally during fetal development. The result is blood flow from the left side of the heart to the right side and then to the pulmonary vasculature, producing pulmonary hypertension. Ventricular septal defects (VSDs) are also common.

Moderate to mild intellectual disability (standardized IQ ranging from 40 to 60) occurs in most persons with Down syndrome, and this condition alone accounts for approximately 10% of all cases of intellectual disability in the United States. In recent years clinical trials designed to test whether specific medications might improve attention and learning in school age-children with Down syndrome have been initiated (see www.clinicaltrials.gov).

Several other medical problems occur in infants and young children with Down syndrome. Conductive and sometimes sensorineural hearing loss, hypothyroidism, and various eye abnormalities are the most important and common. Clinical Commentary 6-1 outlines a plan for routine medical care of infants and children with Down syndrome.

The medical problems seen in children with Down syndrome result in decreased survival rates. Congenital heart defects are the most important single cause of early mortality. In the early 1960s, only about half of children with this disorder survived as long as 5 years. As a result of improvements in corrective surgery, antibiotic treatment, and management of leukemia, the survival rate has increased considerably in the past 40 years. Currently, it is estimated that more than 80% of children with Down syndrome will survive to age 10 years, and more than half survive to 50 years of age. There is convincing evidence that enriched environments and educational interventions can produce significant improvements in intellectual function.

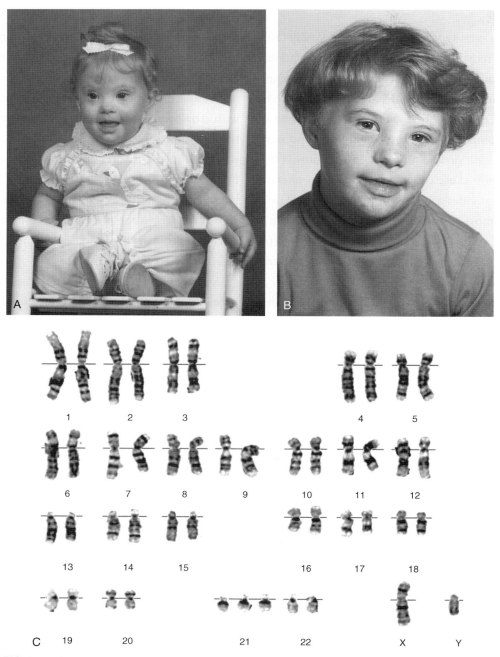

FIG 6-8 **A**, An infant with Down syndrome, illustrating typical features of this disorder: upslanting palpebral fissures, redundant skin of the inner eyelid (epicanthic fold), protruding tongue, and low nasal bridge. **B**, Same girl as in A, 7 years later. Note that the typical features are present but less obviously expressed. **C**, A karyogram of a male with trisomy 21.

Males with Down syndrome are nearly always sterile, with only a few reported cases of reproduction. Many females with Down syndrome can reproduce, although approximately 40% fail to ovulate. A female with Down syndrome has a 50% risk of producing a gamete with two copies of chromosome 21 (which would then produce a trisomic zygote).

However, because about 75% of trisomy 21 conceptions are spontaneously aborted, the risk of producing affected live-born offspring is considerably lower than 50% in women with Down syndrome. Because reproduction is uncommon, nearly all cases of trisomy 21 can be regarded as new mutations.

Approximately 95% of Down syndrome cases are

CLINICAL COMMENTARY 6-1

Anticipatory Guidance and Health Supervision in Children with Down Syndrome

An approach termed *health supervision* and *anticipatory guidance* has evolved for the care and treatment of persons with genetic syndromes and chronic diseases. After a thorough study of the disease in question (including an extensive literature review), basic guidelines are established for the screening, evaluation, and management of patients. If followed by the primary care practitioner or the specialist, these guidelines should help to prevent further disability or illness. We illustrate the health supervision and anticipatory guidance approach with the current guidelines for care of children with Down syndrome.

- As mentioned in the text, AV canals are the most common congenital heart defect seen in newborns with Down syndrome. Surgical correction of this condition is appropriate if it is detected before 1 year of age; after this time, pulmonary hypertension has been present too long for surgery to be successful. Accordingly, it is now recommended that an echocardiogram be performed during the newborn period and no later than 6 months.
- Because Down syndrome patients often have strabismus (deviation of the eye from its normal visual axis) and other eye problems, they should be examined regularly by their physician. If any symptoms or signs are observed, the patient is referred to an ophthalmologist

familiar with Down syndrome. In asymptomatic children, an ophthalmological examination before the age of 4 years is recommended to evaluate visual acuity.
- Hypothyroidism is common, especially during adolescence. Therefore, thyroid hormone levels should be measured annually.
- Sensorineural and conductive hearing loss are both seen in children with Down syndrome. The routine follow-up should include a hearing test at birth and every 6 months until 2 years of age, with subsequent testing as needed.
- Instability of the first and second vertebrae has led to spinal cord injuries in some older Down syndrome patients. It is thus suggested that imaging studies be carried out in children with neurological symptoms and in those planning to participate in athletic activities.
- Referral of infants and children with Down syndrome to preschool programs to provide intervention for developmental disabilities is an important component of routine care.

Similar series of guidelines have been developed for children with trisomy 18, Williams syndrome, and Turner syndrome. In principle, the anticipatory guidance and health supervision approach can be applied to any genetic disease for which there is sufficient knowledge.

---

caused by nondisjunction, and most of the remainder are caused by chromosome translocations (see later discussion). Comparisons of chromosome 21 polymorphisms in parents and offspring have demonstrated that the extra chromosome is contributed by the mother in 90% to 95% of trisomy 21 cases. About 75% of these maternal nondisjunctions occur during meiosis I, and the remainder occur during meiosis II. As discussed in greater detail later, there is a strong correlation between maternal age and the risk of producing a child with Down syndrome.

Mosaicism (see Chapter 4) is seen in approximately 2% to 4% of trisomy 21 live births. These persons have some normal somatic cells and some cells with trisomy 21. This type of mosaicism in a male is designated 47, XY, +21[10]/46, XY [10], with the numbers inside the brackets indicating the number of cells scored with each karyotype. The most common cause of mosaicism in trisomy is a trisomic conception followed by loss of the extra chromosome during mitosis in some embryonic cells. Mosaicism often results in milder clinical expression of the phenotype associated with a chromosome abnormality.

Depending on the timing and the way the mosaicism originated, some persons have **tissue-specific mosaicism**. As the term suggests, this type of mosaicism is confined only to certain tissues. This can complicate diagnosis because cytogenetic analysis is usually based on a single tissue type (usually circulating lymphocytes derived from a blood sample, or, less commonly, fibroblasts derived from a skin biopsy). Mosaicism affecting primarily the germline of a parent can lead to multiple recurrences of Down syndrome in the offspring. This factor helps to account for the fact that the recurrence risk for Down syndrome among mothers younger than 30 years is about 1% (i.e., 10 times higher than the population risk for this age group).

Because of the prevalence and clinical importance of Down syndrome, considerable effort has been devoted to determining which genes on chromosome 21 account for the features of this disorder. A candidate for intellectual disability in Down syndrome is *DYRK1A*, a kinase gene that causes learning and memory defects when it is over-expressed in mice. Another gene located in the critical region, *APP*, encodes the amyloid β precursor protein. A third copy of *APP* is likely to account for the occurrence of Alzheimer disease features in nearly all Down syndrome patients by 40 years of age. Mutations of *APP* cause a small percentage of Alzheimer disease cases (see Chapter 5), and Down syndrome individuals with partial trisomies that do not include the *APP* gene do not develop Alzheimer disease features.

▶ Trisomy 21, which causes Down syndrome, is the most common autosomal aneuploidy seen among live births. The most significant features include intellectual disability, gastrointestinal tract obstruction, congenital heart defects, and respiratory infections. The extra 21st chromosome is contributed by the mother in approximately 90% of cases. Mosaicism is seen in 2% to 4% of Down syndrome cases, and it often accompanies a milder phenotype. Specific genes contributing to the Down syndrome phenotype are being identified.

Trisomy 18

Trisomy 18 (47,XY,+18), also known as Edwards syndrome, is the second most common autosomal trisomy, with a prevalence of about 1 per 6000 live births. It is, however, much more common at conception and is the most common chromosome abnormality among stillborns with congenital malformations. It is estimated that fewer than 5% of trisomy 18 conceptions survive to term.

The Edwards syndrome phenotype is as discernible as Down syndrome, but because it is less common, it is less likely to be recognized clinically. Infants with trisomy 18 have prenatal growth deficiency (weight that is low for gestational age), characteristic facial features, and a distinctive hand abnormality that often helps the clinician to make the initial diagnosis (Fig. 6-9). Minor anomalies of diagnostic importance include small ears with unraveled helices, a small mouth that is often hard to open, a short sternum, and short halluces (first toes). Most babies with trisomy 18 have major malformations.

Congenital heart defects, particularly VSDs, are the most common and occur in 90% of children. Other medically significant congenital malformations include omphalocele (protrusion of the bowel into the umbilical cord), radial aplasia (missing radius bone), diaphragmatic hernia, and, occasionally, spina bifida.

About 50% of infants with trisomy 18 die within the first several weeks of life, and only about 5% to 8% survive to 12 months of age. A combination of factors, including aspiration pneumonia, predisposition to infections and apnea, and congenital heart defects, accounts for the high mortality rate.

Marked developmental disabilities are seen among those trisomy 18 patients who survive infancy. The degree of delay is much more significant than in Down syndrome, and most children are not able to walk independently. However, children with trisomy 18 do progress in their milestones, albeit slowly, and older children learn some communication skills.

More than 95% of patients with Edwards syndrome have complete trisomy 18; only a small percentage have mosaicism. As in trisomy 21, there is a significant maternal age effect, and more than 90% of trisomy 18 cases are the result of an extra chromosome transmitted by the mother.

Trisomy 13

Trisomy 13 (47,XY,+13), also termed Patau syndrome, is seen in about 1 of every 10,000 births. The malformation pattern is quite distinctive and usually permits clinical recognition. It consists primarily of orofacial clefts, microphthalmia (small, abnormally formed eyes), and postaxial polydactyly (Fig. 6-10). Malformations of the central nervous system are often seen, as are heart defects and renal abnormalities. Cutis aplasia (a defect of the skin of the scalp on the posterior occiput) can also occur.

The survival rate is very similar to that of trisomy 18, and about 95% of live-born infants die during the first year of life. Children who survive infancy have significant developmental disability, with skills seldom progressing beyond those of a child of 2 years. However, as in trisomy 18, children with tri-

FIG 6-9   A girl with full trisomy 18 at 3 years **(A)** and 13 years **(B)** of age. She shows the typical facial features of an older child with short palpebral fissures and ear variations. **A** also depicts the overriding of the index finger onto the third finger, a characteristic finding of the hands in the syndrome.

somy 13 do progress somewhat in their development and are able to communicate with their families to some degree.

About 80% of patients with Patau syndrome have full trisomy 13. Most of the remaining patients have trisomy of the long arm of chromosome 13 due to a translocation (see later discussion). As in trisomies 18 and 21, the risk of bearing a child with this condition increases with advanced maternal age. It is estimated that 95% or more of trisomy 13 conceptions are spontaneously lost during pregnancy.

> Trisomies of the 13th and 18th chromosomes are sometimes compatible with survival to term, although 95% or more of affected fetuses are spontaneously aborted. These trisomies are much less common at birth than is trisomy 21, and they produce more serious disease features, with 90% to 95% mortality during the first year of life. As in trisomy 21, there is a maternal age effect, and the mother contributes the extra chromosome in more than 90% of cases.

Trisomies, Nondisjunction, and Maternal Age

The prevalence of Down syndrome among offspring of mothers of different ages is shown in Figure 6-11. Among mothers younger than 30 years of age, the risk is less than 1/1000. It increases to approximately 1/400 at age 35 years, 1/100 at age 40 years, and approximately 1/25 after age 45 years. Most other tri-

FIG 6-10   An 8-year-old girl with full trisomy 13 showing her small eyes and prominent, wide nose.

somies, including those in which the fetus does not survive to term, also increase in prevalence as maternal age increases. This risk is one of the primary indications for prenatal diagnosis (see Chapter 10).

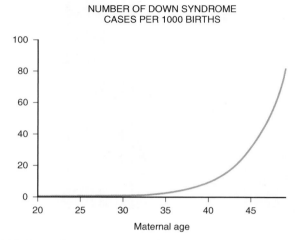

FIG 6-11 The prevalence of Down syndrome among live births in relation to age of the mother. The prevalence increases with maternal age and becomes especially notable after the age of 35 years. (Data from Hook EB, Chambers GM. *Birth defects.* 1977; 23[3A]: 123-141.)

Several hypotheses have been advanced to account for this increase, including the idea that a trisomic pregnancy is less likely to be spontaneously aborted in older women. Direct studies of the frequency of chromosome abnormalities in sperm and egg cells indicate that the pattern is instead due to an increase in nondisjunction among older mothers. Recall that nearly all of a female's oocytes are formed during her embryonic development. (There is recent evidence that a small number of oocytes may be produced later in life.) They remain suspended in prophase I until they are shed during ovulation. Thus, an ovum produced by a 45-year-old woman is itself about 45 years old. This long period of suspension in prophase I might impair normal chromosome disjunction, although the precise nature of this mechanism is not understood.

Many factors have been examined to determine whether they affect the frequency of nondisjunction in women. These include hormone levels, cigarette smoking, autoimmune thyroid disease, alcohol consumption, and radiation (the latter does increase nondisjunction when administered in very large doses to experimental animals). None of these factors has shown consistent correlations with nondisjunction in humans, however, and maternal age remains the only known correlated factor.

Although maternal age is strongly correlated with the risk of Down syndrome, approximately three fourths of Down syndrome children are born to mothers younger than 35 years of age. This is because the great majority of children (more than 90%) are borne by women in this age group.

Numerous studies, including direct analysis of sperm cells, have tested the hypothesis of a paternal age effect for trisomies. The consensus is that such an effect, if it exists at all, is minor. This is probably because spermatocytes, unlike oocytes, are generated throughout the life of the male.

 Nearly all autosomal trisomies increase with maternal age as a result of nondisjunction in older mothers. There is little evidence for a paternal age effect on nondisjunction in males.

Sex Chromosome Aneuploidy

Among live-born infants, about 1 in 400 males and 1 in 650 females have some form of sex chromosome aneuploidy. Primarily because of X inactivation, the consequences of this class of aneuploidy are less severe than those of autosomal aneuploidy. With the exception of the complete absence of an X chromosome, all of the sex chromosome aneuploidies are compatible with survival in at least some cases.

Monosomy of the X Chromosome (Turner Syndrome)

The phenotype associated with a single X chromosome (45, X) was described by Henry Turner in 1938. (An earlier description was given by Otto Ullrich in 1930.) Persons with Turner syndrome are female and usually have a characteristic phenotype, including the variable presence of proportionate short stature, sexual infantilism and ovarian dysgenesis, and a pattern of major and minor malformations. The physical features can include a triangle-shaped face; posteriorly rotated external ears; and a broad, "webbed neck" (Fig. 6-12). In addition, the chest is broad and shield-like in shape. Lymphedema of the hands and feet is observable at birth. Many infants with Turner syndrome have congenital heart defects, most commonly obstructive lesions of the left side of the heart (bicuspid aortic valve in 50% of patients and coarctation [narrowing] of the aorta in 15%-30%). Severe obstructions should be surgically repaired. About 50% of persons with Turner syndrome have structural kidney defects, but they usually do not cause medical problems. There is typically some diminution in spatial perceptual ability, but intelligence is usually normal.

FIG 6-12 A girl with Turner syndrome (45,X). Note the characteristically broad, webbed neck. Stature is reduced, and swelling (lymphedema) is seen in the ankles and wrists.

Girls with Turner syndrome exhibit proportionate short stature and do not undergo an adolescent growth spurt. Mature height is reduced by approximately 20 cm, on average. Growth hormone administration produces increased height somewhat in these girls, and families now commonly choose this therapy. In most persons with Turner syndrome, streaks of connective tissue, rather than ovaries, are seen (gonadal dysgenesis). Lacking normal ovaries,

they do not usually develop secondary sexual characteristics, and most women with this condition are infertile (about 5%-10% have sufficient ovarian development to undergo menarche, and a small number have borne children). Teenagers with Turner syndrome are typically treated with estrogen to promote the development of secondary sexual characteristics. The dose is then continued at a reduced level to maintain these characteristics and to help prevent osteoporosis.

The diagnosis of Turner syndrome is often made in the newborn infant, especially if there is a noticeable webbing of the neck coupled with a heart defect. The facial features are more subtle than in the autosomal abnormalities described previously, but the experienced clinician can often diagnose Turner syndrome on the basis of one or more of the listed clues. If Turner syndrome is not recognized in infancy or childhood, it is often diagnosed later because of short stature and/or amenorrhea.

The chromosome abnormalities in persons with Turner syndrome are quite variable. About 50% of these patients have a 45,X karyotype in their peripheral lymphocytes. At least 30% to 40% have mosaicism, most commonly 45,X/46,XX and less commonly 45,X/46,XY. Patients with mosaicism who have Y chromosomes in some cells are predisposed to neoplasms (gonadoblastomas) in the gonadal streak tissue. About 10% to 20% of patients with Turner syndrome have structural X chromosome abnormalities involving a deletion of some or all of Xp. This variation in chromosome abnormality helps to explain the considerable phenotypic variation seen in this syndrome.

Approximately 60% to 80% of monosomy X cases are caused by the absence of a paternally derived sex chromosome, occurring either during early mitosis in the embryo or during meiosis in the father (i.e., the offspring receives an X chromosome only from the mother). The 45,X karyotype is estimated to occur in 1% to 2% of conceptions, but Turner syndrome is seen in only about 1/2000 to 1/3000 liveborn girls. Thus, the great majority (more than 99%) of 45,X conceptions are lost prenatally. Among those that do survive to term, many have mosaicism, and mosaicism of the placenta alone (**confined placental mosaicism**) is especially common. It is likely that the presence of some normal cells in mosaic fetuses enhances fetal survival.

Molecular analysis has begun to pinpoint specific genes involved in the Turner syndrome phenotype. For example, mutations in the *SHOX* gene, which encodes a transcription factor expressed in embryonic limbs, produce short stature. This gene is located on the distal tip of the X and Y short arms (in a region of the X chromosome that escapes inactivation; see Clinical Commentary 6-2). Thus, it is nor-

mally transcribed in two copies in both males and females. In females with Turner syndrome, this gene is present in only one active copy, and the resulting haploinsufficiency contributes to short stature.

 Most females with Turner syndrome have a 45,X karyotype. Although this disorder is common at conception, it is relatively rare among live births, reflecting a very high rate of spontaneous abortion. Mosaicism, including confined placental mosaicism, appears to increase the probability of survival to term.

CLINICAL COMMENTARY 6-2
XX Males, XY Females, and the Genetic Basis of Sex Determination

During normal meiosis in the male, crossover occurs between the tip of the short arm of the Y chromosome and the tip of the short arm of the X chromosome (Fig. 6-13). These regions of the X and Y chromosomes contain highly similar DNA sequences. Because this resembles the behavior of autosomes during meiosis, the distal portion of the Y chromosome is known as the **pseudoautosomal region**. It spans approximately 2.5 Mb.

Just centromeric of the pseudoautosomal region lies a gene known as *SRY* (sex-determining region on the Y). This gene, which is expressed in embryonic development, encodes a transcription factor that interacts with other genes to initiate the development of the undifferentiated embryo into a male (including Sertoli cell differentiation and secretion of müllerian-inhibiting substance). In particular, the protein product of *SRY* binds to an enhancer element that regulates expression of the *SOX9* gene, which in turn regulates a series of genes that promote male development while repressing ovarian development. *SRY* thus acts as a key regulatory switch in sex determination. When the mouse *Sry* gene is inserted experimentally into a female mouse embryo, a male mouse is produced. Loss-of-function mutations of *SRY* can produce individuals with an XY karyotype but a female phenotype. *SOX9* acts as the next switch in this pathway, and *SOX9* mutations can produce sex reversal (XY females) and campomelic dysplasia (malformations of bone and cartilage).

Approximately 1 of every 20,000 males presents with a phenotype similar to Klinefelter syndrome (without increased height), but chromosome evaluation shows that they have a normal *female* karyotype (46,XX). It has been demonstrated that these XX males have an X chromosome that includes the *SRY* gene. This is a result of a faulty crossover between the X and Y chromosomes during male meiosis, such that the *SRY* gene, instead of remaining on the Y chromosome, is transferred to the X chromosome. The offspring who inherits this X chromosome from his father consequently has a male phenotype. Conversely, an offspring who inherits a Y chromosome that lacks the *SRY* gene is an XY female. These females

have gonadal streaks rather than ovaries and have poorly developed secondary sexual characteristics.

FIG 6-13 The distal short arms of the X and Y chromosomes exchange material during meiosis in the male. The region of the Y chromosome in which this crossover occurs is called the pseudoautosomal region. The *SRY* gene, which triggers the process leading to male gonadal differentiation, is located just outside the pseudoautosomal region. Occasionally, the crossover occurs on the centromeric side of the *SRY* gene, causing it to lie on an X chromosome instead of on the Y chromosome. An offspring receiving this X chromosome will be an XX male, and an offspring receiving the Y chromosome will be an XY female.

Klinefelter Syndrome

Like Down and Turner syndromes, the syndrome associated with a 47,XXY karyotype was identified before the underlying chromosomal abnormality was understood. Described in 1942 by Harry Klinefelter, the syndrome that bears his name is seen in approximately 1/500 to 1/1000 male births. Although Klinefelter syndrome is a common cause of primary hypogonadism in males, the phenotype is less striking than those of the syndromes described thus far. Patients with Klinefelter syndrome tend to be taller than average, with disproportionately long arms and legs (Fig. 6-14). Clinical examination of postpubertal patients reveals small testes (less than 10 ml in volume), and most males with Klinefelter syndrome are sterile as a result of atrophy of the seminiferous tubules. Testosterone levels in adolescents and adults are low. Gynecomastia (breast development) is seen in approximately one third of affected persons and leads to an increased risk of breast cancer, which can be reduced by mastectomy (breast removal). Body hair is typically sparse after puberty, and muscle mass tends to be reduced. In addition, there is a predisposition for learning disabilities and a reduction in verbal IQ. Although intelligence is usually in the normal range, the IQ is on average 10 to 15 points lower than that of the affected person's siblings. Because of the subtlety of this disorder, Klinefelter syndrome is often not diagnosed until after puberty, and the condition is sometimes first ascertained in fertility clinics.

The extra X chromosome is derived maternally in about 50% of Klinefelter cases, and the syndrome increases in incidence with advanced maternal age. Mosaicism, which is seen in about 15% of patients, increases the likelihood of viable sperm production. Individuals with the 48,XXXY and 49,XXXXY karyotypes have also been reported. Because they have a Y chromosome, they have a male phenotype, but the degree of developmental disability and physical abnormality increases with each additional X chromosome.

Testosterone therapy, beginning in midadolescence, can enhance secondary sex characteristics, and it helps to decrease the risk of osteoporosis. There is some evidence that this treatment also improves psychological well-being.

FIG 6-14 A male with Klinefelter syndrome (47,XXY). Stature is increased, gynecomastia may be present, and body shape may be somewhat feminine.

 Males with Klinefelter syndrome (47,XXY) are taller than average, might have reduced IQ, and are usually sterile. Testosterone therapy and mastectomy for gynecomastia are sometimes recommended.

Trisomy X

The 47,XXX karyotype occurs in approximately 1/1000 females and usually has benign consequences. Overt physical abnormalities are rarely seen, but these females sometimes have sterility, menstrual irregularity, or mild cognitive disability. As in Klinefelter syndrome, the 47,XXX karyotype is often first ascertained in fertility clinics. Approximately 90% of cases are the result of nondisjunction in the mother, and, as with other trisomies, the incidence increases among the offspring of older mothers.

Females have also been seen with four, five, or even more X chromosomes. Each additional X chromosome is accompanied by increased intellectual disability and physical abnormality.

47,XYY Syndrome

The final sex chromosome aneuploidy to be discussed is the 47,XYY karyotype. Males with this karyotype tend to be taller than average, and they have a 10- to 15-point reduction in average IQ. This condition, which causes few physical problems, achieved great notoriety when its incidence in the male prison population was discovered to be as high as 1/30, compared with 1/1000 in the general male population. This led to the suggestion that this karyotype might confer a predisposition to violent, criminal behavior. A number of studies have addressed this issue and have shown that XYY males are not inclined to commit violent crimes. There is, however, evidence of an increased incidence of minor behavioral disorders, such as hyperactivity, attention deficit disorder, and learning disabilities.

> The 47,XXX and 47,XYY karyotypes are seen in about 1/1000 females and males, respectively. Each involves a slight degree of reduction in IQ but few physical problems.

ABNORMALITIES OF CHROMOSOME STRUCTURE

In addition to the loss or gain of whole chromosomes, parts of chromosomes can be lost or duplicated as gametes are formed, and the arrangement of portions of chromosomes can be altered. Structural chromosome abnormalities may be **unbalanced** (the rearrangement causes a gain or loss of chromosomal material) or **balanced** (the rearrangement does not produce a loss or gain of chromosome material). Unlike aneuploidy and polyploidy, balanced structural abnormalities often do not produce serious health consequences. Nevertheless, abnormalities of chromosome structure, especially those that are

unbalanced, can produce serious disease in individuals or their offspring.

Alterations of chromosome structure can occur when homologous chromosomes line up improperly during meiosis (e.g., unequal crossover, as described in Chapter 4). In addition, **chromosome breakage** can occur during meiosis or mitosis. Mechanisms exist to repair these breaks, and usually the break is repaired perfectly with no damage to the daughter cell. Sometimes, however, the breaks remain, or they heal in a fashion that alters the structure of the chromosome. The likelihood of chromosome breakage may be increased in the presence of certain harmful agents, called **clastogens**. Clastogens identified in experimental systems include ionizing radiation, some viral infections, and some chemicals, but none have been convincingly demonstrated to cause chromosome abnormalities in humans.

Translocations

A **translocation** is the interchange of genetic material between nonhomologous chromosomes. Balanced translocations represent one of the most common chromosomal aberrations in humans, occurring in 1 of every 500 to 1000 individuals (Table 6-2). There are two basic types of translocations, **reciprocal** and **Robertsonian**.

Reciprocal Translocations

Reciprocal translocations happen when breaks occur in two different chromosomes and the material is mutually exchanged. The resulting chromosomes are called **derivative chromosomes**. The carrier of a reciprocal translocation is usually unaffected because he or she has a normal complement of genetic material. However, the carrier's offspring can be normal, can carry the translocation, or can have duplications and deletions of genetic material.

An example of a reciprocal translocation between chromosomes 3 and 6 is shown in Figure 6-15. The distal half of the short arm of chromosome 6 is translocated to the short arm of chromosome 3, and a small piece of chromosome 3 is translocated to the short arm of chromosome 6. If the translocations occur at 3p13

TABLE 6-2   Prevalence of Chromosomal Abnormalities among Newborns

ABNORMALITY	PREVALENCE AT BIRTH
Autosomal Syndromes	
Trisomy 21	1/700
Trisomy 18	1/6000
Trisomy 13	1/10,000
Unbalanced rearrangements	1/17,000
Balanced rearrangements	
Robertsonian translocations	1/1000
Reciprocal translocations	1/11,000
Sex Chromosome Abnormalities	
47,XXY	1/1000 male births
47,XYY	1/1000 male births
45,X*	1/5000 female births
47,XXX	1/1000 female births
All Chromosome Abnormalities	
Autosomal disorders and unbalanced rearrangements	1/230
Balanced rearrangements	1/500*

*The 45,X karyotype accounts for about half of the cases of Turner yndrome.

A   **Parent**

B   **Offspring**

FIG 6-15   A, The parent has a reciprocal balanced translocation involving the short arms of chromosomes 6 and 3. The distal short arm of the 6 has been translocated to the very distal tip of the 3. A small piece of chromosome 3 is attached to the derivative 6. This person had a child whose chromosomes are depicted in **B**. The child received the derivative chromosome 3 (with part of the 6 short arm attached) and the normal 6; from the other parent, the child received a normal 3 and a normal 6. Therefore, the child had a partial trisomy of the 6 short arm and, presumably, a small deletion of the 3 short arm.

and 6p14, the karyotype is designated 46,XX, t(3;6)(p13;p14). The offspring of this woman received the derivative chromosome 3, termed der (3), and the normal 6; thus, the child had a **partial trisomy** of the distal portion of chromosome 6 (i.e., 6p trisomy). This is a well-established but rather uncommon chromosomal syndrome.

> Reciprocal translocations are caused by two breaks on different chromosomes, with a subsequent exchange of material. Although carriers of balanced reciprocal translocations usually have normal phenotypes, their offspring might have a partial trisomy or a partial monosomy and an abnormal phenotype.

Robertsonian Translocations

In Robertsonian translocations, the short arms of two nonhomologous chromosomes are lost and the long arms fuse at the centromere to form a single chromosome (Fig. 6-16). This type of translocation is confined to the acrocentric chromosomes (13, 14, 15, 21, and 22) and has no effect on a carrier because the short arms of these chromosomes are very small and contain no essential genetic material. Although Robertsonian translocation carriers have only 45 chromosomes in each cell, they are phenotypically unaffected. Their offspring, however, may inherit an extra or missing long arm of an acrocentric chromosome.

Robertsonian translocation

FIG 6-16 In a Robertsonian translocation, shown here, the long arms of two acrocentric chromosomes (13 and 14) fuse, forming a single chromosome.

A common Robertsonian translocation involves fusion of the long arms of chromosomes 14 and 21. The karyotype of a male carrier of this translocation is 45,XY,der(14;21)(q10; q10). This person lacks one normal 14 and one normal 21 and instead has a chromosome derived from a translocation of the entire long arms of chromosomes 14 and 21. During meiosis in this person, the translocation chromosome must still pair with its homologs. Figure 6-17 illustrates the ways these chromosomes can segregate in the gametes formed by the translocation carrier. If **alternate segregation** occurs, then the offspring are either chromosomally normal or have a balanced translocation with a normal phenotype. If one of the **adjacent segregation** patterns occurs, then the gametes are unbalanced and the offspring may have trisomy 14, monosomy 14, monosomy 21, or trisomy 21. (Note that these trisomies and monosomies are genetically the same as trisomies and monosomies produced by nondisjunction, because only the long

arms of these chromosomes contain genetically significant material.) Fetuses with the first three adjacent segregation patterns do not survive to term, and the last pattern results in an infant with three copies of the long arm of chromosome 21 and a Down syndrome phenotype. Robertsonian translocations are responsible for approximately 5% of Down syndrome cases.

It is expected that the three types of conceptions compatible with survival would occur in equal frequencies: One third would be completely normal, one third would carry the translocation but be phenotypically normal, and one third would have Down syndrome. In part because of prenatal loss, the actual fraction of live-born offspring with Down syndrome is less than one third (about 10%-15% for mothers who carry the translocation, and only 1%-2% for fathers who carry it). This recurrence risk, however, is greater than the risk for parents of a child who has the nondisjunction type of Down syndrome (1% for mothers younger than 30 years of age). This difference in recurrence risks demonstrates why it is critical to order a chromosome study whenever a condition such as Down syndrome is suspected.

 Robertsonian translocations occur when the long arms of two acrocentric chromosomes fuse at the centromere. The carrier of a Robertsonian translocation can produce conceptions with monosomy or trisomy of the long arms of acrocentric chromosomes.

Deletions

A **deletion** is caused by a chromosome break and subsequent loss of genetic material. A single break leading to a loss that includes the chromosome's tip is called a **terminal deletion**. An **interstitial deletion** results when two breaks occur and the material between the breaks is lost. For example, a chromosome segment with normal DNA can be symbolized ABCDEFG. An interstitial deletion could produce the sequence ABEFG, and a terminal deletion could produce ABCDE.

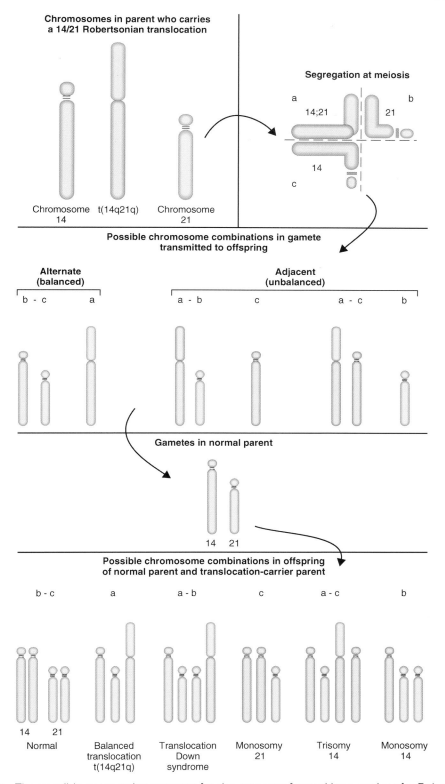

FIG 6-17   The possible segregation patterns for the gametes formed by a carrier of a Robertsonian translocation. Alternate segregation (quadrant *a* alone, or quadrant *b* with quadrant *c*) produces either a normal chromosome constitution or a translocation carrier with a normal phenotype. Adjacent segregation (quadrant *a* with *b*, quadrant *c* alone, quadrant *a* with *c*, or quadrant *b* alone) produces unbalanced gametes and results in conceptions with translocation Down syndrome, monosomy 21, trisomy 14, or monosomy 14, respectively. For example, monosomy 14 is produced when the parent who carries the translocation transmits a copy of chromosome 21 but does not transmit a copy of chromosome 14 (as in the *lower right corner*).

Usually, a gamete containing a chromosome with a deletion unites with a normal gamete to form a zygote. The zygote then has one normal chromosome and a homolog with the deletion. Microscopically visible deletions generally involve multiple genes, and the consequences of losing this much genetic material from even one member of the chromosome pair can be severe. After the three autosomal aneuploidies described earlier, the autosomal deletion syndromes are the most common group of clinically significant chromosome abnormalities.

A well-known example of a chromosome deletion syndrome is the *cri-du-chat* syndrome. This term (French, "cry of the cat") describes the distinctive cry of the child. This cry usually becomes less obvious as the child ages, making a clinical diagnosis more difficult after 2 years of age. Cri-du-chat syndrome is caused by a deletion of the distal short arm of chromosome 5; the karyotype is 46,XY,del (5p). Seen in approximately 1 in 50,000 live births, it is also characterized by intellectual disability (average IQ about 35), microcephaly (small head), and a characteristic but not distinctive facial appearance. Although mortality rates are increased if serious congenital defects are present, most persons with cri-du-chat syndrome now survive to adulthood.

Wolf-Hirschhorn syndrome (Fig. 6-18), caused by a deletion of the distal short arm of chromosome 4, is another well-characterized deletion syndrome. Other well-known deletions include those of 18p, 18q, and 13q. With the exception of the 18p deletion syndrome, each of these disorders is relatively distinctive, and the diagnosis can often be made before the karyotype is obtained. The features of the 18p deletion syndrome are more subtle, and usually this condition is recognized when chromosome analysis is performed for evaluation of developmental disability.

 Microscopically observable chromosome deletions, which may be either terminal or interstitial, usually affect a fairly large number of genes and produce recognizable syndromes.

FIG 6-18 Child with Wolf-Hirschhorn syndrome (46,XX, del[4p]). Note the wide-spaced eyes and repaired cleft lip.

Microdeletion Syndromes

The deletions described thus far all involve relatively large segments of chromosomes, and many of them were described before chromosome banding techniques were developed. With the advent of high-resolution banding, it has become possible to identify microscopically a large number of deletions that were previously too small for detection. In addition, advances in molecular genetics, particularly the FISH and aCGH techniques (see Fig. 6-4), have permitted the detection of deletions that are often too small to be observed microscopically (i.e., <5 Mb).

Prader-Willi syndrome, a disorder discussed in Chapter 4, is a good example of a **microdeletion syndrome**. Although this condition was described in the 1950s, it was not until 1981 that advanced banding techniques detected a small deletion of chromosome bands 15q11-q13 in about 50% of these patients. With the use of molecular techniques, deletions that were too small to be detected cytogenetically were also discovered. In total, about 70% of Prader-Willi cases are caused by microdeletions of 15q.

Because of imprinting, the inheritance of a microdeletion of the paternal chromosome 15 material produces Prader-Willi syndrome, while a micro-deletion of the maternally derived chromosome 15 produces the phenotypically distinct Angelman syndrome (see Chapter 4).

Williams syndrome, which is characterized by mild intellectual disability, supravalvular aortic stenosis (SVAS), multiple peripheral pulmonary arterial stenoses, characteristic facial features, dental anomalies, and hypercalcemia, is another example of a microdeletion syndrome (Fig. 6-19). A series of molecular analyses have identified some of the individual genes responsible for the Williams syndrome phenotype. The gene that encodes elastin, *ELN*, for example, is located in the Williams syndrome critical region and is expressed in blood vessels. Elastin is an important component of the aortic wall (microfibrils, which were discussed in Chapter 4 in the context of Marfan syndrome, are another component). Mutations or deletions of elastin alone result in isolated SVAS without the other features of Williams syndrome. Larger deletions, encompassing additional genes, produce the complete Williams syndrome phenotype. A second gene in the critical region, *LIMK1*, encodes a brain-expressed kinase that may be involved in the visual-spatial cognition defects observed in patients with Williams syndrome. This is supported by observation of patients with partial deletions of the critical region affecting only the *ELN* and *LIMK1* genes. These persons have SVAS and visual-spatial cognitive deficiency but none of the other features of Williams syndrome.

High-resolution banding and molecular genetic techniques have often led to a more precise specification of the critical chromosome region that must be deleted to cause a given syndrome. Wolf-Hirschhorn syndrome, for instance, can be produced by the deletion of only a very small interstitial segment of 4p, just 2 megabases from the telomere. In some instances, specific genes responsible for chromosome abnormality syndromes can be pinpointed. For example, persons with a deletion of 11p can present with a series of features including **W**ilms tumor (a kidney tumor), **a**niridia (absence of the iris), **g**enitourinary abnormalities (Some authorities believe that the "G" should stand for gonadoblastoma rather than genitourinary abnormality), and "mental **r**etardation" (sometimes termed the WAGR syndrome). The genes responsible for the kidney tumor and for aniridia have now each been identified and cloned. Because the WAGR syndrome involves the deletion of a series of adjacent genes, it is sometimes referred to as an example of a **contiguous gene syndrome** (Williams syndrome, discussed previously, is another example of a contiguous gene syndrome). In addition to microdeletions, microduplications can also produce contiguous gene syndromes.

FIG 6-19   A, Girl with Williams syndrome, illustrating typical facial features: broad forehead, short palpebral fissures, low nasal bridge, anteverted nostrils, long philtrum, full cheeks, and relatively large mouth with full lips. **B**, Angiogram illustrating supravalvular aortic stenosis (narrowing of the ascending aorta) (*arrow*). (Courtesy Dr. Mark Keating, Harvard University.)

Some of the microdeletion syndromes, such as the Prader-Willi and Williams syndromes, manifest deletions of a critical region of consistent size (e.g., 4 Mb for Prader-Willi syndrome). Recent studies show that this is caused by the presence of multiple repeated sequences, termed **low-copy repeats** (see Chapter 2), at the deletion boundaries. These repeated sequences promote unequal crossing over (see Chapter 4), which then produces duplications and deletions of the region bounded by the repeat elements.

Several additional examples of microdeletions are given in Table 6-3. Many of these conditions, includ-ing the Prader-Willi, Miller-Dieker, Williams, and velocardiofacial syndromes (Clinical Commentary 6-3), are now diagnosed using the FISH or aCGH tech-niques.

 Microdeletions are a subtype of chromo-some deletion that can be observed only in banded chromosomes or, in some cases, using molecular genetic approaches. Syndromes caused by the deletion of a series of adjacent genes are sometimes called *contiguous gene syndromes*.

TABLE 6-3 Microdeletion Syndromes*

SYNDROME	CLINICAL FEATURES	CHROMOSOMAL DELETION
Prader-Willi	Intellectual disability, short stature, obesity, hypotonia, characteristic facies, small feet	15q11-13
Angelman	Intellectual disability, ataxia, uncontrolled laughter, seizures	15q11-13
Langer-Giedion	Characteristic facies, sparse hair, exostosis, variable intellectual disability	8q24
Miller-Dieker	Lissencephaly, characteristic facies, significant cognitive and psychomotor disability	17p13.3
Velocardiofacial/DiGeorge	Characteristic facies, cleft palate, heart defects, poorly developed thymus	22q11
Smith-Magenis	Intellectual disability, hyperactivity, dysmorphic features, self-destructive behavior	17p11.2
Williams	Developmental disability, characteristic facies, supravalvular aortic stenosis	7q1
Aniridia, Wilms tumor	Intellectual disability, predisposition to Wilms tumor, genital defects	11p13
Deletion 1p36	Intellectual disability, seizures, hearing loss, heart defects, growth failure, distinctive facial features	1p36
Rubinstein-Taybi	Intellectual disability, broad thumbs and great toes, characteristic facial features, vertebral and sternal abnormalities, heart defects	16p13.3
Alagille	Neonatal jaundice, "butterfly" vertebrae, pulmonic valvular stenosis, characteristic facial features	20p12

*For most of these conditions, only some cases are caused by the listed microdeletion; other cases may be caused by single-gene mutations within the same region.

CLINICAL COMMENTARY 6-3

DiGeorge Sequence, Velocardiofacial Syndrome, and Microdeletions of Chromosome 22

The DiGeorge sequence* is characterized by structural or functional defects of the thymus, conotruncal heart defects, hypoparathyroidism (reduced parathyroid function), and secondary hypocalcemia (decreased serum calcium). This pattern of malformations is caused by an alteration of the embryonic migration of neural crest cells to the develop-ing structures of the neck. In the 1980s some children with DiGeorge sequence were found to have a deletion of part of the long arm of chromosome 22, often related to an unbalanced translocation between this and another chromosome. This led to the hypothesis that genes on chromosome 22 were responsible for this condition.

Independent of this work, a condition called the velo-cardiofacial (VCF) syndrome, or Shprintzen syndrome, was described in the late 1970s. This syndrome includes palatal (velum) abnormalities (including cleft palate), a characteristic facial appearance (Fig. 6-20), and, in some cases, heart malformations. In addition, these patients have learning disabilities and developmental delay. Later it was discovered that some persons with VCF have dys-functional T cells (these cells mature in the thymus), and some have all features of DiGeorge sequence. This sug-gested that DiGeorge sequence was somehow related to VCF syndrome.

CLINICAL COMMENTARY 6-3
DiGeorge Sequence, Velocardiofacial Syndrome, and Microdeletions of Chromosome 22 (Continued)

The resemblance between the DiGeorge sequence and VCF syndrome led to the hypothesis that both conditions were caused by abnormalities on chromosome 22. High-resolution chromosome studies, including FISH, of patients with DiGeorge sequence and patients with VCF syndrome revealed small submicroscopic deletions of chromosome 22 in both groups. These analyses also helped to narrow the critical region that causes both conditions. Approximately 80% to 90% of infants with DiGeorge sequence have a 3-Mb microdeletion of the 22q11.2 region, and most VCF patients have the same microdeletion. In addition, 15% to 20% of persons with isolated conotruncal defects exhibit this deletion. Thus, most persons with either DiGeorge sequence or VCF syndrome have a microdeletion of 22q11.2 and are collectively described as having 22q11.2 deletion syndrome. With a prevalence of 1 in 3000 to 4000 live births, this is the most common human microdeletion syndrome.

About 90% of persons with 22q11.2 microdeletions lack the same 3-Mb region, containing about 35 genes. Another 8% have a smaller, 1.5-Mb deletion located within the 3-Mb region. No consistent phenotypic differences are seen between these two groups of patients. Both the 1.5- and 3-Mb regions are flanked by low-copy repeats that are thought to promote unequal crossing over, and thus deletion, in this region. One of the genes located in the deleted region, *TBX1*, encodes a transcription factor that helps to regulate the migration of neural crest cells and the development of facial structures, the thymus, the parathyroid, and the heart. In mouse models, *Tbx1* haploinsufficiency produces many of the features of DiGeorge sequence and VCF syndromes.

This example illustrates how cytogenetic studies can demonstrate potential biological relationships between genetic syndromes. Further studies are under way to characterize the individual genes in this region and how they contribute to the phenotypic variation seen in DiGeorge sequence and VCF syndromes.

FIG 6-20   Face of a boy with 22q11 deletion syndrome. Note the narrow, tall nasal root and nasal bridge and the somewhat smooth philtrum. (Courtesy Dr. Lynne M. Bird, Children's Hospital, San Diego.)

*A **sequence** is defined as a series of alterations that are all due to a single, primary defect (see Chapter 12 for further discussion). In DiGeorge sequence, the primary defect is an abnormality in the migration of neural crest cells, and its secondary alterations are the anomalies of the thymus, parathyroids, and heart.

Subtelomeric Rearrangements

The regions near telomeres of chromosomes tend to have a high density of genes. Consequently, rearrangements of genetic material (e.g., deletions, duplications) in these regions often result in genetic disease. It is estimated that at least 5% of unexplained cases of intellectual disability are caused by **subtelomeric rearrangements**. The most common of these rearrangements is a deletion of several thousand bases of chromosome 1p36, which is seen in approximately one in 5000 live births. This condition, termed monosomy 1p36 syndrome, is associated with significant intellectual disability, developmental delay, seizures, hearing impairment, heart defects, hypotonia, and characteristic facial features (Fig. 6-21).

FIG 6-21   Face of young boy with 1q36 deletion syndrome. Note the horizontal eyebrows, deep-set eyes, broad nasal root, and pointed chin.

Collections of probes have been designed so that FISH analysis of metaphase chromosomes can be undertaken to determine whether a subtelomeric deletion or duplication has occurred in a patient. In most clinical applications aCGH is carried out, hybridizing differentially labeled patient and control DNA samples to microarrays that contain probes corresponding to all human subtelomeric regions. If a subtelomeric region is duplicated or deleted, the patient's DNA will show either excessive or deficient hybridization to the probe corresponding to that region.

> Subtelomeric rearrangements involve deletions or duplications of DNA in the gene-rich regions near telomeres. They can be detected by hybridizing specifically designed FISH probes to metaphase chromosomes or by comparative genomic hybridization of patient and control DNA to microarrays containing subtelomeric probes.

Uniparental Disomy

As discussed earlier, about 70% of cases of Prader-Willi syndrome are caused by microdeletions. Most of the remaining cases involve **uniparental disomy** (*di* = "two"), a condition in which one parent has contributed two copies of a chromosome and the other parent has contributed no copies (Fig. 6-22). If the parent has contributed two copies of one homolog, the condition is termed **isodisomy**. If the parent has contributed one copy of each homolog, it is termed **heterodisomy**. Isodisomy or heterodisomy of an imprinted chromosome can cause diseases such as Prader-Willi syndrome (i.e., the inheritance of two copies from the mother and none from the father means that the offspring receives no active paternal genes in the imprinted region; see Chapter 4). Isodisomy can result in autosomal recessive disease in the offspring of a heterozygous parent if the parent contributes two copies of the chromosome homolog that contains the disease-causing mutation (see Fig. 6-22). The first documented case of uniparental disomy in a human was seen in a patient with cystic fibrosis

whose heterozygous carrier parent had transmitted two copies of chromosome 7 containing a mutated *CFTR* gene, while the other parent transmitted neither copy of chromosome 7.

Uniparental disomy can arise in a number of ways. A trisomic conception can lose one of the extra chromosomes, resulting in an embryo that has two copies of the chromosome contributed by one parent. Disomy can also result from the union of a gamete that contains two copies of a specific chromosome with a gamete that contains no copies of that chromosome (see Fig. 6-22). In the early embryo, cells with uniparental disomy can be produced by mitotic errors, such as chromosome loss with subsequent duplication of the homologous chromosome. In addition to the Prader-Willi and Angelman syndromes and cystic fibrosis, uniparental disomy has been seen in cases of Russell-Silver syndrome, hemophilia A (see Chapter 4), and Beckwith-Wiedemann syndrome (see Chapters 4 and 12).

Duplications

A partial trisomy, or duplication, of genetic material may be seen in the offspring of persons who carry a reciprocal translocation. Duplications can also be caused by unequal crossover during meiosis, as described for the X-linked color vision loci (see Chapter 4) and for Charcot-Marie-Tooth disease (see Chapter 3). Duplications tend to produce less-serious consequences than deletions, again illustrating the principle that a loss of genetic material is more serious than an excess of genetic material.

> Duplications can arise from unequal crossover, or they can occur among the offspring of reciprocal translocation carriers. Duplications generally produce less-serious consequences than do deletions of the same region.

Ring Chromosomes

Deletions sometimes occur at both tips of a chromosome. The remaining chromosome ends can then fuse, forming a **ring chromosome** (Fig. 6-23). The

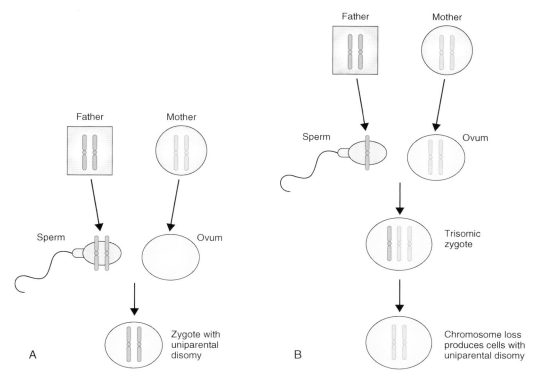

FIG 6-22   Two mechanisms that can produce uniparental disomy. **A,** Parental nondisjunction produces a sperm cell with two copies of a specific chromosome, and maternal nondisjunction produces an ovum with no copies of the same chromosome. The resulting zygote has two copies of the father's chromosome and no copies of the mother's chromosome (in this example the father contributes both chromosomes, but it is also possible that the mother could contribute both chromosomes). **B,** Nondisjunction (in the mother, in this example) results in a trisomic zygote. Loss of the paternal chromosome during mitosis produces embryonic cells that have two copies of the mother's chromosome.

karyotype of a female with a ring X chromosome is 46,X,r(X). If the ring chromosome includes a centromere, it can often proceed through cell division, but its structure can create difficulties. Ring chromosomes are often lost, resulting in monosomy for the chromosome in at least some cells (i.e., mosaicism for the ring chromosome may be seen). Ring chromosomes have been described in at least one case for each of the human autosomes; rings 14 and 22 represent two of the most common ring syndromes in humans.

Inversions

An inversion is the result of two breaks on a chromosome followed by the reinsertion of the intervening fragment at its original site but in inverted order. Thus, a chromosome symbolized as ABCDEFG might become ABEDCFG after an inversion. If the inversion includes the centromere, it is called a **peri-centric inversion**. Inversions that do not involve the

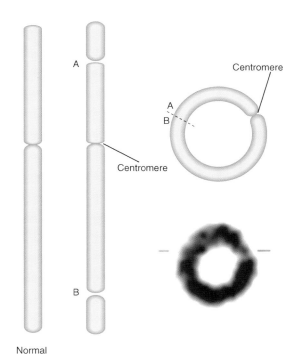

FIG 6-23   Both tips of a chromosome can be lost, leaving sticky ends that attach to each other, forming a ring chromosome. A chromosome 12 ring is shown here.

centromere are termed **paracentric inversions**.

Like reciprocal translocations, inversions are a balanced structural rearrangement. Consequently, they seldom produce disease in the inversion carrier (recall from Chapter 4, though, that an inversion that interrupts the factor VIII gene produces severe hemophilia A). Inversions can interfere with meiosis, however, producing chromosome abnormalities in the offspring of inversion carriers. Because chromosomes must line up in perfect order during prophase I, a chromosome with an inversion must form a loop to line up with its normal homolog (Fig. 6-24). Crossing over within this loop can result in duplications or deletions in the chromosomes of daughter cells. Thus, the offspring of persons who carry inversions often have chromosome deletions or duplications. It is estimated that about 1 in 1000 people carries an inversion and is therefore at risk for producing gametes with duplications or deletions.

Figure 6-24 gives an example of a pericentric inversion on chromosome 8 (46,XX, inv[8]). About 5% of the offspring of persons who carry this inversion receive a deletion or duplication of the distal portion of 8q. This combination results in the recombinant 8 syndrome, which is characterized by cognitive disability, heart defects, seizures, and a characteristic facial appearance.

▶ Chromosome inversions are relatively common structural abnormalities and may be either pericentric (including the centromere) or paracentric (not including the centromere). Parents with inversions are usually normal in phenotype but can produce offspring with deletions or duplications.

FIG 6-24 A pericentric inversion in chromosome 8 causes the formation of a loop during the alignment of homologous chromosomes in meiosis. Crossing over in this loop can produce duplications or deletions of chromosome material in the resulting gamete. The offspring in the lower right received one of the recombinant 8 chromosomes from this parent.

Isochromosomes

Sometimes a chromosome divides along the axis perpendicular to its usual axis of division (Fig. 6-25). The result is an **isochromosome**, a chromosome that has two copies of one arm and no copies of the other. Because the genetic material is substantially altered, isochromosomes of most autosomes are lethal. Most isochromosomes observed in live births involve the X chromosome, and babies with isochromosome Xq (46,X,i[Xq]) usually have features of Turner syndrome. Isochromosome 18q, which produces an extra copy of the long arm of chromosome 18, has been observed in infants with Edwards syndrome phenotype. Although most isochromosomes appear to be formed by faulty division, they can also be created by Robertsonian translocations of homologous acrocentric chromosomes (e.g., a Robertsonian translocation of the two long arms of chromosome 21).

CHROMOSOME ABNORMALITIES AND PREGNANCY LOSS

For a long time it was difficult to detect the early stages of pregnancy with certainty. It was thus possible for a woman to become pregnant but to lose the embryo before knowing of the pregnancy. Sensitive urinary assays of chorionic gonadotropin levels, which increase when the embryo implants in the uterine wall, have allowed researchers to pinpoint accurately the occurrence of pregnancy at this early stage. Follow-up of women in whom implantation was verified in this way has shown that about one third of pregnancies are lost after implantation (the number lost before implantation is unknown). Therefore, spontaneous pregnancy loss is common in humans.

As mentioned earlier, chromosome abnormalities are the leading known cause of pregnancy loss. It is estimated that a minimum of 10% to 20% of conceptions have a chromosome abnormality, and at least 95% of these chromosomally abnormal conceptions are lost before term. Karyotype studies of miscarriages indicate that about 50% of the chromosome abnormalities are trisomies, 20% are monosomies,

Normal X   Isochromosome X

FIG 6-25   *Top,* Normal chromosome division. *Center,* An isochromosome is formed when a chromosome divides along an axis perpendicular to its usual axis of division. This produces one chromosome with only the short arms and another with only the long arms. *Bottom,* A normal X chromosome is compared with an isochromosome of Xq.

and 15% are triploids. The remainder consists of tetraploids and structural abnormalities. Some chromosome abnormalities that are common at conception seldom or never survive to term. For example, trisomy 16 is thought to be the most common trisomy at conception, but it is never seen in live births.

It is possible to study chromosome abnormalities directly in sperm and egg cells. Oocytes are typically obtained from unused material in in vitro fertilization studies. Karyotypes obtained from these cells indicate that at least 20% to 25% of oocytes have missing or extra chromosomes. Human sperm cells can be studied by FISH analysis or after fusing them with hamster oocytes so that their DNA begins mitosis and condenses, allowing easier visualization. The frequency of aneuploidy in these sperm cells is about 3% to 4%. Structural abnormalities (see later discussion) are seen in about 1% of oocytes and 5% of sperm cells, and the incidence increases with advanced paternal age. Undoubtedly, this high rate of chromosome abnormality contributes importantly to later pregnancy loss.

These approaches, while informative, can involve some biases. For example, mothers in whom in vitro fertilization is performed are not a representative sample of the population. In addition, their oocytes have been stimulated artificially, and only those oocytes that could not be fertilized by sperm cells are studied. Thus, the oocytes themselves might not be a representative sample. The sperm cells studied in human-hamster hybrids represent only those that are capable of penetrating the hamster oocyte and again might not be a representative sample.

FISH analysis of aneuploidy can evaluate many cells quite rapidly, giving it an important advantage over the human-hamster technique. In general, the FISH studies have yielded results similar to those of the human-hamster studies, showing that on average, the frequency of disomy is approximately 0.15% for each autosome and 0.26% for the sex chromosomes. These studies have also confirmed a tendency for elevated frequencies of nondisjunction of the sex chromosomes and some of the acrocentric chromosomes, including chromosome 21, in sperm cells.

▶ Pregnancy loss is common in humans, with approximately one third of pregnancies lost spontaneously after implantation. Chromosome abnormalities, which have been studied in sperm and egg cells and in miscarriages and stillbirths, are an important cause of pregnancy loss.

CHROMOSOME ABNORMALITIES AND CLINICAL PHENOTYPES

As we have seen, most autosomal aberrations induce consistent recognizable patterns of multiple malformations, minor anomalies, and phenotypes with variable degrees of developmental disability. Although the individual features are usually nonspecific (e.g., palmar creases can be seen in both Down syndrome and trisomy 18), the general pattern of features is usually distinctive enough to permit a clinical diagnosis. This is especially true of the well-known chromosome syndromes: Down syndrome, Edwards syndrome, Patau syndrome, and Turner syndrome. However, there is considerable phenotypic variability even within these syndromes. No one patient has every feature; most congenital malformations (e.g., heart defects) are seen in only some affected individuals. This phenotypic variability, and the attendant potential for misdiagnosis, underscores the need to order a chromosome analysis (karyotype or aCGH) whenever clinical features suggest a chromosome abnormality.

Usually the biological basis for phenotypic variability is unknown, although mechanisms such as mosaicism, which often leads to milder expression, are being uncovered. The basis of variable expression of chromosome syndromes will be better understood as the individual genes involved in these abnormalities are identified and characterized.

In spite of the variability of chromosome syndromes, it is possible to make several generalizations:

- Most chromosome abnormalities (especially those involving autosomes) are associated with developmental delay in children and intellectual disability in older persons. This reflects the fact that a large number of human genes, perhaps one third or more of the total, participate in the development of the central nervous system. Therefore, a chromosome abnormality, which typically can affect hundreds of genes, is very likely to involve genes that affect nervous system development.
- Most chromosome syndromes involve alterations of facial morphogenesis that produce characteristic facial features. For this reason, the patient

often resembles other persons with the same disorder more than members of his or her own family. Usually the facial features and minor anomalies of the head and limbs are the best aids to diagnosis (see Chapter 12).

- Growth delay (short stature and/or poor weight gain in infancy) is commonly seen in autosomal syndromes.

- Congenital malformations, especially congenital heart defects, occur with increased frequency in most autosomal chromosome disorders. These defects occur in specific patterns. For example, AV canals and VSDs are common in children with Down syndrome. Other congenital heart defects, such as aortic coarctation or hypoplastic (under-developed) left ventricle, are seldom seen in these children but may be seen in those with Turner syndrome.

The most common clinical indications for a chromosome analysis are a newborn with multiple congenital malformations or a child with developmental delay. A summary of clinical situations in which a chromosome evaluation should be considered is given in Box 6-1.

▶ Chromosome abnormalities typically result in developmental delay, intellectual disability, characteristic facial features, and various types of congenital malformations. Despite some overlap of phenotypic features, many chromosome abnormalities can be recognized by clinical examination.

SUMMARY

Chromosome abnormalities are responsible for a proportion of genetic diseases, occurring in approximately 1 of every 150 live births. Cytogenetics is the study of chromosomes and their abnormalities. Technologies used to study chromosomes include karyotype analysis, chromosome banding, fluorescence in situ hybridization (FISH), and comparative genomic hybridization (CGH). Human chromo-

BOX 6-1   Indications for Performing Chromosome Analysis

- Persons with a suspected recognizable chromosome syndrome (e.g., Down syndrome)
- Persons with an unrecognizable pattern of two or more malformations
- Persons with ambiguous genitalia
- Intellectual disability or developmental delay in children who have physical abnormalities
- Parents and children of persons with chromosomal translocations, deletions, or duplications
- Stillborn infants with malformation or with no recognizable reason for fetal death
- Females with proportionate short stature and primary amenorrhea (consider Turner syndrome)
- Males with small testes or significant gynecomastia (consider Klinefelter syndrome)

somes are classified as metacentric, acrocentric, or submetacentric, according to the position of the centromere. Chromosome bands are used to identify individual chromosomes and structural abnormalities in chromosomes. Banding techniques include the use of quinacrine and Giemsa stains and reverse, C-, and NOR-banding. High-resolution banding, using prophase or prometaphase chromosomes, increases the number of observable bands. For FISH, a labeled probe is hybridized to metaphase, prophase, or interphase chromosomes; FISH can be used to test for missing or additional chromosomal material as well as chromosome rearrangements. The CGH technique, in which differentially labeled DNA from test and control sources is hybridized to probes in microarrays, allows for the detection of chromosome duplications and deletions but not balanced rearrangements. Array CGH can detect deletions and duplications shorter than 100 kb and requires small amounts of DNA. Abnormalities of chromosome number include euploidy and aneuploidy. Euploidy refers to cells that have a multiple of 23 chromosomes. Polyploid conditions that have been observed in humans are triploidy and tetraploidy. Aneuploidy refers to cells that contain missing or additional individual chromosomes. Aneuploid conditions consist primarily of monosomies and trisomies. Autosomal monosomies are almost always lethal, but some autosomal trisomies are compatible with survival. Trisomy 21 is the most common autosomal aneuploidy among live births. Nearly all autosomal trisomies increase with maternal age as a result of nondisjunction in older mothers. Chromosome breakage can cause structural chromosomal abnormalities such as translocation, deletion, inversion, duplication, ring chromosome, and isochromosome. Chromosome abnormalities typically result in developmental delay, intellectual disability, characteristic facial features, and various types of congenital malformations. Chromosome abnormalities are also an important cause of pregnancy loss.

IMPORTANT TERMINOLOGY

cytogenetics   细胞遗传学

chromosome abnormalities   染色体畸变

karyotype   核型

chromosome banding   染色体显带技术

fluorescence in situ hybridization (FISH)   荧光原位杂交

comparative genomic hybridization (CGH)   比较基因组杂交

euploid   整倍体

aneuploidy   非整倍体

translocation   易位

derivative chromosome   衍生染色体

deletion   缺失

microdeletion syndrome   微缺失综合征

subtelomeric rearrangement   亚(近)端粒区重排

uniparental disomy   单亲二体

duplication   重复

ring chromosome   环状染色体

inversion   倒位

isochromosome   等臂染色体

REVIEW QUESTIONS

1. Distinguish among haploidy, diploidy, polyploidy, euploidy, and aneuploidy.

2. Explain the uses and relative advantages of FISH, spectral karyotyping, and comparative genomic hybridization (CGH).

3. Describe three ways in which triploidy could arise.

4. Studies of karyotypes obtained by prenatal diagnosis at 10 weeks' gestation (chorionic villus sampling; see Chapter 10) reveal prevalence rates of chromosome abnormalities that differ from those obtained in karyotypes at 16 weeks' gestation (amniocentesis; see Chapter 10). Explain this.

5. Even though conditions such as Down syndrome and Edwards syndrome can usually be diagnosed accurately by clinical examination alone, a karyotype is always recommended. Why?

6. Rank the following, from lowest to highest, in terms of the risk of producing a child with Down syndrome:

45-year-old woman with no previous family history of Down syndrome

25-year-old woman who has had one previous child with Down syndrome

25-year-old male carrier of a 21/14 Robertsonian translocation

25-year-old female carrier of a 21/14 Robertsonian translocation

7. Females with the 49,XXXXX karyotype have been reported. Explain how this karyotype could occur.

8. A man with hemophilia A and a normal woman produce a child with Turner syndrome (45,X). The child has normal factor VIII activity. In which parent did the meiotic error occur?

9. A cytogenetics laboratory reports a karyotype of 46,XY,del(8)(p11) for one patient and a karyotype of 46,XY,dup(8)(p11) for another patient. Based on this information alone, which patient is expected to be more severely affected?

SUGGESTED READINGS AND WEBSITES

1. American Academy of Pediatrics. Committee on Genetics. Health supervision for children with Down syndrome. *Pediatrics.* 2011; 128(2): 393-406.

2. Antonarakis SE, Epstein CJ. The challenge of Down syn-

drome. *Trends Mol Med*. 2006; 12(10): 473-479.

3. Carey JC. Perspectives on the care and management of infants with trisomy 18 and trisomy 13: striving for balance. *Curr Opin Pediatr*. 2012; 24: 672-678.

4. Carey JC. Trisomy 18 and 13 syndromes. In: Cassidy SB, Allanson JE, eds. *Management of Genetic Syndromes*. Hoboken, NJ: Wiley-Liss; 2010: 807-823.

5. Cereda A, Carey JC. The trisomy 18 syndrome. *Orphanet J Rare Dis*. 2012; 7: 81.

6. Curry CJ. Autosomal trisomies. In: Rimoin DL, Pyeritz RE, Korf BR, eds. *Emery and Rimoin's Principles and Practice of Medical Genetics*. 6th ed. Philadelphia: Elsevier; 2013.

7. Gartler SM. The chromosome number in humans. A brief history. *Nat Rev Genet*. 2006; 7(8): 655-660.

8. Gravholt CH. Sex chromosome abnormalities. In: Rimoin DL, Pyeritz RE, Korf BR, eds. *Emery and Rimoin's Principles and Practice of Medical Genetics*. 6th ed. Philadelphia: Elsevier; 2013.

9. Groth KA, Skakkebaek A, Host C, et al. Clinical review: Klinefelter syndrome—a clinical update. *J Clin Endocrinol Metab*. 2013; 98: 20-30.

10. Hunter AGW. Down syndrome. In: Cassidy SB, Allanson JE, eds. *Management of Genetic Syndromes*. Hoboken, NJ: Wiley-Liss; 2010: 309-336.

11. Larney C, Bailey TL, Koopman P. Switching on sex: transcriptional regulation of the testis-determining gene Sry. *Development*. 2014; 141: 2195-2205.

12. Loscalzo ML. Turner syndrome. *Pediatr Rev*. 2008; 29(7): 219-227.

13. McDonald-McGinn DM, Kohut T, Zackai EH. Deletion 22q11.2 (Velo-cardio-facial /DiGeorge syndrome). In: Cassidy SB, Allanson JE, eds. *Management of Genetic Syn-*

dromes. Hoboken, NJ: Wiley-Liss; 2010: 263-284.

14. Nagaoka SI, Hassold TJ, Hunt PA. Human aneuploidy: mechanisms and new insights into an age-old problem. *Nat Rev Genet*. 2012; 13: 493-504.

15. Riggs ER, Wain KE, Riethmaier D, et al. Chromosomal microarray impacts clinical management. *Clin Genet*. 2014; 85: 147-153.

16. Shaffer LG, McGowan-Jordan J, Schmid M, eds. *An International System for Human Cytogenetic Nomenclature (2013)*. Basel: S. Karger; 2013.

17. Spinner NB, Conlin LK, Mulchandani S. Deletions and other structural abnormalities of the autosomes. In: Rimoin DL, Pyeritz RE, Korf BR, eds. *Emery and Rimoin's Principles and Practice of Medical Genetics*. 6th ed. Philadelphia: Elsevier; 2013.

18. Tartaglia NR, Howell S, Sutherland A, et al. A review of trisomy X (47,XXX). *Orphanet J Rare Dis*. 2010; 5: 8.

19. Yamazawa K, Ogata T, Ferguson-Smith AC. Uniparental disomy and human disease: an overview. *Am J Med Genet C Semin Med Genet*. 2010; 154C: 329-334.

20. GeneReviews (a comprehensive series of regularly updated reviews on many genetic conditions including chromosome syndromes): http://www.ncbi.nlm.nih.gov/books/NBK1116/

21. European Cytogenetics Association (a series of URLs for various cytogenetics websites): http://www.biologia.uniba.it/eca/

22. National Association for Down Syndrome (contains many URLs for Down syndrome websites): http://www.nads.org/

23. Support Organization for Trisomy 18, 13, and Related Disorders (S.O.F.T.): http://www.trisomy.org/

(Changyan Ma)

Biochemical Genetics

Each of us is composed of a large number of complex molecules that are hierarchically arranged in space to form cells, tissues, organs, and ultimately a complete human being. These molecules are constructed from individual elements that may be synthesized endogenously or obtained from the environment. Once created, these molecules are not static. In fact, they are perpetually being synthesized, degraded, excreted, and sometimes recycled in a tightly choreographed metabolic dance.

Each metabolic process consists of a sequence of catalytic steps mediated by enzymes encoded by genes. Usually, these genes are replicated with high fidelity, and enzymatic systems continue to work effectively from generation to generation. Occasionally, mutations reduce the efficiency of encoded enzymes to a level at which normal metabolism cannot occur. Such variants of metabolism were recognized by Sir Archibald Garrod at the beginning of the 20th century, based partly on his studies of **alkaptonuria (AKU)**. Garrod recognized that these variants illustrated "chemical individualities," and he called these disorders "inborn errors of metabolism," thus setting the cornerstone for contemporary biochemical genetics.

AKU is a rare disorder in which homogentisic acid (HGA), an intermediate metabolite in phenylalanine and tyrosine metabolism (Fig. 7-1), is excreted in large quantities in urine, causing it to darken on standing. Hence, AKU was classically referred to as "black urine disease." Additionally, an oxidation product of HGA is directly deposited in connective tissues, resulting in abnormal pigmentation and debilitating arthritis.

Garrod proposed in 1902 that AKU was caused by a deficiency of the enzyme that normally splits the aromatic ring of HGA. Fifty years later, it was established that AKU is produced by a failure to synthesize homogentisate1, 2-dioxygenase (HGO). However, it was not until 1996 that scientists identified thegene that is altered in AKU, based on homologytoa gene encoding an HGO enzyme that was isolated from a fungus species. The coding region of *HGO* comprises 14 exons distributed over 54 kb of DNA. Many of the mutations identified in *HGO* encode proteins that show no HGO activity when expressed in vitro. This

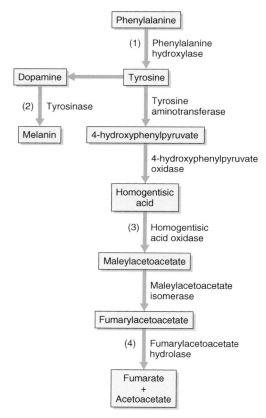

FIG 7-1 Major pathway of phenylalanine metabolism. Different enzymatic defects in this pathway cause classic phenylketonuria (*1*), tyrosinase-negative oculocutaneous albinism (*2*), alkaptonuria (*3*), and tyrosinemia type 1 (*4*).

indicates that AKU is caused by a loss-of-function mutation, confirming the hypothesis put forth by Garrod more than a century ago.

 Almost all biochemical processes of human metabolism are catalyzed by enzymes. Variations of enzymatic activity among humans are common, and a minority of these variants causes disease. These concepts were introduced by Archibald Garrod and exemplified by his studies of alkaptonuria.

VARIANTS OF METABOLISM

Prevalence of Metabolic Disease

Hundreds of different inborn errors of metabolism have been described to date, and most of these are rare. Taken together, however, metabolic disorders account for a substantial percentage of the morbidity and mortality directly attributable to genetic disease (Table 7-1). One survey conservatively estimated that the incidence of **metabolic disorders** is approximately 1 in every 2500 births, or 10% of all monogenic conditions in children. Moreover, we are beginning to understand that different alleles of genes that encode enzymes can alter one's risk for many common diseases, such as diabetes, heart disease, stroke, and cancer.

The diagnosis of a metabolic disorder can be challenging (Clinical Commentary 7-1); thus, the morbidity associated with metabolic defects is probably underestimated. In the 1970s, an often fatal acute metabolic encephalopathy called Reye syndrome was diagnosed in many children. In the following decades, we learned that some children with anencephalopathy indistinguishable from Reye syndrome had a urea cycle defect that produced hyperammonemia (increased levels of circulating ammonia) and death. Recognition of Reye syndrome as a **phenocopy** of a urea cycle defect is important because, in addition to supportive care (supportive care is care that supports the elementary functions of the body, such as maintenance of fluid balance,

oxygenation, and blood pressure, but is not aimed at treating the disease process directly.), the children can now receive direct treatment for the urea cycle defects. Similarly, on postmortem examination, some children who have died from sudden infant death syndrome (SIDS) have been found to have a defect of fatty acid metabolism. These are also treatable disorders, and life-threatening episodes can be avoided with appropriate care.

 Although individual metabolic disorders are rare, their overall direct and indirect contribution to morbidity and mortality is substantial.

Inheritance of Metabolic Defects

Most metabolic disorders are inherited in an autosomal recessive pattern: Only individuals having two mutant alleles are affected. Although a mutant allele produces reduced or no enzyme activity (loss of function), it usually does not alter the health of a heterozygous carrier. Because many of the genes encoding disease-related enzymes have been identified and their mutations characterized, carrier testing and prenatal diagnosis are available for many metabolic disorders. However, testing samples of dried blood for elevated levels of metabolites in the newborn period (e.g., for **phenylketonuria** and **galactosemia**; see Chapter 10) remains the most commonly used population-based screening test for metabolic disorders. Expanded newborn screening that tests for dozens of different disorders by checking for the presence of abnormal metabolites in blood is common. As the technology for rapid and efficient DNA testing of mutant alleles progresses, population-based screening for additional disorders is likely to be incorporated.

Most inborn errors of metabolism are inherited in an autosomal recessive pattern. The carrier state usually is not associated with morbidity. Carrier and diagnostic testing are becoming widely available for many disorders.

TABLE 7-1   Disorders of Metabolism

NAME	PREVALENCE	MUTANT GENE PRODUCT	CHROMOSOMAL LOCATION
Carbohydrate Disorders			
Classic galactosemia	1/35,000 to 1/60,000	Galactose-1-phosphate uridyl transferase	9p13
Hereditary fructose intolerance	1/20,000	Fructose 1,6-bisphosphate aldolase	9q13-q32
Fructosuria	≈1/100,000	Fructokinase	2p23
Hypolactasia (adult)	Common	Lactase	2q21
Diabetes mellitus type 1	1/400 (Europeans)	Multiple	Polygenic
Diabetes mellitus type 2	1/20	Multiple	Polygenic
Maturity-onset diabetes of the young (MODY)	≈1/400	Multiple	Multiple loci
Amino Acid Disorders			
Phenylketonuria	1/10,000	Phenylalanine hydroxylase	12q24
Tyrosinemia (type 1)	1/100,000	Fumarylacetoacetate hydrolase	15q23-25
Maple syrup urine disease	1/180,000	Branched-chain α-ketoacid dehydrogenase (multiple subunits)	Multiple loci
Alkaptonuria	1/250,000	Homogentisic acid oxidase	3q2
Homocystinuria	1/340,000	Cystathionine β-synthase	21q2
Oculocutaneous albinism	1/35,000	Tyrosinase	11q
Cystinosis	1/100,000	CTNS	17p13
Cystinuria	1/7000	SLC3A1 (type 1)	2p
		SLC7A9 (types II & III)	19q13
Lipid Disorders			
MCAD	1/1,000 to 1/15,000	Medium-chain acyl-CoA dehydrogenase	1p31
VLCAD	1/30,000	Very Long-chain acyl-CoA dehydrogenase	17p13.1
SLO	1/10,000	Δ7-sterol reductase	11q12-q13
Organic Acid Disorders			
Methylmalonic acidemia	1/20,000	Methylmalonyl-CoA mutase	6p
Propionic acidemia	Rare	Propionyl-CoA carboxylase	13q32; 3q
Urea Cycle Defects			
Ornithine transcarbamylase deficiency	1/60,000	Ornithine carbamyl transferase	Xp21
Carbamyl phosphate synthetase deficiency	1/300,000	Carbamyl phosphate synthetase I	2p
Argininosuccinic acid synthetase deficiency	1/250,000	Argininosuccinic acid synthetase	9q34
Energy Production Defects			
Cytochrome c oxidase deficiency	Rare	Cytochrome oxidase peptides	Multiple loci
Pyruvate carboxylase deficiency	Rare	Pyruvate carboxylase	11q
Pyruvate dehydrogenase complex (E_1) deficiency	Rare	Pyruvate decarboxylase, $E_1\alpha$	Xp22
NADH-CoQ reductase deficiency	Rare	Multiple nuclear genes	Multiple loci
Heavy Metal Transport Defects			
Wilson disease	1/50,000	ATP7B	13q14
Menkes disease	1/250,000	ATP7A	Xq13
Hemochromatosis	1/200 to 1/400 (Europeans)	HFE	6p21
Acrodermatitis enteropathica	Rare	SLC39A4	8q24

MCAD, Medium-chain acyl-CoA dehydrogenase; *SLO,* Smith-Lemli-Opitz syndrome; *VLCAD,* very long-chain acyl-CoA dehydrogenase.

CLINICAL COMMENTARY 7-1

Diagnosis of a Metabolic Disorder

The presentations of persons with inborn errors of metabolism are highly variable. During gestation, the maternal-placental unit usually provides essential nutrients and prevents the accumulation of toxic substrates. Thus, a fetus is infrequently symptomatic. However, after birth, persons with metabolic disorders can present at ages ranging from the first day of life to adulthood. The presentation may be precipitous and characterized by dramatic alterations in homeostasis and even death. In contrast, the disorder may be insidious, with only subtle changes in function over long periods. For most metabolic disorders, the presymptomatic period and onset of symptoms lie somewhere between these two extremes. The following case illustrates this point.

Anthony is a 9-month-old Latin American boy who comes to the emergency department accompanied by his parents. His parents complain that he has been irritable and vomiting for the last 36 hours, and over the past 12 hours he has become increasingly sleepy. They sought medical attention because it was difficult to awaken Anthony to breast-feed him. Anthony's medical history is unremarkable. He has a healthy 8-year-old sister and had a brother who died in his crib at 7 months of age. An investigation of the brother's death and an autopsy were performed. The findings were consistent with sudden infant death syndrome (SIDS).

Anthony is hospitalized and is noted to be hypoglycemic (low serum glucose level), slightly acidemic (serum pH<7.4), and hyperammonemic (elevated plasma ammonia). Intravenous infusion of glucose transiently improves his level of alertness, but he becomes comatose and dies 5 days later. An autopsy reveals marked cerebral edema (swelling of the brain) and fatty infiltration of the liver consistent with a diagnosis of Reye syndrome. Anthony's mother is concerned that the boys' deaths are related to each other, especially since she is pregnant again. She is counseled that the causes of death are unrelated and neither disorder is likely to recur in her family.

One year later her 6-month-old daughter, Maria, is hospitalized for the third time because of lethargy and weakness. Laboratory studies reveal moderate hypoglycemia, hyperammonemia, and ketonuria (ketones in the urine). Additional studies, including measurement of urine organic acids,* serum amino acids, and free and esterified plasma carnitines, suggest that Maria has a defect of fatty acid oxidation. Therapy is initiated with intravenous glucose, oral carnitine, and the restriction of fats to no more than 20% of her caloric requirements. More specific biochemical and molecular studies confirm that Maria has medium-chain acyl-CoA dehydrogenase (MCAD) deficiency. Molecular studies from preserved tissues that had been collected at autopsy from Maria's deceased brothers indicate that they also had MCAD deficiency. Maria's asymptomatic older sister is similarly affected. Both girls are healthy 2 years later, eating a low-fat diet and using a carnitine supplement. They have a new baby brother who underwent prenatal testing for MCAD and was found to be unaffected.

The disparate presentations of MCAD deficiency in this family (sudden death, acute illness, chronic illness, and asymptomatic) illustrate the phenotypic variability often observed in persons with inborn errors of metabolism, even those sharing an identical mutation. Thus, there might not be a disease-specific pattern of symptoms and findings. Often it is the heightened index of suspicion of care providers that leads to the testing necessary to identify a metabolic disorder. Supportive therapy can be lifesaving and should be initiated before making a diagnosis. Nevertheless, it is imperative that prudent attempts be made to make a specific diagnosis, because it can have important implications for the family (e.g., prenatal testing, presymptomatic therapy). The treatment of MCAD deficiency is completely effective in preventing early death from the toxic effects of accumulated fatty acid intermediates.

---

*Organic acids are carbon-based acids that are products of intermediate metabolism and normally do not accumulate in plasma or urine beyond the buffering capacities of these fluids.

Types of Metabolic Processes

Metabolic disorders have been classified in many different ways, based on the pathological effects of the pathway blocked (e.g., absence of end product, accumulation of substrate); different functional classes of proteins (e.g., receptors, hormones); associated cofactors (e.g., metals, vitamins); and pathways affected (e.g., glycolysis, citric acid cycle). Each of these has advantages and disadvantages, and none of them encompasses all metabolic disorders. However, the classification that most completely integrates our

knowledge of cell biology, physiology, and pathology with metabolic disorders categorizes defects of metabolism by the types of processes that are disturbed.

DEFECTS OF METABOLIC PROCESSES

Almost all biochemical reactions in the human body are controlled by enzymes, which act as **catalysts**. The catalytic properties of enzymes typically increase reaction rates by more than a million-fold. These reactions mediate the synthesis, transfer, use, and degradation of biomolecules to build and maintain the internal structures of cells, tissues, and organs. Biomolecules can be categorized into four primary groups: nucleic acids, proteins, carbohydrates, and lipids. The major metabolic pathways that metabolize these molecules include glycolysis, citric acid cycle, pentose phosphate shunt, gluconeogenesis, glycogen and fatty acid synthesis and storage, degradative pathways, energy production, and transport systems. We now discuss how defects in each of these metabolic pathways can cause human disease.

Carbohydrate Metabolism

Because of the many different applications that they serve in all organisms, carbohydrates are the most abundant organic substance on Earth. Carbohydrates function as substrates for energy production and storage, as intermediates of metabolic pathways, and as the structural framework of DNA and RNA. Consequently, carbohydrates account for a major portion of the human diet and are metabolized into three principal monosaccharides: glucose, galactose, and fructose. Galactose and fructose are converted to glucose before glycolysis. The failure to effectively use these sugars accounts for the majority of the inborn errors of human carbohydrate metabolism.

Galactose

The most common monogenic disorder of carbohydrate metabolism, transferase deficiency galactosemia (classic galactosemia), affects 1 in every 50,000 newborns. It is most commonly caused by mutations in the gene encoding galactose-1-phosphate uridyl transferase (GAL-1-P uridyltransferase) (Fig. 7-2). This gene is composed of 11 exons distributed across 4 kb of DNA, and approximately 70% of galactosemia-causing alleles in people of Western European origin have a single missense mutation in exon 6, p.Q188R. As a result of diminished GAL-1-P uridyl transferase activity, affected persons cannot effectively convert galactose to glucose; consequently, galactose is alternatively metabolized to galactitol and galactonate (see Fig. 7-2). Although galactose and its metabolites accumulate in many tissues, the pathophysiology of classic galactosemia is not well understood.

Classic galactosemia typically manifests in the newborn period with poor sucking, failure to thrive, and jaundice. If galactosemia is left untreated, sepsis, hyperammonemia, and shock leading to death usually follow. Cataracts (opacification of the lens of the eye) are found in about 10% of infants. Newborn screening for galactosemia is widespread, and most affected persons are identified as they begin to develop symptoms. Early identification affords prompt treatment, which consists largely of eliminating dietary galactose. This substantially reduces the morbidity associated with the acute effects of elevated levels of galactose metabolites. Long-term disabilities may include poor growth, developmental delay (developmental delay is the delayed attainment of age-appropriate motor, speech, and/or cognitive milestones; the outcomes of developmental delay range from normal to profound intellectual disability.), speech problems, and ovarian failure in females. These sequelae are thought to be caused by endogenous production of galactose. The effects of prospective dietary therapy on the prevalence of these long-term sequelae are less clear. Early studies suggested that there was no effect, but as more longitudinal data become available, it appears that patients treated early in life with dietary therapy may have a normal cognitive outcome.

Galactosemia can also be caused by mutations in the genes encoding galactokinase or uridine diphosphate galactose-4-epimerase (UDP-galactose-4-epimerase) (see Fig. 7-2). Deficiency of galactokinase is associated with the formation of cataracts but does not cause growth failure, intellectual disability, or hepatic disease. Dietary restriction of galactose is also the treatment for galactokinase deficiency. Deficiency of UDP-galactose-4-epimerase can be limited to red blood cells and leukocytes, causing no ill effects, or it can be systemic and produce symptoms similar to those of classic galactosemia. Treatment is aimed at reducing the dietary intake of galactose, but not as severely as in patients with classic galactosemia, because some galactose must be provided to produce UDP-galactose for the synthesis of some complex carbohydrates.

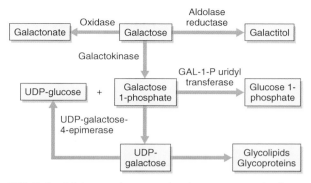

FIG 7-2 Major pathways of galactose metabolism. The most common enzymatic abnormality producing galactosemia isa defect of GAL-1-P uridyl transferase. Defects of galactokinase or of UDP-galactose 4-epimerase are much lesscommon causes of galactosemia. *GAL*, Galactose; *UDP*, uridine diphosphate.

▶ Galactosemia is one of the most common inherited disorders of carbohydrate metabolism. Newborn screening for galactosemia is widespread. Early identification allows prompt treatment, which consists largely of eliminating dietary galactose. Mutations in the gene that encodes GAL-1-P uridyl transferase are the most common cause of galactosemia.

Fructose

Three autosomal recessive defects of fructose metabolism have been described. The most common is caused by mutations in the gene encoding hepatic fructokinase. This enzyme catalyzes the first step in the metabolism of dietary fructose, the conversion to fructose-1-phosphate (Fig. 7-3). Inactivation of hepatic fructokinase results in asymptomatic fructosuria (presence of fructose in the urine).

In contrast, hereditary fructose intolerance (HFI) results in poor feeding, failure to thrive, hepatic and renal insufficiency, and death. HFI is caused by a deficiency of fructose 1,6-bisphosphate aldolase in the liver, kidney cortex, and small intestine. Infants and adults with HFI are asymptomatic unless they ingest fructose or sucrose (a sugar composed of fructose and glucose). Infants who are breast-fed become symptomatic after weaning, when fruits and vegetables are added to their diet. Affected infants may

survive into childhood because they avoid foods they consider noxious, thereby self-limiting their intake of fructose. The prevalence of HFI may be as high as 1 in 20,000 births, and, since the cloning of the gene encoding fructose-1-phosphate aldolase, differences in the geographic distribution of mutant alleles have been found.

Deficiency of hepatic fructose 1,6-bisphosphatase (FBPase) causes impaired gluconeogenesis, hypoglycemia (reduced level of circulating glucose), and severe metabolic academia (serum pH<7.4). Affected infants commonly present for treatment shortly after birth, although cases diagnosed later in childhood have been reported. If patients are adequately supported beyond childhood, growth and development appear to be normal. A handful of mutations have been found in the gene encoding FBPase, some of which encode mutant proteins that are inactive in vitro.

▶ Asymptomatic deficiency of fructokinase is the most common defect of fructose metabolism. Hereditary fructose intolerance is less prevalent but is associated with much more severe problems.

Glucose

Abnormalities of glucose metabolism are the most common errors of carbohydrate metabolism. However, the causes of these disorders are heterogeneous and include both environmental and genetic factors. Historically, disorders associated with elevated levels of plasma glucose (hyperglycemia) have been classified into three categories: type 1 diabetes mellitus (T1DM), type 2 diabetes mellitus (T2DM), and maturity-onset diabetes of the young (MODY), of which there are many subtypes. T1DM is associated with reduced or absent levels of plasma insulin and usually manifests in childhood. DM type 2 is characterized by insulin resistance and, most commonly, adult onset. A more detailed discussion of T1DM and T2DM can be found in Chapter 5.

Substantial advances in understanding of the pathophysiology of common diabetes have been achieved by identifying mutations that cause rare

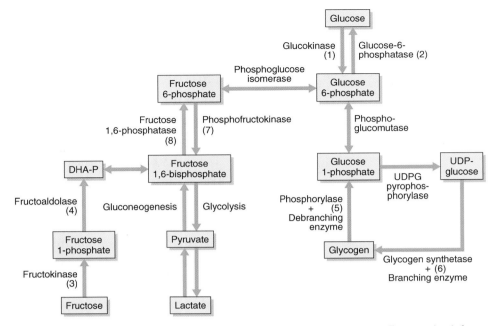

FIG 7-3 Summary of glucose, fructose, and glycogen metabolism. Enzymatic defects in this pathway cause hyperglycemia (*1*), Von Gierke disease (*2*), fructosuria (*3*), hereditary fructose intolerance (*4*), Cori disease (*5*), Anderson disease (*6*), Tarui disease (*7*), and fructose1,6-bisphosphatase (FBPase) deficiency (*8*). *UDP*, Uridine diphosphate.

monogenic forms of hyperglycemia. Mutations in the insulin receptor gene have been associated with a disorder characterized by insulin resistance and acanthosis nigricans (hypertrophic skin with a corrugated appearance). These mutations can decrease the number of insulin receptors on a cell's surface, or they can decrease the insulin-binding activity level or the insulin-stimulated tyrosine kinase activity level. Mutations in mitochondrial DNA and in the genes encoding insulin and glucokinase have also been associated with hyperglycemic disorders.

 Studies of rare, monogenic forms of diabetes define the pathways that may be disturbed in the more common forms of diabetes mellitus.

Lactose

The ability to metabolize lactose (a sugar composed of glucose and galactose) depends, in part, on the activity of an intestinal brush-border enzyme called lactase-phlorizin hydrolase (LPH). In most mammals, LPH activity diminishes after infants are weaned from maternal milk. However, the persistence of intestinal LPH activity is a common autosomal recessive trait

in human populations, with an incidence ranging from 5% to 90%. The geographic distribution of lactase persistence is concordant with areas of high milk intake, such as northwestern Europe and certain parts of Africa. The persistent ability for adults to use dairy products as a source of vitamin D had a selective advantage in these populations.

Lactase nonpersistence (i.e., adult-type hypolactasia or lactose intolerance) is common in most tropical and subtropical countries. Persons with lactase nonpersistence can experience nausea, bloating, and diarrhea after ingesting lactose. Thus, in many regions where reduced lactase activity is prevalent, the lactose in dairy products is often partially metabolized (e.g., by lactobacilli in the preparation of yogurt) before consumption. The role of lactase nonpersistence as a cause of abdominal pain and symptoms of irritable bowel syndrome is controversial.

LPH is encoded by the lactase gene (*LCT*) on chromosome 2. In European populations, adult LPH expression is regulated by a polymorphism located in an upstream gene named *minichromosome maintenance 6* (*MCM6*). However, in sub-Saharan African, Central Asian, and Arabian peninsular populations in which lactase persistence is common, this polymorphism is found at low frequency or is absent. Lactase persistence in these populations is caused by different polymorphisms that appear to increase transcription of *LCT*. These polymorphisms appear to have arisen relatively recently in human evolution and have increased in incidence as a result of natural selection independently in populations in Europe and Africa. In each case, the selective force appears to have been a local adaptive response to the higher fitness afforded by the ability to consume dairy products.

Mutations that abolish lactase activity altogether cause congenital lactase deficiency and produce severe diarrhea and malnutrition in infancy. Such mutations are very rare.

Glycogen

Carbohydrates are most commonly stored as glycogen in humans. Consequently, enzyme deficiencies that lead to impaired synthesis or degradation of glycogen are also considered disorders of carbohydrate metabolism. Defects of each of the proteins involved in glycogen metabolism have been identified (Table 7-2). These cause different forms of glycogen storage disorders and are classified numerically according to the chronological order in which their enzymatic basis was described. The two organs most severely affected by glycogen storage disorders are the liver and skeletal muscle. Glycogen storage disorders that affect the liver typically cause hepatomegaly (enlarged liver) and hypoglycemia (low plasma glucose level). Glycogen storage disorders that affect skeletal muscle

cause exercise intolerance, progressive weakness, and cramping. Some glycogen storage disorders, such as Pompe disease, can also affect cardiac muscle, causing cardiomyopathy and early death. Treatment of some glycogen storage disorders by enzyme replacement (e.g., giving active forms of the enzyme intravenously) can improve, and in some cases prevent, symptoms and therefore preserve function and prevent early death.

 Each disorder of glycogen metabolism is uncommon, yet taken together these defects account for substantial morbidity. Early intervention can prevent severe disabilities and early death.

Amino Acid Metabolism

Proteins play the most diverse roles of the major biomolecules (e.g., providing mechanical support, coordinating immune responses, generating motion). Indeed, nearly all known enzymes are proteins. The fundamental structural units of proteins are amino acids. Some amino acids can be synthesized endogenously (nonessential), and others must be obtained from the environment (essential). Many defects of the metabolism of amino acids have been described.

Phenylalanine

Defects in the metabolism of phenylalanine (an essential amino acid) cause the hyperphenylalaninemias, some of the most widely studied of all inborn errors of metabolism. These disorders are caused by mutations in genes that encode components of the

TABLE 7-2	Glycogen Storage Disorders	
TYPE	**DEFECT**	**MAJOR AFFECTED TISSUES**
Ia (Von Gierke)	Glucose-6-phosphatase	Liver, kidney, intestine
Ib	Microsomal glucose-6-phosphate transport	Liver, kidney, intestine, neutrophils
II (Pompe)	Lysosomal acid β-glucosidase	Muscle, heart
IIIa (Cori)	Glycogen debranching enzyme	Liver, muscle
IIIb	Glycogen debranching enzyme	Liver
IV (Anderson)	Branching enzyme	Liver, muscle
V (McArdle)	Muscle phosphorylase	Muscle
VI (Hers)	Liver phosphorylase	Liver
VII (Tarui)	Muscle phosphofructokinase	Muscle

phenylalanine hydroxylation pathway (see Fig. 7-1). Elevated levels of plasma phenylalanine disrupt essential cellular processes in the brain such as myelination and protein synthesis, eventually producing severe intellectual disability. Most cases of hyperphenylalaninemia are caused by mutations of the gene that encodes phenylalanine hydroxylase (PAH), resulting in classic phenylketonuria (PKU). Hundreds of different mutations have been identified in PAH, including substitutions, insertions, and deletions. The prevalence of hyperphenylalaninemia varies widely among groups from different geographic regions; PKU ranges from 1 in every 10,000 people of European origin to 1 in every 90,000 in those of African ancestry. Less commonly, hyperphenylalaninemia is caused by defects in the synthesis of tetrahydrobiopterin, a cofactor necessary for the hydroxylation of phenylalanine, or by a deficiency of dihydropteridine reductase.

Treatment of most hyperphenylalaninemias is aimed at restoring normal blood phenylalanine levels by restricting dietary intake of phenylalanine-containing foods (Box 7-1). However, phenylalanine is an essential amino acid, and adequate supplies are necessary for normal growth and development. A complete lack of phenylalanine is fatal. Thus, a fine balance must be maintained between providing enough protein and phenylalanine for normal growth and preventing the serum phenylalanine level from rising too high. Persons with PKU clearly benefit from lifelong treatment. Thus, once PKU is diagnosed, the person must follow a phenylalaninerestricted diet for life. Sapropterin dihydrochloride, a form of tetrahydrobiopterin (BH4) can help BH-4 responsive PKU patients.

Hyperphenylalaninemia in a pregnant woman results in elevated phenylalanine levels in the fetus. This can cause poor growth, birth defects, micro-cephaly, and intellectual disability in the fetus (regardless of the fetus's genotype). Thus, it is important that women with PKU receive appropriate pregnancy counseling. Optimally, they should maintain a low-phenylalanine diet at conception and throughout pregnancy.

 Hyperphenylalaninemias are the most common defects of amino acid metabolism. Classic PKU is caused by mutations in the gene that encodes phenylalanine hydroxylase. Hyperphenylalaninemias are treated by restricting dietary intake of phenylalanine-containing foods.

Tyrosine

The amino acid tyrosine is the starting point of the synthetic pathways leading to catecholamines, thyroid hormones, and melanin pigments, and it is incorporated into many proteins. Elevated levels of serum tyrosine can be acquired (e.g., severe hepatocellular dysfunction), or they can result from an inborn error of catabolism, of which there are several. Hereditary tyrosinemia type 1 (HT1) is the most common metabolic defect of tyrosine and is caused by a deficiency of fumarylacetoacetate hydrolase (FAH), which catalyzes the last step in tyrosine catabolism (see Fig. 7-1). Accumulation of FAH's substrate, fumarylacetoacetate, and its precursor, maleylacetoacetate, is thought to be mutagenic and toxic to the liver. Consequently, HT1 is characterized by dysfunction of the renal tubules, acute episodes of peripheral neuropathy, progressive liver disease leading to cirrhosis, and a high risk for developing liver cancer (hepatocellular carcinoma).

Management of HT1 includes supportive care, dietary restriction of phenylalanine and tyrosine, and administration of 2-(nitro-4-trifluoro-methylbenzoyl)-1,3-cyclohexanedione (NTBC) or nitisinone, an inhibi-

---

BOX 7-1   Dietary Management of Inborn Errors of Metabolism

The most important component of therapy for many inborn errors of metabolism is manipulation of the diet. This commonly includes restriction of substrates that are toxic, such as carbohydrates (e.g., in galactosemia, diabetes mellitus), fats (e.g., in MCAD deficiency), and amino acids (e.g., in PKU, MSUD, urea cycle defects); avoidance of fasting; replacement of deficient cofactors (e.g., B vitamins, carnitine); or using alternative pathways of catabolism to eliminate toxic substances. Because many metabolic disorders are diagnosed in infants whose nutri-

BOX 7-1   Dietary Management of Inborn Errors of Metabolism (Continued)

tional requirements change quickly (sometimes weekly), it is imperative to provide infants with diets that provide adequate calories and nutrients for normal growth and development. Thus, the responsibility for maintaining a special diet begins with the parents of an affected child and shifts to the child when he or she is capable of managing independently. For most persons with metabolic diseases, a special diet must be maintained for life. This results in many unique challenges that are often unforeseen by families and care providers alike. Consequently, it is important that support and guidance be provided by clinical dietitians, gastroenterologists, psychologists, genetic counselors, and biochemical geneticists.

For example, newborns with PKU are fed a low-phenylalanine diet to prevent the effects of hyperphenylalaninemia on the brain. Breast milk contains too much phenylalanine to be used as the only source of nutrients. Therefore, many infants are fed an expensive low-phenylalanine formula that is available only by prescription, a medical food.* Small quantities of breast milk can be mixed with the formula, although the breast milk must be pumped and carefully titrated to avoid giving the infant too much phenylalanine. Serum phenylalanine levels are measured frequently, and adjustments must be made to the diet to compensate for an infant's growth and varying individual tolerances for phenylalanine. These interventions can disrupt mother-infant bonding and distort a family's social dynamics.

As a child with PKU grows older, low-protein food substitutes are introduced to supplement the formula (e.g., low-protein breads and pasta). To put this in perspective, consider that a 10-year-old child with PKU might ingest 300 to 500 mg of phenylalanine per day. Thus, three or four slices of regular bread would meet a child's nutritional needs and dietary phenylalanine limit because of the relatively high protein content of grains. Low-protein foods make the diet more substantive and varied. Indeed, seven slices of low-protein bread contain the phenylalanine equivalent of one piece of regular bread. Yet, many of these foods have an odor, taste, texture, or appearance that differs distinctively from foods containing normal amounts of protein. The intake of many fruits, fats, and carbohydrates is less restricted (see table at the right). However, phenylalanine is found unexpectedly in many food items (e.g., gelatin, beer). In fact, the FDA requires manufacturers to label products containing aspartame (a common artificial sweetener that contains phenylalanine) with a warning for persons with PKU.

Teenagers with PKU sometimes have difficulty socializing with their peers because their dietary restrictions limit food choices at restaurants, sporting events, and parties. Adults with PKU must consume more medical food than they did during childhood due to their size and protein requirements. Women with PKU must be on a severely restricted low-phenylalanine diet during pregnancy because hyperphenylalaninemia is a known teratogen (see text).

Inborn errors of metabolism are chronic diseases that are often treated by substantially modifying the diet. This can require considerable changes in lifestyle, precipitating financial and emotional hardships of which health-care providers need to be aware.

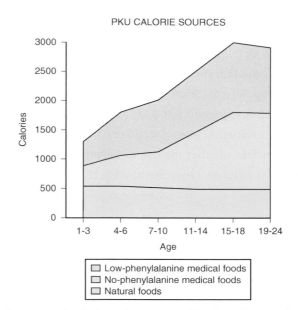

Sources of calories of persons with phenylketonuria (PKU) at different ages. The amount of no-protein medical foods and low-protein medical foods eaten increases with age as the need for energy and protein increases. (Courtesy Kathleen Huntington and Diane Waggoner, Oregon Health and Science University.)

Phenylalanine Content of Some Common Foods

FOOD	MEASURE	PHENYLALANINE (mg)
Turkey, light meat	1 cup	1662
Tuna, water-packed	1 cup	1534
Baked beans	1 cup	726
Lowfat milk (2% fat)	1 cup	393
Soy milk	1 ounce	46
Breast milk	1 ounce	14
Broccoli (raw)	3 tablespoons	28
Potato (baked)	2 tablespoons	14
Watermelon	1/2 cup	12
Grapefruit (fresh)	1/4 fruit	13
Beer	6 ounces	11
Gelatin dessert	1/2 cup	36

*U.S. Public Law 100-290 defines a medical food as a food that is formulated to be consumed or administered enterally under the supervision of a physician and that is intended for the specific dietary management of a disease or condition for which distinctive nutritional requirements, based on recognized scientific principles, are established by medical evaluation.

tor of an enzyme upstream of FAH (4-hydroxyphenylpy-ruvate dioxygenase). Use of NTBC, combined with a low-tyrosine diet, has produced marked improvement in children with HT1. The long-term effects of NTBC are still unclear, but children who have been treated for more than 20 years appear to be doing well. Liver transplantation can be curative but is typically reserved for persons who fail to respond to NTBC or who develop a malignancy. In a mouse model of HT1, gene therapy (see Chapter 10) has been used to repopulate the liver with cells that exhibit stable long-term expression of FAH (FAH+ hepatocytes). Because some FAH-hepatocytes remain in these livers, it is unclear whether the risk of hepatocellular carcinoma is reduced. Gene therapy for HT1 in humans might someday replace life-long dietary and pharmacologic treatment.

Mutations in FAH have been identified in many families. A splice-site mutation is quite common in French-Canadians, and its high frequency is probably the result of founder effect (see Chapter 3). This mutation results in an in-frame deletion of an exon, which removes a series of critically important amino acids from FAH. Missense and nonsense mutations of *FAH* have also been found in persons with HT1.

Tyrosinemia type 2 (oculocutaneous tyrosinemia) is caused by a deficiency of tyrosine aminotransferase. It is mainly characterized by corneal erosions and thickening of the skin on the palms and the soles. Tyrosinemia type 3 is associated with reduced activity of 4-hydroxyphenylpyruvatedioxygenase. Only a few affected persons have been reported.

▶ Deficiency of FAH causes HT1. Accumulation of the substrates of FAH leads to neurological, kidney, and liver dysfunction. Although liver transplantation has been the cornerstone of treatment for HT1, the use of drugs that block the production of FAH has proved effective.

Branched-Chain Amino Acids

Approximately 40% of the preformed amino acids required by mammals are branched-chain amino acids (BCAAs) such as valine, leucine, and isoleucine.

BCAAs can be used as a source of energy through an oxidative pathway that uses an α-ketoacid as an intermediate. Decarboxylation of α-ketoacids is mediated by a multimeric enzyme complex called branched-chain α-ketoacid dehydrogenase (BCKAD). The BCKAD complex is composed of at least four catalytic components and two regulatory enzymes, which are encoded by six genes. A deficiency of any one of these six components produces a disorder known as maple syrup urine disease (MSUD), so named because the urine of affected persons has an odor reminiscent of maple syrup.

The prevalence of MSUD in the general population is low, but MSUD is relatively common in the Mennonite community of Lancaster County, Pennsylvania, where approximately1 in every 7 persons is a heterozygous carrier. All of these carriers have the same disease-causing mutation of *E1* , one of the loci encoding a catalytic component of BCKAD, and all are descendants of a couple who emigrated from Europe in the 18th century. This is another example of founder effect in a small, relatively isolated population (see Chapter 3).

Untreated patients with MSUD accumulate BCAAs and their associated ketoacids, leading to progressive neurodegeneration and death in the first few months of life. Treatment of MSUD consists of dietary restriction of BCAAs to the minimum required for normal growth. Despite treatment, episodic deterioration is common, and supportive care is required during these crises. Because increasing BCKAD activity by only a few percentage points can alter the course of disease substantially, therapy with thiamine, a cofactor of BCKAD, is used to treat these patients. Gene therapy for MSUD is also being investigated.

▶ Maple syrup urine disease is caused by defects in branched-chain α-ketoacid dehydrogenase. Accumulation of BCAAs causes progressive neurodegeneration and death. Treatment consists of restricting dietary intake of BCAAs to a minimal level.

Early detection of amino acid defects, coupled with prompt intervention, can prevent severe physical impairment and death. Moderate increases of enzyme activity can dramatically alter the course of some aminoacidopathies, making them good candidates for somatic cell gene therapy.

Lipid Metabolism

Lipids (Greek, *lipos*, "fat") are a heterogeneous group of biomolecules that are insoluble in water and highly soluble inorganic solvents (e.g., chloroform). They provide the backbone for phospholipids and sphingolipids, which are components of all biological membranes. Lipids such as cholesterol are also constituents of steroid hormones; they act as intracellular messengers and serve as an energy substrate. Elevated serum lipid levels (hyperlipidemia) are common and result from defective lipid transport mechanisms. Errors in the metabolism of fatty acids (hydrocarbon chains with a terminal carboxylate group) are much less common. However, characterizing hyperlipidemias (see Chapter 5), errors of fatty acid metabolism, and defects of cholesterol production and use has been a powerful approach for understanding the biochemical basis of lipid catabolism.

During fasting and prolonged aerobic exercise, fatty acids are mobilized from adipose tissue and become a major substrate for energy production in the liver, skeletal muscle, and cardiac muscle. Major steps in this pathway include the uptake and activation of fatty acids by cells, transport across the outer and inner mitochondrial membranes, and entry into the β-oxidation spiral in the mitochondrial matrix (Fig. 7-4). Defects in each of these steps have been described in humans, although defects of fatty acid oxidation (FAO) are the most common.

Fatty Acids

The most common inborn error of fatty acid metabolism results from a deficiency of medium-chain acyl-coenzyme A dehydrogenase (MCAD). MCAD deficiency is characterized by episodic hypoglycemia, which is often provoked by fasting (see Clinical

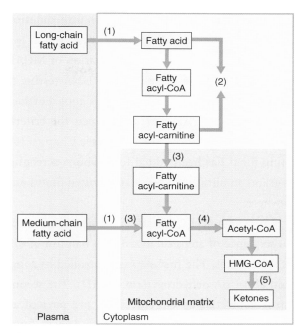

FIG 7-4 Summary of fatty acid metabolism: (*1*) fatty acid entry into a cell, (*2*) activation and transesterification, (*3*) mitochondrial uptake, (*4*) oxidation via β-oxidation, (*5*) formation of ketone bodies. Note that medium-chain fatty acids can traverse the mitochondrial membrane without carnitine mediated transport. *CoA*, Coenzyme A.

Commentary 7-1). Commonly, a child with MCAD deficiency presents with vomiting and lethargy after a period of diminished oral intake due to a minor illness (e.g., upper respiratory illness, gastroenteritis). Fasting results in the accumulation of fatty acid intermediates, a failure to produce ketones in sufficient quantities to meet tissue demands, and the exhaustion of glucose supplies. Cerebral edema and encephalopathy result from the indirect and direct effects of fatty acid intermediates in the central nervous system. Death often follows unless a usable energy source such as glucose is provided promptly. Between these episodes, children with MCAD deficiency often have normal examinations. Treatment consists of the avoidance of fasting, ensuring an adequate source of calories, and providing supportive care during periods of nutritional stress.

To date, most of the reported MCAD patients are of northwestern European origin, and the majority have an A-to-G missense mutation, c.985A>G, that results in the substitution of glutamate for lysine.

Additional substitution, insertion, and deletion mutations have been identified but are much less common. The molecular characterization of MCAD has made it possible to offer direct DNA testing as a reliable and inexpensive diagnostic tool. Furthermore, because MCAD deficiency meets the criteria established for newborn screening (see Chapter 10), testing for it has been added to newborn screening programs in all fifty states of the United States and elsewhere.

Long-chain acyl-CoA fatty acids are metabolized in a sequence of steps catalyzed by a handful of different enzymes. The first step is controlled by long-chain acyl-CoA dehydrogenase (LCAD). The second step is catalyzed by enzymes that are part of an enzyme complex called the mitochondrial trifunctionalprotein (TFP). One of the enzymes of the TFP is long-chain L-3-hydroxyacyl-CoA dehydrogenase (LCHAD).

LCHAD deficiency is one of the most severe of the FAO disorders. The first cases reported manifested with severe liver disease ranging from fulminant neonatal liver failure to a chronic, progressive destruction of the liver. Over the last 10 years, the phenotype has expanded to include cardiomyopathy, skeletal myopathy, retinal disease, peripheral neuropathy, and sudden death. Its clinical and biochemical characteristics clearly differentiate it from other FAO disorders. Treatment consists of avoidance of fasting, a low-fat diet, supplementation with medium-chain triglycerides, and carnitine supplementation in some cases.

In the last decade, a number of women pregnant with a fetus affected with LCHAD deficiency have developed a severe liver disease called acute fatty liver of pregnancy (AFLP) and HELLP syndrome (**h**emolysis, **e**levated **l**iver function tests, **l**ow **p**latelets). It is hypothesized that failure of the fetus to metabolize free fatty acids results in the accumulation of abnormal fatty acid metabolites in the maternal liver and placenta. Accumulation in the liver might cause the abnormalities observed in women with AFLP and HELLP. Accumulation in the placenta might cause intrauterine growth retardation and increase the probability of preterm delivery, both of which are common in children with LCHAD deficiency.

Cholesterol

Elevated levels of plasma cholesterol have been associated with various conditions, most notably atherosclerotic heart disease. It has been demonstrated that substantially reduced levels of cholesterol can adversely affect growth and development. The final step of cholesterol biosynthesis is catalyzed by the enzyme Δ7-sterol reductase (DHCR7). For years it has been noted that persons with an autosomal recessive disorder called Smith-Lemli-Opitz (SLO) syndrome have reduced levels of cholesterol and increased levels of 7-dehydrocholesterol (a precursor of DHCR7). SLO is characterized by various congenital anomalies of the brain, heart, genitalia, and hands (Fig. 7-5). It is unusual in this respect because most inborn errors of metabolism do not cause congenital malformations.

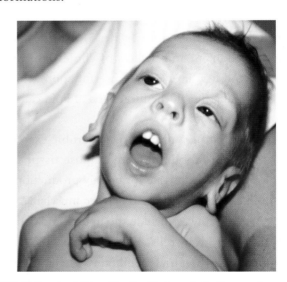

FIG 7-5 A child with Smith-Lemli-Opitz syndrome. Note the broad nasal root, upturned nasal tip, and inner epicanthal folds that are characteristic of this disorder. (From Jones K. *Smith's Recognizable Patterns of Human Malformation*. 6th ed. Philadelphia: Saunders; 2006: 116.)

In 1998, SLO was discovered to be caused by mutations in the *DHCR7* gene, and to date more than 100 different mutations in *DHCR7* have been found. Most of these are missense mutations that result in substitutions of a highly conserved residue of the protein. Population screens for mutant

DHCR7 alleles suggest that the carrier frequency in populations of European ancestry is 3% to 4%. This high frequency suggests the incidence of SLO should be much higher than is commonly observed. One explanation is that some pregnancies with affected fetuses result in miscarriages or that SLO is undetected in some mildly affected patients. Supplementing the diet of SLO children with cholesterol can ameliorate their growth and feeding problems, although its effect on cognitive development is less clear.

 The clinical presentation of children with defects of lipid metabolism varies from slow deterioration to sudden death. MCAD deficiency is the most common of these disorders. Most affected persons can be diagnosed by biochemical analysis of a drop of dried blood at birth.

Steroid Hormones

Cholesterol is the precursor for several major classes of steroid hormones including glucocorticoids (e.g., cortisol), mineralocorticoids (e.g., aldosterone), androgens (e.g., testosterone),and estrogens (Fig. 7-6). The actions of these steroid hormones are typically mediated by binding to an intracellular receptor, and these receptor-ligand complexes have myriad effects on a wide range of physiological processes. Defects in the synthesis of steroid hormones or their receptors can cause a wide variety of clinical abnormalities.

Congenital adrenal hyperplasia (CAH) consists of a group of genetically heterogeneous autosomal recessive disorders of cortisol biosynthesis. Approximately 95% of cases of CAH are caused by mutations in *CYP21A2*, the gene that encodes21-hydroxylase, and are characterized by cortisol deficiency, variable deficiency of aldosterone, and an excess of

FIG 7-6 Summary of steroid synthesis. Enzymes involved in the production of cortisol, aldosterone, and testosterone are indicated. (Modified from Turnpenny P. *Emery's Elements of Medical Genetics*. 13th ed. Philadelphia: Churchill Livingstone; 2007.)

androgens. The overall incidence of 21-hydroxylase deficiency is about 1 in 15,000; therefore, the carrier frequency is about 1in every 60 persons. However, the incidence of CAH varies widely among different ethnic groups. For example, among the Yupik of Alaska the incidence is 1 in 280.

The clinical severity of CAH varies widely and depends on the extent of residual 21-hydroxylase activity. The severe or classic form is typified by overproduction of cortisol precursors and thus excess adrenal androgens. In addition, aldosterone deficiency leads to loss of salt. In the milder forms, sufficient cortisol is produced, but there is still an over production of androgens. Female infants with CAH typically have ambiguous genitalia (Fig. 7-7) at birth due to in utero exposure to high concentrations of androgens, and CAH is the most common cause of ambiguous genitalia in 46,XX infants. Boys with CAH have normal genitalia at birth, so the age of diagnosis depends on the severity of aldosterone deficiency. Most boys have the salt-losing form of CAH and typically present between 7 and 14 days of age in adrenal crisis manifested as weight loss, lethargy, dehydration, hyponatremia (decreased plasma

Na$^+$ concentration), and hyperkalemia (increased plasma K$^+$ concentration). If CAH is left untreated, death soon follows. Adrenal crisis is less common in girls because their ambiguous genitalia typically leads to early diagnosis and intervention.

Boys who do not have a salt-losing form of CAH present at 2 to 4 years of age with premature virilization. Persons with nonclassic or mild CAH do not have cortisol deficiency but manifest symptoms in late childhood or adulthood caused by increased androgen levels including premature pubertal development, hirsutism (increased hair growth in women in areas where hair is usually thin), amenorrhea or oligomenorrhea, polycystic ovaries, or acne.

Treatment of CAH consists of replacing cortisol, suppressing adrenal androgen secretion, and providing mineralocorticoids to return electrolyte concentrations to normal. The surgical management of children born with ambiguous genitalia is complex and somewhat controversial, but most girls with CAH identify as female, and feminizing surgery during the first year of life is standard. In pregnancies in which the fetus is at risk for classic CAH, steroids are administered to the mother to suppress the fetal overproduction of androgens and reduce the incidence of ambiguous genitalia in affected female infants.

CYP21A2 is located on chromosome 6p21 within the major histocompatibility complex (MHC; see Chapter 9). More than 75% of mutant *CYP21A2* alleles are caused by gene conversion (gene conversion is a process in which two different DNA segments recombine in such a way that one segment is altered to become identical to the other.) in which deleterious mutations are transferred to *CYP1A2*. These mutations result in a protein product that lacks normal 21-hydroxylase activity.

FIG 7-7 A 46,XX infant with congenital adrenal hyperplasia. The external genitalia are virilized, with rugation and partial fusion of the labial folds. No gonads were palpable, and auterus and ovaries were visualized by ultrasonography. (Courtesy Melissa Parisi, University of Washington.)

 Congenital adrenal hyperplasia is a relatively common defect of cortisol synthesis that causes masculinization of the genitalia in females and premature virilization in males. It is commonly caused by diminished activity of 21-hydroxylase.

Steroid Hormone Receptors

Defects of most steroid hormone receptors are rare. For example, defects of the estrogen receptor have been found in a small number of persons in whom failed epiphyseal closure results in tall stature. Mutations in the gene that encodes the glucocorticoid receptor can produce hereditary resistance to the actions of cortisol.

In contrast, mutations in the X-linked gene that encodes the androgen receptor (AR) are relatively common. These mutations commonly result in complete or partial androgen in sensitivity syndromes (CAIS or PAIS) in 46,XY persons. CAIS was formerly called "testicular feminization syndrome" and is characterized by typical female external genitalia at birth, absent or rudimentary müllerian structures (i.e., fallopian tubes, uterus, and cervix), a short vaginal vault, inguinal or labial testis, and reduced or absent secondary sexual characteristics. Persons with PAIS can have ambiguous external genitalia, varied positioning of the testes, and absent or present secondary sexual characteristics. Nearly all affected persons are infertile.

CAIS and PAIS are transmitted in an X-linked recessive pattern. More than 95% of persons with CAIS have mutations in the *AR* gene, and to date, hundreds of different mutations have been found. Most of these mutations are predicted to impair androgen binding or binding of the androgen receptor to DNA. Expansion of a polyglutamine tract in the androgen receptor causes a completely different genetic disorder called spinal bulbar muscular atrophy (see Chapter 4).

The Hemoglobin Disorders

Hemoglobin disorders are the most common group of single-gene diseases: an estimated 7% of the world's population carries one or more mutations of the genes involved in hemoglobin synthesis. Because almost all of the types of mutation described in this chapter have been observed in the hemoglobin disorders, these diseases serve as an important illustration of the clinical consequences of mutation.

The hemoglobin molecule is a **tetramer** composed of four polypeptide chains, two labeled α and two labeled β. The β chains are encoded by a gene on chromosome 11, and the α chains are encoded by two genes on chromosome 16 that are very similar to each other. Typically, an individual has two normal β genes and four normal α genes (Fig. 7-8). Ordinarily, tight regulation of these genes ensures that roughly equal numbers of α and β chains are produced. Each of these **globin** chains is associated with a **heme** group, which contains an iron atom and binds with oxygen. This property allows hemoglobin to perform the vital function of transporting oxygen in erythrocytes (red blood cells).

The hemoglobin disorders can be classified into two broad categories: structural abnormalities, in which the hemoglobin molecule is altered, and thalassemias, a group of conditions in which either the α- or the β-globin chain is structurally normal but reduced in quantity. Another condition, hereditary persistence of fetal hemoglobin (HPFH), occurs when fetal hemoglobin, encoded by the α-globin genes and by two β-globin-like genes called ${}^{A}\gamma$ and ${}^{G}\gamma$ (see Fig. 7-8), continues to be produced after birth (normally, γ-chain production ceases and β-chain production begins at the time of birth). HPFH does not cause disease but instead can compensate for a lack of normal adult hemoglobin.

A large array of different hemoglobin disorders

FIG 7-8 The α-globin gene cluster on chromosome 16 and the β-globin gene cluster on chromosome 11. The β-globin cluster includes the ε-globin gene, which encodes embryonic globin, and the γ-globin genes, which encode fetal globin. The ψβ gene is not expressed. The α-globin cluster includes the ζ-globin gene, which encodes embryonic α-globin.

TABLE 7-3   Summary of the Major Hemoglobin Disorders

DISEASE	MUTATION TYPE	MAJOR DISEASE FEATURES
Sickle cell disease	β-globin missense mutation	Anemia, tissue infarctions, infections
HbH disease	Deletion or abnormality of three of the four α-globin genes	Moderately severe anemia, splenomegaly
Hydrops fetalis (Hb Barts)	Deletion or abnormality of all four α-globin genes	Severe anemia or hypoxemia, congestive heart failure; stillbirth or neonatal death
β^0-Thalassemia	Usually nonsense, frameshift, or splice-site donor or acceptor mutations; no β-globin produced	Severe anemia, splenomegaly, skeletal abnormalities, infections; often fatal during first decade if untreated
β^+-Thalassemia	Usually missense, regulatory, or splice-site consensus sequence or cryptic splice-site mutations; small amount of β-globin produced	Features similar to those of β^0-thalassemia but often somewhat milder

have been identified. The discussion that follows is a greatly simplified presentation of the major forms of these disorders. The hemoglobin disorders, the mutations that cause them, and their major features are summarized in Table 7-3.

Sickle Cell Disease

Sickle cell disease, which results from an abnormality of hemoglobin structure, is seen in approximately 1 in 400 to 1 in 600 African American births. It is even more common in parts of Africa, where it can affect up to 1 in 50 births, and it is also seen occasionally in Mediterranean and Middle Eastern populations. Sickle cell disease is typically caused by a single missense mutation that effects a substitution of valine for glutamic acid at position 6 of the β-globin polypeptide chain (Fig. 7-9). In homozygotes, this amino acid substitution alters the structure of hemoglobin molecules such that they form aggregates, causing erythrocytes to assume a characteristic sickle shape under conditions of low oxygen tension (see Fig. 7-9, A). These conditions are experienced in

FIG 7-9   A, Erythrocytes from patients with sickle cell disease assume a characteristic shape under conditions of low oxygen tension. **B,** Compare with normal erythrocytes.

capillaries, the tiny vessels whose diameter is smaller than that of the erythrocyte. Normal erythrocytes (see Fig. 7-9, B) can squeeze through capillaries, but sickled erythrocytes are less flexible and are unable to do so. In addition, the abnormal erythrocytes tend to stick to the vascular endothelium (the innermost lining of blood vessels).

The resultant vascular obstruction produces localized hypoxemia (lack of oxygen), painful sickling crises, and infarctions of various tissues, including bone, spleen, kidneys, brain, and lungs (an infarction is tissue death due to hypoxemia). Premature destruction of the sickled erythrocytes decreases the number of circulating erythrocytes and the hemoglobin level, producing **anemia**. The spleen becomes enlarged (splenomegaly), but infarctions eventually destroy this organ, producing some loss of immune function. This contributes to the recurrent and sometimes fatal bacterial infections (especially pneumonia) that are commonly seen in persons with sickle cell disease. About 10% of persons with sickle cell disease experience a stroke before age 20 years. In North America, it is estimated that the life expectancy of persons with sickle cell disease is reduced by about 30 years.

Sickle cell disease, which causes anemia, tissue infarctions, and multiple infections, is the result of a single missense mutation that produces an amino acid substitution in the β-globin chain.

Thalassemia

The term *thalassemia* is derived from the Greek word *thalassa* ("sea"); **thalassemia** was first described in populations living near the Mediterranean Sea, although it is also common in portions of Africa, the Mideast, India, and Southeast Asia. In contrast to sickle cell disease, in which a mutation alters the structure of the hemoglobin molecule, the mutations that cause thalassemia reduce the quantity of either α globin or β globin. Thalassemia can be divided into two major groups, α-thalassemia and β-thalassemia, depending on the globin chain that is reduced in quantity. When one type of chain is decreased in number, the other chain type, unable to participate

in normal tetramer formation, tends to form molecules consisting of four chains of the excess type only. These are termed **homotetramers**, in contrast to the **heterotetramers** normally formed by α and β chains. In α-thalassemia, the α-globin chains are deficient, so the β chains (or γ chains in the fetus) are found in excess. They form homotetramers that have a greatly reduced oxygen-binding capacity, producing hypoxemia. In β-thalassemia, the excess α chains form homotetramers that precipitate and damage the cell membranes of red blood cell precursors (i.e., the cells that form erythrocytes). This leads to premature erythrocyte destruction and anemia.

Most cases of α-thalassemia are caused by deletions of the α-globin genes. The loss of one or two of these genes has no clinical effect. The loss or abnormality of three of the α genes produces moderately severe anemia and splenomegaly (HbH disease). Loss of all four α genes, a condition seen primarily among Southeast Asians, produces hypoxemia in the fetus and *hydrops fetalis* (a condition in which there is a massive buildup of fluid). Severe hydrops fetalis often causes stillbirth or neonatal death.

The α-thalassemia conditions are usually caused by deletions of α-globin genes. The loss of three of these genes leads to moderately severe anemia, and the loss of all four is fatal.

Persons with a β-globin mutation in one copy of chromosome11 (heterozygotes) are said to have β-thalassemia minor, a condition that involves little or no anemia and does not ordinarily require clinical management. Those in whom both copies of the chromosome carry a β-globin mutation develop either β-thalassemia major (also called Cooley's anemia) or a less-serious condition, β-thalassemia intermedia. β-Globin may be completely absent (β^0-thalassemia), or it may be reduced to about 10% to 30% of the normal amount (β^+-thalassemia). Typically, β^0-thalassemia produces a more severe disease phenotype, but because disease features are caused by an excess of α-globin chains, patients with β^0-thalassemia are less severely affected when they also have α-globin mutations that reduce the quantity of α-globin chains.

β-thalassemia major are not seen clinically until the age of 2 to 6 months. These patients develop severe anemia. If the condition is left untreated, substantial growth retardation can occur. The anemia causes bone marrow expansion, which in turn produces skeletal changes, including a protuberant upper jaw and cheekbones and thinning of the long bones (making them susceptible to fracture). Splenomegaly (Fig. 7-10) and infections are common, and patients with untreated β-thalassemia major often die during the first decade of life. β-thalassemia can vary considerably in severity, depending on the precise nature of the responsible mutation.

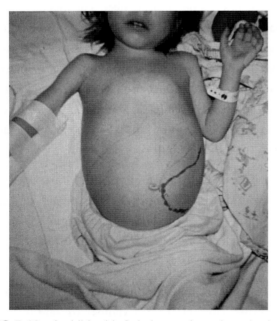

FIG 7-10   A child with β-thalassemia major who has severe splenomegaly.

In contrast to α-thalassemia, gene deletions are relatively rare in β-thalassemia. Instead, most cases are caused by single base mutations. Nonsense mutations, which result in premature termination of translation of the β-globin chain, usually produce β^0-thalassemia. Frameshift mutations also typically produce the β^0 form. In addition to mutations in the β-globin gene itself, alterations in regulatory sequences can occur. β-globin transcription is regulated by a promoter, two enhancers, and an upstream region known as the **locus control region (LCR)**

(see Fig. 7-8). Mutations in these regulatory regions usually result in reduced synthesis of mRNA and a reduction, but not complete absence, of β-globin (β^+-thalassemia). Several types of splice-site mutations have also been observed. If a point mutation occurs at a donor or acceptor site, normal splicing is destroyed completely, producing β^0-thalassemia. Mutations in the surrounding consensus sequences usually produce β^+-thalassemia. Mutations also occur in the cryptic splice sites found in introns or exons of the β-globin gene, which causes these sites to be available to the splicing mechanism. These additional splice sites then compete with the normal splice sites, producing some normal and some abnormal β-globin chains. The result is usually β^+-thalassemia.

> Many different types of mutations can produce β-thalassemia. Nonsense, frameshift, and splice-site donor and acceptor mutations tend to produce more severe disease. Regulatory mutations and those involving splice-site consensus sequences and cryptic splice sites tend to produce less severe disease.

Hundreds of different β-globin mutations have been reported. Consequently, most patients with β-thalassemia are not homozygotes in the strict sense: they usually have a *different* β-globin mutation on each copy of chromosome 11 and are termed **compound heterozygotes** (Fig. 7-11). Even though the mutations differ, each of the two β-globin genes is altered, producing a disease state. It is common to apply the term *homozygote* loosely to compound heterozygotes.

Patients with sickle cell disease or β-thalassemia major are sometimes treated with blood transfusions and with chelating agents that remove excess iron introduced by the transfusions. Prophylactic administration of antibiotics and antipneumococcal vaccine help to prevent bacterial infections in patients with sickle cell disease, and analgesics are administered for pain relief during sickling crises. Bone marrow transplantation, which provides donor stem cells

FIG 7-11 **A,** True homozygotes have two alleles that are identical in DNA sequence. Here, the homozygote has two copies of a single-base mutation, shown by the *asterisk* in the same position in the DNA sequence. Both mutations (alleles 1 and 2) have a loss-of-function effect, giving rise to a recessive disease. **B,** The same effect is seen in a compound heterozygote, which has two different mutations (*asterisks*) in two different locations in the gene's DNA sequence. Each allele has a loss-of-function effect, again causing a recessive disease.

that produce genetically normal erythrocytes, has been performed on patients with severe β-thalassemia or sickle cell disease. However, it is often impossible to find a suitably matched donor, and the mortality rate from this procedure is still fairly high (approximately 5% to 30%, depending onthe severity of disease and the age of the patient). A lack of normal adult β-globin can be compensated for by reactivating the genes that encode fetal β-globin (the γ-globin genes, discussed previously). Agents such as hydroxycarbamide and butyrate can reactivate these genes and are being investigated. Also, β-thalassemia is a strong candidate for gene therapy (see Chapter 10).

Peroxisomal Enzymes

Peroxisomes are organelles that contain more than 50 enzymes that catalyze synthetic and degradative metabolic functions related mainly to lipid metabolism. Disorders of peroxisomes are typically divided into two groups: peroxisome biogenesis disorders (PBDs) and the single peroxisomal enzyme deficiencies (PEDs).

The PBD group comprises four disorders: Zellweger syndrome, neonatal adrenoleukodystrophy, infantile Refsum disease, and rhizomelic chondrodysplasia punctata type 1. Zellweger syndrome is the most severe of these disorders and manifests in newborns as severe hypotonia, progressive disease of the white matter of the brain, a distinctive facial appearance, and typically death in infancy. Children with neonatal adrenoleukodystrophy have similar but less-severe symptoms along with seizures. Infantile Refsum disease is less severe than Zellweger syndrome and neonatal adrenoleukodystrophy, yet affected children still have developmental delay, learning disabilities, hearing loss, and visual impairment.

PBDs are caused by mutations in PEX genes that encode peroxins. These proteins are necessary both for peroxisome biogenesis and for importing proteins of the peroxisomal matrix and membrane. To date, mutations in more than a dozen different peroxin-encoding genes have been discovered, and for many of these genes, mutations can cause Zellweger syndrome, neonatal adrenoleukodystrophy, or infantile Refsum disease.

Nearly a dozen different PEDs have been described to date, and persons with these enzyme defects have widely disparate clinical characteristics depending on which peroxisomal function is primarily impaired. One of the most common is X-linked adrenoleukodystrophy (ALD), which involves faulty β-oxidation of very long chain fatty acids (VLCFA). ALD is subdivided into several disorders, depending in part on age of onset. The most common of these are childhood cerebral ALD or CCALD and adrenomyeloneuropathy (AMN).CCALD typically manifests between the ages of 3 and 10 years with progressive cognitive and behavioral deterioration that leads to profound disability. AMN causes similar but less severe neurological symptoms but has a much later age of onset and slower rate of progression. Unlike many X-linked recessive disorders, 40% to 50% of women who are heterozygous for ALD develop AMN-like symptoms.

> Peroxisomal defects cause a wide variety of neurological problems in children and adults. These range from relatively mild and slowly progressive to severe and life threatening.

Degradative Pathways

Most biomolecules are dynamic, perpetually being recycled as part of the normal metabolic state of a cell. Existing molecules are degraded into their constituents to produce substrates for building new molecules. The byproducts of energy production, substrate conversions, and anabolism also need to be processed and eliminated. Errors in these degradative pathways result in the accumulation of metabolites that would otherwise have been recycled or eliminated.

Lysosomal Storage Disorders

The lysosomal storage disorders are the prototypical inborn errors of metabolism: Disease results from the accumulation of substrate. Enzymes within lysosomes catalyze the stepwise degradation of sphingolipids, glycosaminoglycans (mucopolysaccharides), glycoproteins, and glycolipids. Accumulation (storage) of undegraded molecules results in cell, tissue, and organ dysfunction. Most of the lysosomal disorders are caused by enzyme deficiencies, although some are caused by the inability to activate an enzyme or to transport an enzyme to a subcellular compartment where it can function properly. Many of the lysosomal storage disorders are found with uncommonly high prevalence in various ethnic populations as a result of founder effect, genetic drift, and possibly natural selection (see Chapter 3).

Mucopolysaccharidosis

The **mucopolysaccharidosis** (MPS disorders) are a heterogeneous group of conditions caused by a reduced ability to degrade one or more glycosaminoglycans (e.g., dermatansulfate, heparan sulfate, keratan sulfate, chondroitin sulfate).These glycosaminoglycans are degradation products of proteoglycans found in the extracellular matrix. Ten different enzyme deficiencies cause six different MPS disorders, which share many clinical features (Table 7-4), but these disorders can be distinguished from each other by clinical, biochemical, and molecular analyses. Assays that measure enzyme activity in fibroblasts, leukocytes, serum, or dried blood spots are available for each MPS disorder, and prenatal testing after amniocentesis or chorionic villus sampling (see Chapter 10) is possible. Except for the X-linked Hunter syndrome, all of the MPS disorders are inherited in an autosomal recessive fashion.

All MPS disorders are characterized by chronic and progressive multisystem deterioration, which causes hearing, vision, joint, and cardiovascular dysfunction (Fig. 7-12). Hurler, severe Hunter, and Sanfilippo syndromes are characterized by intellectual disability, and normal cognition is observed in other MPS disorders.

Deficiency of iduronidase (MPS I) is the prototypic MPS disorder. It produces a spectrum of phenotypes that have been traditionally delimited into three groups—Hurler, Hurler-Scheie, and Scheie syndromes—which manifest severe, moderate, and mild disease, respectively. MPS I disorders cannot be distinguished from each other by measuring enzyme activity; therefore, the MPS I phenotype is usually assigned on the basis of clinical criteria. The iduronidase gene has been cloned, and eventually genotype-phenotype correlations may lead to earlier and more accurate classification.

Hunter syndrome (MPS II) is caused by a deficiency of iduronate sulfatase. It is categorized into

TABLE 7-4   Mucopolysaccharidosis*

NAME	MUTANT ENZYME	CLINICAL FEATURES
Hurler-Scheie (MPS-I)	α-L-Iduronidase	Coarse face, hepatosplenomegaly, corneal clouding, dysostosis multiplex,† intellectual disability
Hunter (MPS-II)	Iduronate sulfatase	Coarse face, hepatosplenomegaly, dysostosis multiplex, intellectual disability, behavioral problems
Sanfilippo A MPS-IIIA	Heparan-N-sulfamidase	Behavioral problems, dysostosis multiplex, intellectual disability
Sanfilippo B MPS-IIIB	α-N-Acetylglucosaminidase	Behavioral problems, dysostosis multiplex, intellectual disability
Sanfilippo C MPS-IIIC	Acetyl-CoA: α-glucosaminide N-acetyltransferase	Behavioral problems, dysostosis multiplex, intellectual disability
Sanfilippo D MPS-IIID	N-Acetylglucosamine-6-sulfatase	Behavioral problems, dysostosis multiplex, intellectual disability
Morquio A MPS-IVA	N-Acetylglucosamine-6-sulfatase	Short stature, bony dysplasia, hearing loss
Morquio B MPS-IVB	β-Galactosidase	Short stature, bony dysplasia, hearing loss
Maroteaux-Lamy MPS-VI	Aryl sulfatase B	Short stature, corneal clouding, cardiac valvular disease, dysostosis multiplex
Sly MPS-VII	β-Glucuronidase	Coarse face, hepatosplenomegaly, corneal clouding, dysostosis multiplex

*Hunter syndrome is an X-linked recessive disorder; the remaining MPS disorders are autosomal recessive.
†Dysostosis multiplex is a distinctive pattern of changes in bone, including a thickened skull, anterior thickening of the ribs, vertebral abnormalities, and shortened and thickened long bones.

FIG 7-12   **A,** A boy with a mutation in α-L-iduronidase, which causes Hurler syndrome. Note his coarse facial features, crouched stance, thickened digits, and protuberant abdomen. **B,** Transgenic mice with a targeted disruption of α-L-iduronidase. Progressive coarsening of the face is apparent as 8-week-old mice (*left*) grow to become 52-week-old mice (*right*). (Courtesy Dr. Lorne Clarke, University of British Columbia.)

mild and severe phenotypes based on clinical assessment. The onset of disease usually occurs between 2 and 4 years of age. Affected children develop coarse facial features, short stature, skeletal deformities, joint stiffness, and intellectual disability. The gene that encodes iduronate sulfatase is composed of 9 exons spanning 24 kb. Twenty percent of all identified mutations are large deletions, and most of the remainder are missense and nonsense mutations.

Symptomatic treatment has been the standard of care for MPS for many years. More recently, restoration of endogenous enzyme activity has been accomplished by either bone marrow transplantation (BMT) or enzyme replacement with recombinant enzyme. BMT has become the mainstay of treatment for persons with Hurler syndrome and has been shown to improve the coarse facial features, upper airway obstruction, and cardiac disease. It also appears to mitigate neurological deterioration, although the long-term outcomes are still being investigated. BMT has been less successful for other MPS disorders. BMT is, in general, also associated with substantial morbidity and mortality. Enzyme replacement for Hurler syndrome was approved by the U.S. Food and Drug Administration in 2003 and has been shown to improve hepatosplenomegaly and

respiratory disease. Early studies of enzyme replacement in Hunter syndrome (MPS II) and Maroteaux-Lamy syndrome (MPS VI) are promising. Enzyme replacement for Morquio A syndrome was recently approved by the FDA.

 Defects of glycosaminoglycan degradation cause a heterogeneous group of disorders called mucopolysaccharidosis (MPS disorder). All MPS disorders are characterized by progressive multisystem deterioration causing hearing, vision, joint, and cardiovascular dysfunction. These disorders can be distinguished from each other by clinical, biochemical, and molecular studies.

Sphingolipidoses (Lipid Storage Diseases)

Defects in the degradation of sphingolipids (sphingolipidoses) result in their gradual accumulation, which leads to multiorgan dysfunction (Table 7-5). Deficiency of the lysosomal enzyme glucosylceramidase (also known as glucocerebrosidaseor β-glucosidase), causes an accumulation of glucosylceramide that results in Gaucher disease. This condition is characterized by visceromegaly (enlarged visceral organs), multiorgan failure, and debilitating

TABLE 7-5 Lysosomal Storage Disorders*

NAME	MUTANT ENZYME	CLINICAL FEATURES
Tay-Sachs	β-Hexosaminidase A	Hypotonia, spasticity, seizures, blindness
Gaucher (type 1; nonneuropathic)	β-Glucosidase	Splenomegaly, hepatomegaly, bone marrow infiltration, brain usually spared
Niemann-Pick, type 1A	Sphingomyelinase	Hepatomegaly, corneal opacities, brain deterioration
Fabry	α-Galactosidase	Paresthesia of the hands and feet, corneal dystrophy, hypertension, renal failure, cardiomyopathy
G_{M1} gangliosidosis (infantile)	β-Galactosidase	Organomegaly, dysostosis multiplex,[†] cardiac failure
Krabbe	galactosylceramidase	Hypertonicity, blindness, deafness, seizures, (galactosylceramide-specific) atrophy of the brain
Metachromatic leukodystrophy	Aryl sulfatase A	Ataxia, weakness, blindness, brain atrophy (late-infantile)
Sandhoff	β-Hexosaminidase (total)	Optic atrophy, spasticity, seizures
Schindler	α-N-Acetylgalactosaminidase	Seizures, optic atrophy, retardation
Multiple sulfatase deficiency	Aryl sulfatase A, B, C	Retardation, coarse facial features, weakness, hepatosplenomegaly, dysostosis multiplex

*Of the lysosomal storage disorders included in this table, Fabry syndrome is X-linked recessive and the remainder are autosomal recessive.

[†]Dysostosis multiplex is a distinctive pattern of changes in bone, including a thickened skull, anterior thickening of the ribs, vertebral abnormalities, and shortened and thickened long bones.

skeletal disease. Gaucher disease has traditionally been divided into three subtypes, which can be distinguished by their clinical features. Type 1is most common and does not involve the central nervous system. Type 2 is the most severe, often leading to death within the first 2 years of life. Type 3 Gaucher disease is intermediate between the other two forms. In practice, the clinical phenotypes overlap, and the spectrum of Gaucher is so broad that it ranges from death in utero to persons who remain a symptomatic even in old age.

The extent to which specific organs are affected by Gaucher disease determines a person's clinical course. Splenomegaly, hepatomegaly, and pulmonary disease are shared among all three clinical types of Gaucher disease. Splenomegaly is associated with anemia, leukopenia, and thrombocytopenia, and splenic infarction can cause abdominal pain. Hepatomegalycan cause liver dysfunction, but cirrhosis and hepatic failure are uncommon.

Gaucher disease is caused by more than 400 different mutations in *GBA*, the gene that encodes glucosylceramidase. The frequency of alleles that cause type 1 Gaucher disease is particularly high in Ashkenazi Jews, in whom the five most common alleles account for 97% of all mutations. Persons with the same genotype can have very different clinical outcomes. However, persons with at least one p.*N370S* allele, the most common allele, do not develop primary neurological disease and tend to have a milder outcome in general.

Traditionally, treatment of persons with Gaucher disease was largely supportive (e.g., splenectomy for hypersplenism, blood transfusions for anemia). However, enzyme replacement can improve symptoms resulting from spleen, liver, and bone involvement in type 1 Gaucher disease. The effectiveness of enzyme replacement to treat neurological symptoms remains limited as the enzyme cannot pass through the blood-brain barrier. Some persons with severe involvement, particularly chronic neurological conditions, benefit from BMT.

Enzymes that function in lysosomes are targeted and transported into the lysosomal space by spe-

cific pathways. Targeting is mediated by receptors that bind mannose-6-phosphate recognition markers attached to the enzyme (i.e., a posttranslational modification). The synthesis of these recognition markers is deficient in I-cell disease (mucolipidosis II), so named because the cytoplasm of fibroblasts from affected persons was found by light microscopy to contain inclusions. These inclusions represent partially degraded oligosaccharides, lipids, and glycosaminoglycans. As a consequence of recognition marker deficiency, newly synthesized lysosomal enzymes are secreted into the extracellular space instead of being correctly targeted to lysosomes. Persons with I-cell disease have coarse facial features, skeletal abnormalities, hepatomegaly, corneal opacities, intellectual disability, and early death. There is no specific treatment for I-cell disease.

Many different lysosomal enzymes catalyze the degradation of sphingolipids, glycosaminoglycans, glycoproteins, and glycolipids. Deficiency of a lysosomal enzyme causes accumulation of substrate, visceromegaly, organ dysfunction, and early death if untreated. Genes encoding many of the lysosomal enzymes have been cloned, and treatment with bone marrow transplantation and enzyme replacement is effective for some conditions.

Urea Cycle Disorders

The primary role of the urea cycle is to prevent the accumulation of nitrogenous wastes by incorporating nitrogen into urea, which is subsequently excreted by the kidney. Additionally, the urea cycle is responsible for the de novo synthesis of arginine. The urea cycle consists of five major biochemical reactions (Fig. 7-13); defects in each of these steps have been described in humans.

Deficiencies of carbamyl phosphate synthetase (CPS), ornithine transcarbamylase (OTC), argininosuccinic acid synthetase (ASA), and argininosuccinase (AS) result in the accumulation of urea precursors such as ammonium and glutamine.

FIG 7-13 Schematic diagram of the urea cycle. *AS*, Argininosuccinase; *ASA*, argininosuccinic acid synthetase; *CoA*, coenzyme A; *CPS*, carbamyl phosphate synthetase; *NAGS*, *N*-acetylglutamatesynthetase; *OTC*, ornithine transcarbamylase.

Consequently, the clinical presentations of persons with CPS, OTC, ASA, and AS deficiencies are similar, producing progressive lethargy and coma and closely resembling the clinical presentation of Reye syndrome. Affected persons present in the neonatal period or at any time thereafter, and there is wide interfamilial variability in severity. In contrast, arginase deficiency causes a progressive spastic quadriplegia and intellectual disability. Differential diagnosis of these disorders is based on biochemical testing.

Each of these disorders, except OTC deficiency, is inherited in an autosomal recessive pattern. Although OTC deficiency is an X-linked disorder, women can be symptomatic carriers depending, in part, on the fraction of hepatocytes in which the normal allele is inactivated. The goal of therapy for each disorder is to prevent hyperammonemia by providing sufficient calories with a low-protein diet to maintain normal growth and development. Affected persons often require ammonia scavenging drugs such as glycerol phenylbutyrate, sodium phenylbutyrate, or sodium benzoate as well as supplementation with citrulline or arginine. Acute hyperammonemiais treated with hemodialysis and intravenous sodium phenylacetate and sodium benzoate.

OTC deficiency, an X-linked condition, is the most prevalent of the urea cycle disorders and thus has been intensively studied. A variety of exon dele-

tions and missense mutations have been described, and mutations that affect RNA processing have been observed.

 The urea cycle consists of five major biochemical reactions that convert nitrogenous waste products to urea, which is subsequently excreted by the kidney. Enzymatic defects in this pathway lead to the accumulation of urea precursors, progressive neurological impairment, and death if untreated. The genes that cause most of these disorders have been cloned, including the most common observed defect, X-linked ornithine transcarbamylase (OTC) deficiency.

Energy Production

Energy for cellular activities can be produced from many different substrates, including glucose, ketones, amino acids, and fatty acids. Catabolism of these substrates requires their stepwise cleavage into smaller molecules (via processes such as the citric acid cycle or β-oxidation), followed by passage of hydrogen ions through the oxidative phosphorylation (OXPHOS) system. Alternatively, some substrates are processed anaerobically.

The OXPHOS system consists of five multiprotein complexes that transfer electrons to O_2. These complexes are composed of more than 100 polypeptides and are located in the inner mitochondrial membrane. Thirteen of these polypeptides are encoded by the mitochondrial genome (see Fig. 4-32), and the remainder are encoded by nuclear genes. Thus, assembly and function of the OXPHOS system require ongoing signaling and transport between the nucleus and the mitochondrion. OXPHOS regulation is mediated by a wide variety of factors, including O_2 supply, hormone levels, and metabolite-induced transcription control.

More than 20 clinical disorders characterized by OXPHOS defects are caused by substitutions, insertions, or deletions in the mitochondrial genome and are maternally inherited (see Chapter 4). In addition, nuclear genes that can cause mitochondrial DNA (mtDNA) deletions or depletion of mtDNA have been isolated, and these disorders are inherited in an autosomal recessive pattern. Mutations in genes affecting the OXPHOS system produce very complex phenotypes as a consequence of the varying metabolic requirements of different tissues and systems at different developmental stages.

Electron transfer flavoprotein (ETF) and ETF-ubiquinoneoxidoreductase (ETF-QO) are nuclear-encoded proteins through which electrons can enter the OXPHOS system. Inherited defects in either of these proteins cause glutaric acidemia type II, which is characterized by hypotonia, hepatomegaly, hypoketotic or nonketotic hypoglycemia, and metabolic acidemia. Most affected persons present in the neonatal period or shortly thereafter, and despite aggressive therapy, affected children often die within months.

In most tissues, the metabolism of pyruvate proceeds through pyruvate dehydrogenase, the citric acid cycle, and the OXPHOS system. However, in tissues with high glycolytic activity and a reduced or absent OXPHOS capacity, the end products of metabolism are pyruvate and lactic acid (see Fig. 7-3). Lactate is produced by the reduction of pyruvate, and the bulk of circulating lactate is usually absorbed by the liver and converted to glucose. Defects in the pathways of

pyruvate metabolism produce lactic acidemia. The most common of such disorders is a deficiency of the pyruvate dehydrogenase (PDH) complex. It may be caused by mutations in the genes encoding one of five components of the PDH complex: E_1, E_2, E_3, X-lipoate, or PDH phosphatase. These disorders are characterized by varying degrees of lactic acidemia, developmental delay, and abnormalities of the central nervous system. It has been suggested that the facial features of some children with PDH deficiency resemble those of children with fetal alcohol syndrome (see Clinical Commentary 12-5 in Chapter 12). It has also been proposed that acetaldehyde from the circulation of mothers with alcoholism inhibits PDH in the fetus, creating a phenocopy of PDH deficiency.

 The phenotype produced by defects of energy metabolism is complex because of the varying oxidative demands of different tissues and organs. Once the condition is diagnosed, the goal of treatment is to use alternative pathways of energy production.

Transport Systems

The efficient movement of molecules between compartments (e.g., organelles, cells, the environment), and hence across a barrier, often requires a macromolecule that connects the compartments and mediates transport through the barrier. Abnormalities of these transport systems have myriad effects, depending on whether altered barrier integrity or the accumulation of substrate has a greater impact on normal physiology.

Cystine

Cystine is the disulfide derivative of the amino acid cysteine. Abnormal cystine transport can produce two diseases: cystinuria and cystinosis. Both disorders are inherited in an autosomal recessive fashion.

Abnormal cystine transport between cells and the extracellular environment causes cystinuria, one of the most common inherited disorders of metabolism. Although cystinuria produces substantial morbidity, early death is uncommon. Cystinuria is a genetically heterogeneous disorder caused by a defect of dibasic amino acid transport affecting the epithelial cells of the gastrointestinal tract and renal tubules. As a result, cystine, lysine, arginine, and ornithine are excreted in urine in quantities higher than normal. Cystine is the most insoluble of the amino acids; therefore, elevated urinary cystine predisposes to the formation of renal calculi (kidney stones). Complications of chronic nephrolithiasis (presence of kidney stones) include infection, hypertension, and renal failure. Treatment of cystinuria consists largely of rendering cystine more soluble. This is accomplished by administering pharmacological amounts of water (4-6 L/d), alkalinizing the urine, and using chelating agents such as penicillamine.

Based on amino acid excretion studies, cystinuria has been divided into three phenotypes. Type I cystinuria has been associated with missense, nonsense, and deletion mutations in a gene termed *soluble carrier family 3, member 1 amino acid transporter* (*SLC3A1*). Types II and III cystinuria are caused by mutations in a gene called *SLC7A9*. *SLC3A1* and *SLC7A9* encode the heavy and light subunits of the amino acid transporter $b^{0,+}$ located on the brush-border plasma membrane of epithelial cells in the proximal tubules of the kidney. In vitro studies of mutant SLC3A1 and SLC7A9 protein have demonstrated a marked reduction in transport activity, providing direct evidence for the role of these proteins in cystinuria.

Cystinosis is a rare disorder caused by a diminished ability to transport cystine across the lysosomal membrane. This produces an accumulation of cystine crystals in the lysosomes of most tissues. Affected persons are normal at birth but develop electrolyte disturbances, corneal crystals, rickets, and poor growth by the age of 1 year. Renal glomerular damage is severe enough to necessitate dialysis or transplantationwithin the first decade of life. Transplanted kidneys function normally, but chronic complications such as diabetes mellitus, pancreatic insufficiency, hypogonadism, myopathy, and blindness occur. Until recently, treatment was largely sup-

portive, including renal transplantation. However, cysteine depleting agents such as cysteamine have proved successful in slowing renal deterioration and improving growth. Long acting slow release cysteamine was recently approved by the FDA. Cystinosis is caused by mutations in the gene, *CTNS*, encoding an integral lysosomal membrane protein.

 The phenotype of transport defects is partly contingent on the degree of barrier disruption as well as the compartments through which normal traffic is compromised. Abnormal cystine transport between cells and the extracellular environment causes cystinuria, renal disease, and hypertension. Cystinosis is produced by a defect of cystine efflux from the lysosome; it leads to severe chronic disabilities and, if untreated, death.

Heavy Metals

Many of the enzymes controlling metabolic processes require additional factors (cofactors) to function properly and efficiently. These cofactors are commonly trace elements such as ions of heavy metals (metals that are more dense than those in the first two groups of the periodic table). At least 12 trace elements are essential to humans. For example, a zinc ion acts as a cofactor in carbonic anhydrase, placing a hydroxide ion next to carbon dioxide to facilitate the formation of bicarbonate. Although an adequate supply of trace elements is critical for normal metabolism, excessive amounts of circulating and/or stored heavy metals are highly toxic. Accordingly, a complex series of transport and storage proteins precisely control heavy metal homeostasis. Abnormalities of these proteins cause progressive dysfunction of various organs, often leading to premature death if untreated. Human disorders that disrupt the normal homeostasis of copper (Wilson disease, Menkes disease, occipital horn syndrome), iron (hereditary hemochromatosis; Clinical Commentary 7-2), and zinc (hereditary acrodermatitis enteropathica) have been described.

CLINICAL COMMENTARY 7-2
Hereditary Hemochromatosis

The term hemochromatosis refers to all disorders characterized by excessive iron storage. A subgroup of these disorders are hereditary and can be caused by mutations in one of several different genes. The most common form of hereditary hemochromatosis (HH) is an autosomal recessive disorder of iron metabolism in which excessive iron is absorbed in the small intestine and then accumulates in a variety of organs such as the liver, kidney, heart, joints, and pancreas. It was described by von Recklinghausen, the same physician who described neurofibromatosis 1, in 1889. Approximately 1 of every 8 northern Europeans is a carrier for HH, and 1 of every 200 to 400 persons is a homozygote. Although the penetrance of the disease-causing genotype is incomplete (as discussed later), HH is one of the most common genetic disorders observed in people of European ancestry. Its prevalence is much lower in Asian and African populations.

The most common symptom of HH is fatigue, although the clinical presentation of patients with HH can vary considerably. Additional findings include joint pain, diminished libido, diabetes, increased skin pigmentation, cardiomyopathy, liver enlargement, and cirrhosis. Abnormal serum iron parameters can identify most men at risk for iron overload, but HH is not detected in many premenopausal women. The most sensitive diagnostic test for HH is a liver biopsy accompanied by histochemical staining for hemosiderin (a form of stored iron).

As early as the 1970s, an increased frequency of the human leukocyte antigen HLA-A3 allele in HH patients indicated that an HH gene might be located near the major histocompatibility region (MHC) on chromosome 6p. Subsequent linkage studies confirmed this hypothesis in the late 1970s, but it was not until 1996 that the HH gene was cloned. The HH gene is a widely expressed HLA class I-like gene, *HFE*. The gene product is a cell-surface protein that binds to the transferrin receptor (transferring carries iron molecules), overlapping the binding site for transferrin and inhibiting transferrin-mediated iron uptake. However, this does not directly affect iron transport from the small intestine. Instead, this interaction is thought to be involved in a cell's ability to sense iron levels. This function is disrupted in persons with mutations in *HFE*, resulting in excessive iron absorption from the small intestine and iron overload. Thus, hemochromatosis is not caused by a defect of an iron transport protein but rather by a defect in the regulation of transport.

A single missense mutation that results in the substitution of a tyrosine for cysteine in a β2-microglobulin-binding domain accounts for 85% of all HH-causing mutations. A single ancestral haplotype predominates in Europeans, suggesting that there was a selective advantage conferred by having at least one copy of the HH gene. Because iron deficiency affects one third of the world's population and is significantly less common in HH heterozygotes, it is likely that this explains the higher incidence of HH in many populations.

Treatment of HH consists of reducing the accumulated iron in the body. This is accomplished by serial phlebotomy or by the use of an iron-chelating agent such as deferoxamine. Depending on the quantity of iron stored, return to a normal level of iron can take a few years. However, iron reduction prevents further liver damage, cures the cardiomyopathy, returns skin pigmentation to normal, and might improve the diabetes. Persons who have not developed irreversible liver damage have a nearly normal life expectancy.

The estimated penetrance of HH depends on a person's age, sex, and whether the presence of disease is measured by histological findings such as hepatic fibrosis or clinical symptoms. Most men who are homozygous for an HH-causing mutation do not develop clinical symptoms, and those who do are seldom symptomatic before the age of 40 years. An even smaller fraction of homozygous women develop clinical symptoms. If symptoms are seen, they typically occur 20 years or so later than in men because iron accumulation in women is tempered by iron losses during menstruation, gestation, and lactation (Fig. 7-14).

FIG 7-14 Comparison of hemosiderin stain of normal liver **(A)** with hemosiderin stain of livers from persons affected with hemochromatosis **(B, C,** and **D).** Note the varying degree of increased deposition of hemosiderin in livers of HH homozygotes. This damages the liver, impairs its function, and can lead to cirrhosis and liver cancer.

Copper

Copper is absorbed by epithelial cells of the small intestine and is subsequently distributed by various chaperone proteins that shuttle it to different places in the cell (e.g., cytoplasmic enzymes that use copper as a cofactor, enzymes in the mitochondria). Some copper is transported to the liver to be incorporated into proteins that distribute it to other parts of the body (e.g., brain). Excess copper in hepatocytes is secreted into bile and excreted from the body.

Menkes disease (MND) is an X-linked recessive disorder described in 1962 by John Menkes, who studied five male siblings, all of whom died before 3 years of age. MND is characterized by intellectual disability, seizures, hypothermia, twisted and hypopigmented hair (pili torti), loose skin, arterial rupture, and death in early childhood. In MND patients, copper can be absorbed by the gastrointestinal epithelium but cannot be exported effectively from these cells into the blood stream. Consequently, when the intestinal cells slough, the trapped copper is excreted from the body. The lack of available copper leads to an overall deficiency of copper.

Copper is a required cofactor in tyrosinase, lysyl oxidase, superoxide dismutase, cytochrome c oxidase, and dopamine β-hydroxylase. Reduced availability of copper leads to impaired enzyme function, explaining the major clinical features of MND. For example, lysyl oxidase is required for cross-linking collagen and elastin; therefore, ineffectual crosslinking leads to weakened vascular walls and laxity of the skin. Treatment of MND consists of restoring copper levels in the body to normal. Because copper cannot be absorbed via the gastrointestinal tract in MND patients, it must be administered by an alternative route such as subcutaneous injections. Patients treated this way have demonstrated some clinical improvement. However, none of the abnormalities is completely corrected or prevented. Based on studies in an animal model of MND, the brindled mouse, it has been proposed that treatment for MND would be most effective if it were started in mid-gestation. Consequently, prenatal therapy is being investigated.

In contrast to MND, in which a deficiency of copper causes disease, Wilson disease (WND) results from an excess of copper caused by defective excretion of copper into the biliary tract. This causes progressive liver disease and neurological abnormalities. WND, an autosomal recessive disorder, was first described by Kinnear Wilson in 1912 and was called hepatolenticular degeneration because of end-stage destruction of the liver and brain. Only in the 1940s did it become clear that these findings were due to the accumulation of copper. Further progress in understanding the defect underlying WND was not made until the 1990s.

Patients with WND usually present with acute or chronic liver disease in childhood. If WND is left untreated, the liver disease is progressive, resulting in liver insufficiency, cirrhosis, and failure. Adults commonly develop neurological symptoms such as dysarthria (the inability to correctly articulate words) and diminished coordination. Accumulation of copper can also cause arthropathy (inflammation of the joints), cardiomyopathy (abnormal function of the heart muscle), kidney damage, and hypoparathyroidism (diminished secretion of or response to parathormone). Deposition of copper in Descemet's membrane (at the limbus of the cornea) produces a characteristic finding in the eye (the Kayser-Fleischer ring), which is observed in 95% of all WND patients and 100% of WND patients with neurological symptoms.

Biochemical testing can be used to confirm the diagnosis of WND. Findings include decreased serum ceruloplasmin, increased serum nonceruloplasmin copper, increased urinary copper excretion, and increased deposition of copper in the liver. The most sensitive indicator of WND is the reduced incorporation of isotopes of copper into cells cultured in vitro. Treatment of WND consists of reducing the load of accumulated copper through the use of chelating agents such as penicillamine and trientine. Zinc salts are effective chelating agents for maintenance of copper levels.

In 1993 the gene responsible for MND, *ATP7A*, was cloned. It encodes an adenosine triphosphatase with six tandem copies of a heavy-metal-binding sequence homologous to previously identified bacterial proteins that confer resistance to toxic heavy metals. The high sequence conservation between human and bacterial binding sequences indicated that *ATP7A* has an important role in regulating heavy-metal ion transport. *ATP7A* is expressed in a variety of tissues but not the liver, suggesting that a similar gene that is expressed in the liver might cause WND. Portions of the *ATP7A* gene were used as a probe to test for the presence of a similar gene on chromosome 13 (the known location of a *WND* gene, revealed by linkage analysis). This strategy led to the cloning in 1993 of *ATP7B*, the gene that, when mutated, causes WND. The protein product is highly homologous (76% amino acid homology) to that of *ATP7A*. In contrast to *ATP7A*, *ATP7B* is expressed predominantly in the liver and kidney, which are major sites of involvement in WND.

The ATP7A protein is usually localized to the Golgi network within a cell, where it supplies copper to various enzymes. When copper levels in an epithelial cell of the small intestine exceed a certain concentration, ATP7A redistributes to the plasma membrane and pumps copper into the bloodstream. When copper levels drop, ATP7A returns to the Golgi network. Thus, it mediates the efflux of copper into the bloodstream. ATP7A is also an important transporter of copper across the blood-brain barrier.

A variety of missense, nonsense, and splice site mutations in *ATP7A* have been found in MND patients. Approximately15% to 20% of the mutations in *ATP7A* are large deletions. Several mutations of splice sites in *ATP7A* have been associated with another disorder called the occipital horn syndrome (also known as X-linked cutis laxa or Ehlers-Danlos syndrome type IX), which is characterized by mild intellectual disability, bladder and ureteric diverticula (cul-de-sac-like herniations through the wall), skin and joint laxity, and ossified occipital (the most posterior bone of the calvarium) horns. These mutations permit the production of a small amount of normal protein and prevent development of severe neurological symptoms.

ATP7B plays a similar role as an effector of copper transport. However, it moves between the Golgi network and either endosomes or the cell membrane of hepatocytes, and it controls the excretion of copper into the biliary tree. ATP7B also aids in the incorporation of copper into ceruloplasmin. Several hundred different mutations have been described inpatients with WND. A single missense mutation accounts for about 40% of disease-causing alleles in persons of northern European ancestry.

 Wilson disease (WND) is an autosomal recessive disorder characterized by progressive liver disease and neurological abnormalities. Menkes disease (MND) is an X-linked recessive disorder characterized by intellectual disability, seizures, and death in early childhood. Accumulation of excess copper causes disease in WND, and MND results from a lack of copper and impaired enzyme function. WND and MND are caused by mutations in the highly homologous genes, *ATP7B* and *ATP7A*, respectively.

Zinc

Acrodermatitis enteropathica (AE) is caused by a defect in the absorption of zinc from the intestinal tract. Persons with AE experience growth retardation, diarrhea, dysfunction of the immune system, and a severe dermatitis (inflammation of the skin) that typically affects the skin of the genitals and buttocks, around the mouth, and on the limbs (Fig. 7-15). Children usually present after weaning, and AE can be fatal if it is not treated with high doses of supplemental zinc, which is curative. AE is caused by mutations in *SLC39A4*, which encodes a putative zinc-transporter protein expressed on the apical membrane of the epithelial cell of the small intestine. It is unknown whether persons with AE can still absorb small amounts of zinc through a mutant form of this transporter or whether another transporter exists that can also transport zinc when it is given in high doses.

FIG 7-15 A child with acrodermatitis enteropathica caused by mutations in *SLC39A4*, encoding a protein necessary for intestinal absorption of zinc. The resulting deficiency of zinc produces a characteristic scaly, red rash around the mouth, genitals, buttocks, and limbs. (Courtesy Dr. Virginia Sybert, University of Washington.)

SUMMARY

Almost all biochemical processes of human metabolism are catalyzed by enzymes. Variations of enzymatic activity among humans are common, and a minority of these variants cause disease. These concepts were introduced by Archibald Garrod and exemplified in his studies of alkaptonuria. Although individual metabolic disorders are rare, their overall direct and indirect contribution to morbidity and mortality is substantial. Most inborn errors of metabolism are inherited in an autosomal recessive pattern. Galactosemia is one of the most common inherited disorders of carbohydrate metabolism. Hyperphenylalaninemias are the most common defects of amino acid metabolism. Classic phenylketonuria is caused by mutations in the gene that encodes phenylalanine hydroxylase. Hyperphenylalaninemias are treated by restricting dietary intake of phenylalanine-containing foods. The clinical presentation of children with defects of lipid metabolism varies from slow deterioration to sud-

den death. Medium-chain acyl-CoA dehydrogenase (MCAD) deficiency is the most common of these disorders. Sickle cell disease, which causes anemia, tissue infarctions, and multiple infections, is the result of a single missense mutation that produces an amino acid substitution in the β-globin chain. The α-thalassemia conditions are usually caused by deletions of α-globin genes. The loss of three of these genes leads to moderately severe anemia, and the loss of all four is fatal. Many different types of mutations can produce β-thalassemia. Nonsense, frameshift, and splice-site donor and acceptor mutations tend to produce more severe disease. Regulatory mutations and those involving splice-site consensus sequences and cryptic splice sites tend to produce less severe disease. Defects of glycosaminoglycan degradation cause a heterogeneous group of disorders called mucopolysaccharidosis (MPS) disorders. The urea cycle consists of five major biochemical reactions that convert nitrogenous waste products to urea, which is subsequently excreted by the kidney. Enzymatic defects in this pathway lead to the accumulation of urea precursors, progressive neurologic impairment, and death if untreated. The phenotypes produced by defects of energy metabolism are complex because of the varying oxidative demands of different tissues and organs. The phenotypes of transport defects are partly contingent on the degree of barrier disruption as well as the compartments through which normal traffic is compromised.

IMPORTANT TERMINOLOGY

alkaptonuria (AKU)   尿黑酸尿症
metabolic disorder   代谢性疾病
phenocopy   拟表型
phenylketonuria (PKU)   苯丙酮尿症
galactosemia   半乳糖血症
catalyst   催化剂
hemoglobin disorder   血红蛋白病
tetramer   四聚体
sickle cell disease   镰状细胞病
thalassemia   地中海贫血
mucopolysaccharidosis (MPS disorders)   黏多醣
  贮积症

REVIEW QUESTIONS

1. Garrod found alkaptonuria to be more common in the offspring of consanguineous matings. Explain this finding. In general, what is the association between the coefficient of relationship and the prevalence of an inborn error of metabolism?

2. If many metabolic reactions can proceed in the absence of an enzyme, explain how diminished or absent enzyme activity can produce disease.

3. Despite the low prevalence of most metabolic disorders, why is it important to understand the pathogenesis of inborn errors of metabolism?

4. Describe three types of metabolic processes and give examples of disorders disturbing each of them.

5. Galactosemia is diagnosed in a 1-week-old neonate, yet enzymatic activity of GAL-1-P uridyl transferase is normal. Interpret these results and explain how mutations of different genes can produce a similar phenotype.

6. The prevalence of PKU varies from 1 in 10,000 to less than 1 in 100,000. Explain how prevalence rates of inborn errors of metabolism can vary so widely among different ethnic groups.

7. An 18-year-old woman comes to your office for prenatal counseling. She had a younger brother who died from a defect of mitochondrial fatty acid oxidation when he was a few months old. What is her risk of having an affected child? Explain your answer.

8. An 8-year-old girl develops hyperammonemia and is critically ill. Biochemical testing performed on a liver biopsy confirms that she has OTC deficiency. Which genetic test would you order next? Why?

9. Disorders of the OXPHOS system are commonly associated with elevated blood lactic acid levels. Explain this finding.

10. Polymorphisms that affect metabolism presumably have been maintained by selection because they offer heterozygotes a slight advantage. Provide an example of how these polymorphisms might have been advantageous to a group of hunter-gatherers 10,000 years ago.

SUGGESTED READINGS AND WEBSITES

1. Allen KJ, Gurrin LC, Constantine CC, et al. Iron-overload-related disease in HFE hereditary hemochromatosis. *N Engl J Med.* 2008; 358(3): 221-230.

2. Barton JC. Hemochromatosis and iron overload: from bench to clinic. *Am J Med Sci.* 2013; 346: 403-412.

3. Berry GT. Galactosemia: when is it a newborn screening emergency? *Mol Genet Metab.* 2012; 106: 7-11.

4. Bosch AM. Classical galactosemia revisited. *J Inherit Metab Dis.* 2006; 29: 516-525.

5. Gahl WA. Chemical individuality: concept and outlook. *J Inherit Metab Dis.* 2008; 31: 630-640.

6. Haberle J, Boddaert N, Burlina A, et al. Suggested guidelines for the diagnosis and management of urea cycle disorders. *Orphanet J Rare Dis.* 2012; 7: 1-30.

7. Hollak CEM, Wijburg FA. Treatment of lysosomal storage disorders: successes and challenges. *J Inherit Metab Dis.* 2014; 37: 587-598.

8. Mayatepek E, Hoffmann B, Meissner T. Inborn errors of carbohydrate metabolism. *Best Pract Res Clin Gastroenterol.* 2010; 24: 607-618.

9. McCabe LL, McCabe ERB. Expanded newborn screening: implications for genomic medicine. *Annu Rev Med.* 2008; 59: 163-175.

10. Ranciaro A, Campbell MC, Hirbo JB, et al. Genetic origins of lactase persistence and the spread of pastoralism in Africa. *Am J Hum Genet.* 2014; 94: 496-510.

11. Rosencrantz R, Schilsky M. Wilson disease: pathogenesis and clinical considerations in diagnosis and treatment. *Semin Liver Dis.* 2011; 31: 245-259.

12. Scriver CR, Sly WS, Childs B, et al. *The Metabolic and Molecular Bases of Inherited Disease.* New York: McGraw-Hill; 2001.

13. Scriver CR. The PAH gene, phenylketonuria, and a paradigm shift. *Hum Mutat.* 2007; 28: 831-845.

14. Vockley J, Andersson HC, Antshel KM, et al. Phenylalaninehydroxylase deficiency: diagnosis and management guideline. *Genet Med.* 2014; 16: 188-200.

15. White PC, Bachega TA. Congenital adrenal hyperplasia due to 21hydroxylase deficiency: from birth to adulthood. *Semin Reprod Med*. 2012; 30: 400-409.

16. Wilcken B. Fatty acid oxidation disorders: outcome and long-term prognosis. *J Inherit Metab Dis*. 2010; 33: 501-506.

(Anbing Shi)

Chapter 8

Cancer Genetics

Present evidence indicates that approximately one in four deaths is now due to cancer and that invasive cancer will be diagnosed in more than half of the population at some point in their lives. Many cancers are increasing in incidence, largely as a result of the increased average age of our population.

As shown in this chapter, the causes of cancer are a mixture of environmental and genetic alterations that occur in our tissues. Inherited predisposition plays a role in some families. Dramatic advances in molecular biology and genetics have now clarified the basic molecular elements of cancer and provide a schematic outline of the cellular events leading to cancer. This understanding will be crucially important in the control of cancer, providing the beginnings of a base of knowledge that should lead to significantly improved therapies and preventive strategies.

"Cancer" is a collection of disorders that share the common feature of uncontrolled cell growth. This leads to a mass of cells termed a **neoplasm** (Greek, "new formation"), or **tumor**. The formation of tumors is called **tumorigenesis**. Several key events must occur if cells are to escape the usual constraints that prevent uncontrolled proliferation. Additional growth signals must be produced and processed, and cells must become resistant to signals that normally inhibit growth. Because these abnormal characteristics would typically trigger the process of programmed cell death (**apoptosis**), cells must somehow disable this process. The growing cell mass (tumor) requires nourishment, so a new blood supply must be obtained through **angiogenesis** (the formation of new blood vessels). Additional inhibitory signals must be overcome for the tumor to achieve a **malignant** state, in which neoplasms invade nearby tissues and metastasize (spread) to more distant sites in the body. The capacity to invade and metastasize distinguishes malignant from **benign** neoplasms.

Tumors are classified according to the tissue type in which they arise. Major types of tumors include those of epithelial tissue (**carcinomas**, the most common tumors), connective tissue (**sarcomas**), lymphatic tissue (**lymphomas**), glial cells of the central nervous system (**gliomas**), and hematopoietic organs (**leukemias**). The cells that compose a tumor are usually derived from a single ancestral cell, making them a single clone (**monoclonal**).

Many of the basic biological features of **carcinogenesis** (cancer development) are now understood. Throughout our lives, many of our cells continue to grow and differentiate. These cells form, for example, the epithelial layers of our lungs and colons and the precursor cells of our immune systems. Relatively undifferentiated stem cells produce large numbers of progeny cells to repopulate and renew our worn defensive layers. Through integration of information provided by a complex array of biochemical signals, the new cells eventually stop dividing and terminally differentiate into a cell type appropriate for their role in the body (Fig. 8-1). Alternatively, if the cell is abnormal or damaged, it may undergo apoptosis.

FIG 8-1 In response to environmental signals, a cell might continue to divide or it might differentiate or die (apoptosis).

Occasionally one of these cells fails to differentiate and begins to divide without restraint. The descendants of such cells can become the founders of neoplasms, capable of further transformation into invasive, metastatic cancer. We wish to understand in detail what has gone wrong in these cells, to detect them early, and ultimately to intervene in their development so as to eliminate them.

> ▶ Cells in the body are programmed to develop, grow, differentiate, and die in response to a complex system of biochemical signals. Cancer results from the emergence of a clone of cells freed of these developmental programming constraints and capable of inappropriate proliferation.

CAUSES OF CANCER

Genetic Considerations

Genetic alterations of cell regulatory systems are the primary basis of carcinogenesis. We can create cancer in animal models by damaging specific genes. In cell culture systems, we can reverse a cancer phenotype by introducing normal copies of the damaged genes into the cell. Most of the genetic events that cause cancer occur in somatic cells. The frequency of these events can be altered by exposure to mutagens, thus establishing a link to environmental **carcinogens** (cancer-causing agents). However, these genetic events are not transmitted to future generations because they occur in somatic, rather than germline, cells.

Even though they are *genetic* events, they are not *inherited*.

It is also possible for **cancer-predisposing mutations** to occur in germline cells. This results in the transmission of cancer-causing genes from one generation to the next, producing families that have a high incidence of specific cancers (Fig. 8-2). Such "cancer families," although rare, demonstrate that inheritance of a damaged gene can cause cancer. In these families, inheritance of one mutant allele seems sufficient to cause a specific form of cancer. Most individuals who inherit the mutant allele will develop a tumor. This is because each of their cells now carries the altered gene and thus has already taken the first step down the cancer pathway. The childhood cancer of the eye, retinoblastoma, is a good example. As discussed in Chapter 4, those who inherit a mutant version of the retinoblastoma gene have approximately a 90% chance of developing one or more retinoblastoma tumors.

Although the transmission of cancer as a single-gene disorder is relatively uncommon, there is good evidence for more frequent clustering of some cancer types in families. For many kinds of cancer, such as those of the breast and colon, the diagnosis of the cancer in a first-degree relative implies at least a two-fold increase in one's risk of developing the cancer. It is very likely that the inheritance of altered forms of specific genes is at least partly responsible for this increased risk.

The extent to which each of these mechanisms—inherited germline mutations versus mutations occurring in somatic cells—contributes to human

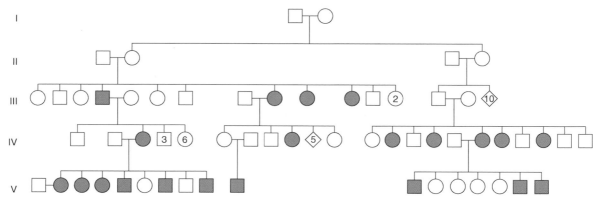

FIG 8-2   A familial colon cancer pedigree. *Darkened symbols* represent individuals with diagnosed colon cancer.

cancer is an important question. If inherited predispositions are significant determinants of a person's risk of acquiring a specific form of cancer, it should be possible to identify those whose risk is elevated. More intensive screening of defined high-risk groups could result in early detection and intervention, leading to better prognoses for patients and lowered morbidity and mortality.

▶ The basic cause of cancer is damage to specific genes. Usually, mutations in these genes accumulate in somatic cells over the years, until a cell accumulates a sufficient number of errors to initiate a tumor. If damage occurs in cells of the germline, however, an altered form of one of these genes can be transmitted to progeny and predispose them to cancer. The increased risk of cancer in such persons is due to the fact that each of their cells now carries the first step in a multistep cancer pathway.

Environmental Considerations

What is the role of the nongenetic environment in carcinogenesis? At the level of the cell, cancer seems intrinsically genetic. Tumor cells arise when certain changes, or mutations, occur in genes that are responsible for regulating the cell's growth. However, the frequency and consequences of these mutations can be altered by a large number of environmental factors. It is well documented, for example, that many chemicals that cause mutation in experimental animals also cause cancer and are thus carcinogens. Furthermore, other environmental agents can enhance the growth of genetically altered cells without directly causing new mutations. Thus, it is often the interaction of genes with the environment that determines carcinogenesis; both play key roles in this process.

Two additional lines of argument support the idea that exposure to environmental agents can significantly alter a person's risk of cancer. The first is that a number of environmental agents with carcinogenic properties have been identified. For example, epidemiological studies and laboratory experiments have shown that cigarette smoke causes lung and other types of cancer. Roles for other environmental agents in specific cancers are also well documented (e.g., uranium dust in lung cancer among miners, asbestos exposure in lung cancer and mesothelioma).

The second line of argument is based on epidemiological comparisons among populations with differing lifestyles. Many kinds of cancer have quite different frequencies in different populations. Breast cancer, for example, is prevalent among northern Europeans and European Americans but relatively rare among women in developing countries. It is usually difficult to determine whether such dissimilarities reflect differences in lifestyle or in gene frequencies.

Examination of genetically similar populations under differing lifestyles, however, provides an opportunity to evaluate the genetic and environmental components of cancer. Epidemiological studies among migrant Japanese populations have yielded important findings with respect to colon cancer. This type of cancer was, until recently, relatively rare in the Japanese population living in Japan, with a lifetime risk of 0.5%, but it is 10 times more common in the United States. Stomach cancer, on the other hand, is common in Japan but relatively rare in the United States. These statistics in themselves cannot distinguish environmental from genetic influences in the two populations. However, because large numbers of Japanese have immigrated, first to Hawaii and then to the U.S. mainland, we can observe what happens to the rates of stomach and colon cancer among the immigrants. It is important to note that many of the Japanese immigrants maintained a genetic identity, marrying largely among themselves. Among the first-generation Japanese in Hawaii, the incidence of colon cancer rose several-fold— not yet as high as in the U.S. mainland, but higher than in Japan. Among second-generation Japanese Americans on the U.S. mainland, the colon cancer rate rose to 5%, equal to the U.S. average. At the same time, stomach cancer has become relatively rare among Japanese Americans.

These observations strongly suggest an important role for environment or lifestyle in the etiology of colon cancer. In each case, diet is a likely culprit: A high-fat, low-fiber diet in the United States is thought to increase the risk of colon cancer, whereas techniques used to preserve and season the fish commonly eaten in Japan are thought to increase the risk of stomach cancer. It is also interesting that the incidence of colon cancer in Japan has increased dramatically during the past several decades, as the Japanese population has adopted a diet more similar to that of North America and Europe.

Are we then to assume that genetic factors play no role in colon cancer? The fact remains that in the North American environment some people will get colon cancer and others will not. This distinction can result from differences within this environment (e.g., dietary variation) as well as differences in genetic predisposition: inherited genes that increase a person's probability of developing cancer. To account for the difference in colon cancer incidence between Japanese living in the U.S. and those living in Japan, it is argued that environmental features in Japan render the predisposing genes less penetrant. Furthermore, a genetic component is strongly suggested by the several-fold increase in risk to a person when a first-degree relative has colon cancer. It is likely, then, that cancer risk is a composite of both genetics and environment, with interaction between the two components.

▶ Environmental factors are known to play important roles in carcinogenesis. However, a person's overall cancer risk depends on a combination of inherited factors and environmental components.

CANCER GENES

Genetic Control of Cell Growth and Differentiation

Cancers form when a clone of cells loses the normal controls over growth and differentiation. More than 100 cancer-causing genes that encode proteins par-

ticipating in this regulation have now been identified. Characterization of the biochemical activities and interactions of these gene products has revealed an increasingly detailed picture of the normal regulation of cell growth and differentiation and the ways these processes become deregulated by the events of carcinogenesis.

Many features of this fundamental process are now well understood (Fig. 8-3). One component of cell regulation is mediated by external signals coming to the cell through **growth factors** (e.g., platelet-derived growth factor, epidermal growth factor, steroid hormones) produced in other cells. Each growth factor interacts with specific **growth factor receptors** located on the cell surface. Binding of a growth factor activates the receptor, triggering molecules that send messages to the cell's nucleus in the process of **signal transduction**. These signal transduction molecules include **protein kinases**, such as src tyrosine kinase, mitogen-activated protein kinase (MAPK), and jun kinase (JunK), which can alter the activity of target

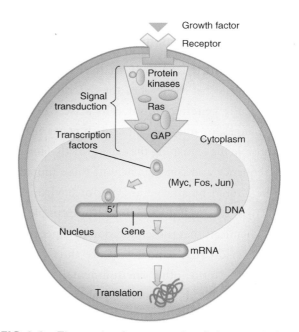

FIG 8-3 The major features of cellular regulation. External growth factors (proteins and steroid hormones such as epidermal growth factor) bind to membrane-spanning growth factor receptors on the cell surface, activating signal transduction pathways in which genes such as *RAS* participate. Components of the signal-transduction pathway in turn interact with nuclear transcription factors, such as Myc and Fos, which can bind to regulatory regions in DNA. *mRNA*, Messenger RNA.

proteins by tagging them at a specific site with a phosphate molecule (phosphorylation). The ultimate stage of the signal transduction pathway is regulation of DNA transcription in the nucleus. Components of the signal transduction cascade interact with nuclear transcription factors that regulate the activity of specific genes whose protein products influence cellular growth and proliferation. Genes that encode these transcription factors include *MYC*, *FOS*, and *JUN*.

After several rounds of cell division, cells normally receive signals that tell them to stop growing and to differentiate into specialized cells. The signals may come from polypeptides, from steroid hormones, from direct contact with adjacent cells, or from internal programs that define the number of cell divisions that are allowed. The signals are transduced to the nucleus of the recipient cell. Here, by altering the transcription patterns of genes that govern the steps of the cell cycle, they repress genes that promote cell division and induce genes that inhibit entry into the cell division cycle.

The regulation of cell growth is accomplished by substances that include: (1) growth factors that transmit signals from one cell to another; (2) specific receptors for the growth factors; (3) signal transduction molecules that activate a cascade of phosphorylating reactions within the cell; and (4) nuclear transcription factors. The cell integrates and interprets the host of signals it receives from its environment. Decisions to grow and divide, or to stop growing and differentiate, result from processing of these signals.

A cancer cell can emerge from within a population of growing cells through the accumulation of mutations in these genes. Although such mutations occur only rarely, these cells can fail to respond to differentiation signals and continue to divide instead of undergoing their normal differentiation program. Furthermore, cancers seem usually to result from a progressive series of events that incrementally increase the extent of deregulation within a cell lineage. Eventually, a cell emerges whose descendants multiply without appropriate restraints. Further changes give these cells the capacity to invade adjacent tissues and form metastases. Each of these changes involves mutations, and the requirement for more than one mutation has been characterized as the **multi-hit concept of carcinogenesis**. An example of this concept is given by colorectal cancer, in which several genetic events are required to complete the progression from a benign growth to a malignant neoplasm (see later discussion).

Mutations can occur in any of the steps involved in regulation of cell growth and differentiation. Accumulation of such mutations within a cell lineage can result in a progressive deregulation of growth, eventually producing a tumor cell.

The Inherited Cancer Gene versus the Somatically Altered Gene

Although "cancer families" have long been recognized, it was not until the early 1970s that we began to understand the relationship between the inherited genetic aberrations and the carcinogenic events that occur in somatic tissue. In 1971, A. G. Knudson's analysis of **retinoblastoma**, a disease already mentioned as a model of inherited cancer, led him to a hypothesis that opened a new window into the mechanism of carcinogenesis. In the inherited form of retinoblastoma (see Chapter 4), an affected individual usually has an affected parent, and there is a 50% chance of genetic transmission to each of the offspring. In the sporadic (noninherited) form, neither parent is affected, nor is there additional risk to other progeny. A key feature distinguishing the two forms is that inherited retinoblastoma is usually bilateral (affecting both eyes), whereas sporadic retinoblastoma usually involves only a single tumor and therefore affects only one eye (unilateral).

Knudson reasoned that at least two mutations may be required to create a retinoblastoma. One of the mutations would alter the retinoblastoma gene; if this happened in the germline, it would be present in all cells of a child who received the mutant allele. The second mutation would be an additional, unspecified genetic event occurring in an already-altered cell. The hypothesis of a second event was required to explain why only a tiny fraction of the retinoblasts of a person who has inherited a mutant retinoblastoma gene actually give rise to tumors. Knudson's hypothesis is known as the **two-hit model of carcinogenesis**.

Familial retinoblastoma would thus be caused by the inheritance of one of the genetic "hits" as a **constitutional** mutation (i.e., a mutation present in all cells of the body). Persons who inherited one hit would require only one additional mutational event in a single retinoblast for that cell to seed a tumor clone. In sporadic cases, on the other hand, both mutations would have to occur somatically in the developing fetus (Fig. 8-4). This is a highly improbable combination of rare events, even considering the several million cells of the target tissue. The child who developed a retinoblastoma by this two-

hit somatic route would be unlikely to develop more than one tumor. The child inheriting a mutant retinoblastoma gene, however, would need only a single, additional genetic hit in a retinoblast for a tumor clone to develop. Knudson argued that such an event was likely to occur in several of the retinoblasts of each carrier of the inherited mutant gene, thus explaining the bilaterality of inherited retinoblastoma.

If the first event in the two-hit model is an inherited mutation, what is the nature of the second hit? Extensive molecular analysis of the region of chromosome 13 that contains the retinoblastoma-causing gene, *RB1*, showed that the second hit, like the first one, is a loss-of-function mutation. Several mechanisms, including point mutation, deletion, and hypermethylation of the *RB1* promoter region (associated with decreased transcription; see Chapters 3 and 4), can produce this effect. The second hit, which occurs in the fetus during the period in which retinoblasts are rapidly dividing and proliferating, has removed the

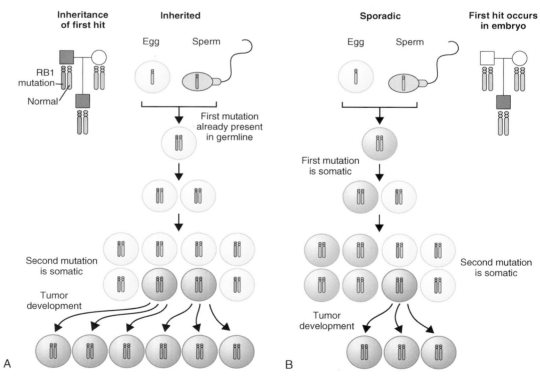

FIG 8-4   A, Persons inheriting an *RB1* mutation are heterozygous for the mutation in all cells of their body. The second hit occurs during embryonic development and typically affects more than one retinoblast, resulting in multiple tumors. **B,** In somatic retinoblastoma, both copies of the *RB1* gene must be disabled in the same retinoblast to cause tumor formation. Each process leads to homozygosity for the mutant *RB1* allele and thus to tumor development.

remaining nor- mal allele of this gene. This implies that a cell with one mutant *RB1* allele and one normal *RB1* allele cannot form a tumor. Thus, the product of the normal gene, even when present only in a single copy, prevents tumor formation.

An important corollary of this two-hit hypothesis is that the genes in which inherited mutations cause familial cancer syndromes may be the same as those that generate common cancers by **somatic mutation**. *By understanding the nature of the mutant alleles inherited in rare cancer families, therefore, we will come to understand more about the somatic pathway to common cancer as well.* Indeed, somatic loss-of-function mutations of both copies of the *RB1* gene are seen frequently in many types of tumors, including small-cell lung carcinoma, breast carcinoma, glioblastoma (a brain tumor), and osteosarcoma.

 Alfred Knudson's two-hit theory of carcinogenesis in retinoblastoma became the paradigm for a model to describe how inheritance of an altered gene predisposes the gene carrier to cancer. The theory states that a cell can initiate a tumor only when it contains two damaged alleles; therefore, a person who inherits one copy of a mutant retinoblastoma gene must experience a second, somatic mutation in one or more retinoblasts in order to develop one or more retinoblastomas. Two somatic mutations can also occur in a single retinoblast of a nonpredisposed fetus, producing sporadic retinoblastoma. Understanding mutated genes that are inherited in families can increase our understanding of the somatic pathway to common cancers.

MAJOR CLASSES OF CANCER GENES

Cancer-causing genes can be classified into three major categories: those that normally inhibit cellular proliferation (tumor suppressors), those that activate proliferation (oncogenes), and those that participate in DNA repair.

Tumor Suppressor Genes

The *RB1* gene was the first identified example of a **tumor suppressor gene**, a class of genes that control cell division and thus help to prevent tumors (Table 8-1). Characteristic of tumor suppressors is the somewhat perplexing feature that inherited mutations are *dominant* alleles at the level of the individual (i.e., heterozygotes usually develop the disease), but they are *recessive* alleles at the level of the cell (heterozygous cells do not form tumors). This apparent contradiction is resolved by realizing that in individuals who have inherited the first hit, a second hit that occurs in any one cell will cause a tumor. Because there are several million target retinoblasts in the developing fetus, heterozygous persons form, on the average, several retinoblasts homozygous for an *RB1* mutation. Each of these can lead to a retinoblastoma. Thus, it is the strong predisposition to tumor formation (i.e., the first hit) that is inherited as an autosomal dominant trait. The incomplete penetrance of the retinoblastoma mutation (90%) is explained by the fact that some people who inherit the disease-causing mutation do not experience a second hit in any of their surviving retinoblasts.

A general property of tumor suppressors is that they normally block the uncontrolled cellular proliferation that can lead to cancer. Often, this is done by participating in pathways that regulate the cell cycle. For example, the protein encoded by *RB1* (pRb) is active when it is relatively unphosphorylated but is down-regulated when it is phosphorylated by cyclin-dependent kinases (CDKs) just before the S phase of the cell cycle (see Chapter 2). In its active, hypophosphorylated state, pRb binds to members of the E2F transcription complex, inactivating them (Fig. 8-5). E2F activity is required for progression into S phase, so its inactivation by pRb halts the cell cycle. pRb thus serves as a cell-cycle brake that is normally released only when pRb is inactivated through phosphorylation by CDKs. This allows the cell to proceed through its mitotic cycle until pRb is activated again through removal of the phosphate groups. A loss-of-function mutation in *RB1*, a deletion of the gene, or hyper-

TABLE 8-1 **Examples of Tumor Suppressor Genes and DNA Repair Genes and Their Roles in Inherited Cancer**

GENE (RELATED GENES IN PARENTHESES)	FUNCTION OF GENE PRODUCT	DISEASE CAUSED BY GERMLINE MUTATIONS
Tumor Suppressor Genes		
RB1(p107, p130)	Cell cycle brake; binds to E2F transcription factor complex	Retinoblastoma; osteosarcoma
APC	Interacts with β-catenin in Wnt signaling pathway	Familial adenomatous polyposis
SMAD4	Transmits signals from TGFβ	Juvenile polyposis
NF1	Down-regulates RAS protein	Neurofibromatosis type 1
NF2	Cytoskeletal protein regulation	Neurofibromatosis type 2
TP53	Transcription factor; induces cell cycle arrest or apoptosis	Li–Fraumeni syndrome
VHL	Regulates multiple proteins, including p53 and NFκB	Von Hippel–Lindau disease (renal cysts and cancer)
WT1	Zinc finger transcription factor; binds to epidermal growth factor gene	Wilms tumor
CDKN2A (p14, p16)	CDK4 inhibitor	Familial melanoma
PTEN	Phosphatase that regulates PI3K signaling pathway	Cowden syndrome (breast and thyroid cancer)
CHEK2	Phosphorylates p53 and BRCA1	Li–Fraumeni syndrome
PTCH	Sonic hedgehog receptor	Gorlin syndrome (basal cell carcinoma, medulloblastoma)
CDH1	E-cadherin; regulates cell–cell adhesion	Gastric carcinoma
DPC4	Transduces transforming growth factor-β signals	Juvenile polyposis
TSC2	Down-regulates mTOR (mammalian target of rapamycin)	Tuberous sclerosis
DNA Repair Genes		
MLH1	DNA mismatch repair	HNPCC
MSH2	DNA mismatch repair	HNPCC
BRCA1	Interacts with BRCA2/RAD51 DNA repair protein complex	Familial breast and ovarian cancer
BRCA2	Interacts with RAD51 DNA repair protein	Familial breast and ovarian cancer
ATM	Protein kinase; phosphorylates BRCA1 in response to DNA damage	Ataxia telangiectasia; conflicting evidence for direct involvement in breast cancer
XPA	Nucleotide excision repair	Xeroderma pigmentosum

methylation of its 5′ region can lead to its permanent inactivation. Without this brake on the cell cycle, the cell can proceed through numerous uncontrolled divisions.

Loss-of-function mutations of other inhibitory factors can also lead to an unregulated cell cycle. A number of tumor suppressor genes encode **CDK inhibitors** (see Fig. 8-5), which inactivate CDKs and thus prevent them from phosphorylating target proteins such as pRb. Tumor suppressors can also control cell proliferation through their effects on transcription or on cell-cell interactions (some examples are discussed later). Again, mutations in these genes can lead to unrestricted cell division and ultimately to cancer.

▶ The discovery that retinoblastoma results when both alleles of the same locus on chromosome 13 are inactivated in the same retinoblast led to the concept of tumor suppressor genes. The products of such genes suppress tumor formation by controlling cell growth and can do so even if a cell contains only one normal version of the gene. Loss-of-function mutations that inactivate both copies of a cell's tumor suppressor gene can lead to uncontrolled cellular proliferation.

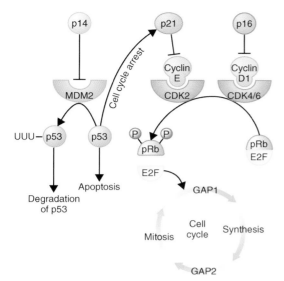

FIG 8-5 Regulation of the cell cycle is accomplished by a complex series of interactions among activators and repressors of the cycle. pRb acts as a master brake on the cell cycle by binding the E2F transcription complex, halting the cycle before S phase begins. The cyclin D-CDK4 complex inactivates pRb by phosphorylating it, thereby releasing the E2F complex and allowing the cell to progress through S phase. CDK inhibitors such as p16 and p21 inactivate CDKs, thus acting as another brake on the cycle. p53, acting through p21, can either halt the cell cycle or induce apoptosis in response to DNA damage. *CDK*, Cyclin-dependent kinase.

Because of the pivotal role of tumor suppressors in preventing tumor formation, their study is of considerable medical significance. By understanding how cancer is naturally suppressed by the body, we can ultimately develop more effective medical therapies for tumor prevention and treatment.

Oncogenes

Oncogenes (i.e., "cancer genes") are a second category of genes that can cause cancer. Most oncogenes originate from **proto-oncogenes**, which are genes involved in the four basic regulators of normal cell growth mentioned previously (growth factors, growth factor receptors, signal transduction molecules, and nuclear transcription factors). When a mutation occurs in a proto-oncogene, it can become an oncogene, a gene whose excessively active product can lead to unregulated cell growth and differentiation. When a cell proceeds from regulated to unregulated growth, the cell is said to have been **transformed.**

Unlike tumor suppressor genes, oncogenes are usually dominant at the cellular level: Only a single copy of a mutated oncogene is required to contribute to the multistep process of tumor progression. Whereas tumor suppressors are typically disabled by deletions or loss-of-function mutations, oncogenes are typically activated by gain-of-function mutations, **gene amplification** (i.e., increased numbers of the gene through trisomy or other mechanisms), hypomethylation of the oncogene's 5′ region (which increases transcription), or chromosome rearrangements that upregulate the oncogene (e.g., the Philadelphia chromosome translocation, Chapter 6). Most tumor suppressor genes are known to exhibit **germline mutations** that can cause inherited cancer syndromes (e.g., retinoblastoma, Li-Fraumeni syndrome). In contrast, although oncogenes are commonly found in sporadic tumors, germline oncogene mutations that cause inherited cancer syndromes are uncommon (a few exceptions are noted later in the discussion). These and other differences are summarized in Table 8-2.

In this section, we review three approaches that have been used to identify specific oncogenes: retroviral definition, transfection experiments, and mapping in tumors.

▶ Proto-oncogenes encode products that control cell growth and differentiation. When mutated or amplified, they can become oncogenes, which can cause cancer. Most oncogenes act as dominant gain- of-function mutations that lead to the deregulation of cell cycle control. In contrast to tumor suppressor genes, most oncogenes do not exhibit germline mutations that cause inherited cancer syndromes. Instead, somatic mutations are seen that lead to sporadic cancers.

It has long been known that certain types of viruses can cause cancer. Especially significant are **retroviruses,** a type of RNA virus that is capable of using reverse transcriptase to transcribe its RNA into DNA. In this way, the RNA genome of the retrovirus is converted

TABLE 8-2   Comparison of Key Features of Tumor Suppressor Genes and Oncogene

FEATURE	TUMOR SUPPRESSOR GENES	ONCOGENES
Function of normal version	Regulates cell growth and proliferation; some can induce apoptosis	Promotes cell growth and proliferation
Mutation (at cell level)	Recessive (both copies of gene inactivated)	Dominant (only one copy of gene mutated)
Effect of mutation	Loss of function	Gain of function
Germline mutations resulting in inherited cancer syndromes	Seen in most tumor suppressor genes	Seen in only a few oncogenes

to DNA, which can be inserted into a chromosome of a host cell. Some retro-viruses carry altered versions of growth-promoting genes into cells. These growth-promoting genes are oncogenes, which were first identified through the study of retroviruses that cause cancer in chickens. When the retrovirus invades a new cell, it can transfer the oncogene into the genome of the new host, thus transforming the cell and initiating cancer.

A number of gene products that affect cell growth or differentiation have been identified through the study of oncogenes carried by transforming retroviruses. For example, retrovirus studies identified the gene encoding the receptor molecule for epidermal growth factor (EGF), through the *ERBB* oncogene. These studies also identified the *RAS* (rat sarcoma) oncogenes, which are altered in at least 25% of human cancers. Transforming retroviruses have also identified the nuclear transcription factor genes, *MYC*, *JUN*, and *FOS*, as other molecular components capable of initiating cell transformation. Table 8-3 provides some examples of proto-oncogenes.

Oncogenes have also been identified in experiments in which material from human tumor cells was transferred to nontumor cells (**transfection**), causing transformation of the recipients. A classic experiment began with the transfer of DNA from a human bladder-cancer cell line into mouse cells. A few recipient cells became fully transformed. Cloning and examination of the human-specific DNA sequences present in the transformed mouse cells revealed that the transforming gene was a mutant allele of the same *RAS* oncogene previously identified by retroviral studies. Thus, the same oncogene that could be transferred by retroviruses also occurs natu-

rally, as a proto-oncogene, in the human genome.

Characterization of the protein product of mutant forms of *RAS* has revealed an important mechanism for the regulation of signal transduction. The RAS protein normally cycles between an *active* form bound to **guanosine triphosphate** (**GTP**) and an *inactive* form bound to **guanosine diphosphate** (**GDP**). The biochemical consequence of RAS mutations is a RAS protein that is unable to shift from the active GTP form, which stimulates growth, to the inactive GDP form. The mutant RAS protein cannot extinguish its growth signal, contributing to excessive cell division.

A third approach for identifying oncogenes derives from the common observation of **chromosomal rearrangements**, such as translocations, in some types of tumor cells (see Chapter 6). A well-known example is the Philadelphia chromosome, in which a translocation between chromosomes 9 and 22 places the *ABL* proto-oncogene next to the *BCR* gene, which enhances tyrosine kinase activity and produces chronic myelogenous leukemia. Another translocation, t(15;17) (q22;q11.2-12), is seen in acute promyelocytic leukemia (APL) and fuses two genes together: the retinoic acid receptor alpha (*RARA*) gene on chromosome 17 and the promyelocytic leukemia (*PML*) gene on chromosome 15. The fusion product (PML-RARα) interferes with the ability of the normal RARα protein to induce terminal differentiation of myeloid cells. (Interestingly, retinoic acid was already in use as a therapeutic agent for APL.) The fusion product also impairs the function of the PML protein, which acts as a tumor suppressor by helping to initiate apoptosis in damaged cells.

TABLE 8-3   Examples of Oncogenes and Their Roles in Cancer[*]

ONCOGENE	FUNCTION	ASSOCIATED TUMOR
Growth Factor Genes		
HST	Fibroblast growth factor	Stomach carcinoma
SIS	β subunit of platelet-derived growth factor	Glioma (brain tumor)
KS3	Fibroblast growth factor	Kaposi sarcoma
Growth Factor Receptor Genes		
RET[†]	Receptor tyrosine kinase	Multiple endocrine neoplasia; thyroid carcinoma
ERBB	Epidermal growth factor receptor	Glioblastoma (brain tumor); breast carcinoma
ERBA	Thyroid hormone receptor	Acute promyelocytic leukemia
NEU (ERBB2)	Receptor protein kinase	Neuroblastoma; breast carcinoma
MET[†]	Receptor tyrosine kinase	Hereditary papillary renal carcinoma; hepatocellular carcinoma
KIT[†]	Receptor tyrosine kinase	Gastrointestinal stromal tumor syndrome
Signal Transduction Genes		
HRAS	GTPase	Carcinoma of colon, lung, pancreas
KRAS	GTPase	Melanoma, thyroid carcinoma, acute monocytic leukemia, colorectal carcinoma
NRAS	GTPase	Melanoma
BRAF	Serine/threonine kinase	Malignant melanoma; colon cancer
ABL	Protein kinase	Chronic myelogenous leukemia; acute lymphocytic leukemia
CDK4[†]	Cyclin-dependent kinase	Malignant melanoma
Transcription Factor Genes		
NMYC	DNA-binding protein	Neuroblastoma; lung carcinoma
MYB	DNA-binding protein	Malignant melanoma; lymphoma; leukemia
FOS	Interacts with JUN oncogene to regulate transcription	Osteosarcoma

[*]For additional examples, see Croce CM. Oncogenes and cancer. *N Engl J Med.* 2008;358(5):502-511 and Garraway and Lander. Lessons from the cancer genome. *Cell.* 2013;153:17-37.
[†]*CDK4, KIT, MET,* and *RET* are proto-oncogenes in which germline mutations can give rise to inherited cancer syndromes.

▶ Retroviruses are capable of inserting oncogenes into the DNA of a host cell, thus transforming the host into a tumor-producing cell. The study of such retroviral transmission has identified a number of specific oncogenes. The transfection of oncogenes from tumor cells to normal cells can cause transformation of the normal cells. Some oncogenes were identified when specific rearrangements of chromosomal material were found to be associated with certain cancers. Because these translocations alter genes vital to cellular growth control, the sites of such rearrangements can be investigated to identify new oncogenes.

The identification of oncogenes has greatly increased our understanding of some of the underlying causes of cancer. In addition, oncogenes provide important targets for cancer therapy because of their key role in carcinogenesis. For example, the *ERBB2* oncogene, mentioned earlier and also known as *HER2/NEU*, is amplified in approximately 20% to 30% of invasive breast carcinomas. Its amplification which can be identified by fluorescent in situ hybridization (FISH) or array comparative genomic hybridization (CGH) (see Chapter 6), is associated with aggressive cancer. The protein product of *HER2/NEU* is a growth factor receptor located on the surfaces of breast cancer cells. Identification of the oncogene and its product contributed to the development of a drug, trastuzumab, which binds to the amplified gene product, effectively downregulating it and helping to treat this form of breast cancer. Similar drugs have been developed to counter the effects of the upregulated *ABL* oncogene in chronic myelogenous leukemia, an upregulated epidermal growth factor receptor gene in non-small-cell lung cancer, and several others.

DNA Repair Genes, Chromosome Integrity, and Tumorigenesis

Tumor cells typically are characterized by widespread mutations, chromosome breaks, and aneuploidy. This condition, termed **genomic instability**, contributes to tumorigenesis because mutations and chromosome defects can activate oncogenes or deactivate tumor suppressor genes. Genomic instability can occur because of defects in the proteins required for accurate cell division or in proteins responsible for DNA repair. It is also associated with hypomethylation of DNA, a common feature of many tumors. These defects are in turn the result of mutations. Sometimes, these mutations are inherited, resulting in relatively rare inherited cancer syndromes (see Table 8-1). More often, they arise in somatic cells and contribute to common, noninherited cancers.

There are a number of ways various types of genomic instability can give rise to cancer. Some breast cancers are caused by defective repair of double-stranded breaks that occur in DNA (e.g., from radiation exposure). This can result from mutations in genes such as *BRCA1*, *BRCA2*, or *ATM*. An inherited form of colon cancer, discussed later, can result from faulty DNA **mismatch repair** (so named because single-base mutations can lead to a DNA molecule in which base pairs are not complementary to each other: a mismatch). Xeroderma pigmentosum, an inherited condition that is characterized in part by multiple skin tumors (see Chapter 3), is the result of impaired nucleotide excision repair. Defects in proteins responsible for chromosome separation during mitosis (e.g., spindle fibers) can give rise to the multiple aneuploidies typically seen in tumor cells. Aneuploidy can contribute to tumorigenesis by creating extra copies of oncogenes or by deleting tumor suppressor genes.

Genomic instability, which can result from defects in DNA repair, is often observed in tumor cells and is characterized by widespread mutations, chromosome breaks, and aneuploidy. These alterations can cause cancer when they affect pathways that regulate cellular proliferation.

Genetic Alterations and Cancer Cell Immortality

Even after a tumor cell has escaped regulation by tumor suppressors or DNA repair proteins, it must overcome one more hurdle to unlimited proliferation: the intrinsic limitation on the number of cell divisions allowed to each cell. Ordinarily, a cell is restricted to about 50 to 70 mitotic divisions. After reaching this number, the cell typically becomes **senescent** and cannot continue to divide. Recent research has provided new insights on the mechanisms that count the number of cell divisions and has illustrated new ways tumor cells can circumvent the counting system.

Each time a cell divides, the telomeres of chromosomes shorten slightly because DNA polymerase cannot replicate the tips of chromosomes. Once the telomere is reduced to a critical length, a signal is transmitted that causes the cell to become senescent. This process would place severe limitations on the proliferating cells in a tumor, preventing further clonal expansion. Many tumor cells overcome the process by activating a gene that encodes **telomerase**, a reverse transcriptase that replaces the telomeric segments that are normally lost during cell division. Activation of this enzyme, which is rarely present in normal cells but is found in 85% to 90% of tumor cells, is part of a process that allows a tumor cell to continue to divide without the restraint ordinarily imposed by telomere shortening. This uninhibited division allows the tumor to become large, and, by allowing continued DNA replication, it permits the accumulation of additional mutations that can further contribute to the aggressiveness of the tumor cell. Recent whole-genome sequencing studies have shown that somatic mutations in the promoter region of the *TERT* gene (which encodes a component of telomerase) are seen in 70% of melanomas. These mutations increase the expression of *TERT* and are likely to contribute to increased telomerase activity in melanoma cells.

 Normally, progressive shortening of telomeres limits the number of divisions of a cell to about 50 to 70. Tumor cells overcome this limitation by activating telomerase, which replaces the telomere segments that are lost during each cell division. This appears to help tumor cells escape the restraint of cellular senescence.

IDENTIFICATION OF INHERITED CANCER-CAUSING GENES

Although the methods described in the previous section have been successful in identifying many oncogenes, they are not well suited to the identification of tumor suppressor genes. These methods require dominant expression of the mutant phenotype, which is characteristic of oncogenes, whereas mutant tumor suppressor alleles seem to have a primarily recessive phenotype at the level of the cell. Alternative approaches to the identification of these tumor suppressor genes were necessary. The first, and most common, of these approaches is linkage mapping in families with hereditary cancer, where the chromosomal segment bearing a cancer-causing mutation can be identified by linkage with polymorphic markers. This approach has been used to identify mutations that cause inherited forms of breast and colon cancer (discussed later).

A second approach takes advantage of the frequent chromosomal losses associated with revealed tumor suppressor genes. As already described, **inherited tumor** suppressor mutations typically result in persons who are heterozygous for the mutation in all of their cells (a first hit). However, the tumor suppressor mutation is a recessive allele at the cellular

level: There are two hits, resulting in the loss of both normal copies of the tumor suppressor gene. Often an inherited mutant allele is unmasked in tumor cells by a deletion of part or all of the other copy of the homologous chromosome that carried the normal allele. Therefore, the observation that a specific chromosome segment is deleted in a tumor suggests a map location for the inherited mutation.

The deleted chromosome regions in tumors can be pinpointed by examining a series of closely linked marker polymorphisms, such as STRs, in the region and determining which of the markers that are heterozygous in the patient's constitutional DNA have become homozygous in tumor DNA (i.e., which markers have lost an allele in the process of tumorigenesis). This **loss of heterozygosity** in tumor DNA indicates that the normal tumor suppressor gene, as well as polymorphic markers surrounding it, has been lost, leaving only the abnormal copy of the tumor suppressor gene (see Fig. 8-4 and 8-6). This approach was used, for example, to help narrow the locations of the retinoblastoma gene on the long arm of chromosome 13 and of a gene for Wilms tumor (nephroblastoma) on 11p. Deleted regions in tumor DNA can also be identified by array CGH (see Chapter 6) or whole-genome sequencing (see Chapter 3). After a loss of heterozygosity is identified in a chromosome region, the DNA sequences within this region can be tested to identify the tumor-causing mutation(s).

A third approach for identifying inherited cancer-causing variants is through genome-wide association studies (GWAS). As discussed in Chapter 8, a GWAS is carried out by comparing the frequencies of thousands to millions of SNPs, typically assayed on a microarray, in a large series of cases and matched disease-free controls. If a SNP shows a significantly different frequency in the two groups, it is likely to be within or near a gene that contributes to cancer susceptibility. This approach has been especially effective in identifying additional risk loci for common cancers such as those of the breast, colon, and prostate. Typically, these SNPs individually raise (or lower) the risk of cancer only modestly, by 5% to 20%. However, when a cancer risk profile is based on multiple cancer-associated SNPs, significant information about an individual's cancer risk can be derived.

As exome and whole-genome sequencing has become more affordable, this technology has been used increasingly to carry out case-control and family-based studies to identify cancer-causing genes. Because sequencing identifies all variants in the exome or genome, it is much more likely to pinpoint a specific cancer-causing variant than is a microarray-based study. Many of these variants are rare in populations, so large samples of cases and controls are needed to provide adequate evidence that the variant is likely to cause cancer. Families with multiple affected members can prove useful when analyzing rare variants because the principles of linkage can be used to show that a cancer-causing variant is transmitted along with a cancer phenotype within a family.

In many sequencing studies, the DNA sequence from tumor samples is compared with DNA sequences from tissues unaffected by the tumor (e.g., white blood cells or buccal cells). DNA from the unaffected tissue represents the patient's germline genetic constitution, while the DNA from a tumor is likely to have undergone non-inherited somatic mutations that contribute to tumorigenesis. Genes that consistently show elevated levels of somatic mutations in a specific tumor type become candidates as cancer-causing loci. Many thousands of tumor DNA samples have now been analyzed using this approach, revealing dozens of additional cancer-causing genes.

FIG 8-6　**A,** *A* and *B* represent two microsatellite (STR) polymorphisms that have been assayed using DNA from a cancer patient's normal cells (*N*) and tumor cells (*T*). In normal cells, the patient is heterozygous for both marker loci. Deletion of the long arm from one of the paired chromosomes in tumor cells results in loss of heterozygosity (LOH) for locus *B* (i.e., the band corresponding to allele *B1* is missing, with only a faint signal due to residual traces of normal cells in the tumor specimen). LOH is a signpost for a tumor-suppressor gene near the deleted locus. **B,** Loss of heterozygosity in breast tumor cells revealed by a SNP microarray. Each dot represents the genotype of one SNP typed in a collection of one person's tumor cells. Each SNP has three possible genotypes: AA, AB, or BB. A region of more than 20 Mb on chromosome 2 has no heterozygous SNPs (genotype AB), illustrating a loss of heterozygosity in this region (and thus the presence of a likely tumor suppressor gene, with only the mutated copy expressed in these cells). (**A,** Courtesy Dr. Dan Fults, University of Utah Health Sciences Center.)

The techniques outlined here (linkage analysis, loss of heterozygosity analysis, GWAS, and DNA sequencing) have identified hundreds of genes that are mutated in various cancers. Some of these genes contribute directly to a growth advantage in tumors and are considered primary causes of cancer. Approximately 150 such **driver genes** have been described. A much larger number of genes undergo somatic mutations during tumorigenesis, but these genes do not directly confer a growth advantage to cells. These are termed **passenger genes**. The *RB1* gene, which normally acts as a "brake" on cell division, is an example of a well-known driver gene.

> Cancer-associated genes can be detected through linkage analysis or by showing that one homolog of a chromosome (or a part of it) is missing in DNA from a tumor. GWAS and exome or whole-genome sequencing are also used to identify cancer-causing genes. These approaches have identified driver genes, which give cells a growth advantage leading to cancer, as well as passenger genes, which are mutated in cancer but do not confer a growth advantage. Confirmation of the etiological role of a possible cancer-causing gene is obtained by showing the consistent presence of mutations in the gene in DNA from affected patients.

Neurofibromatosis Type 1

The initial evidence for mapping the neurofibromatosis type 1 gene (*NF1*) to chromosome 17 came from linkage studies in families. Subsequently, chromosomal translocations were discovered in the karyotypes of two unrelated patients with neurofibromatosis, each of whom had a breakpoint on chromosome 17q at a location indistinguishable from the map location of the *NF1* gene. These translocations were assumed to have caused neurofibromatosis in these persons by disrupting the *NF1* gene. Located only 50 kb apart, the breakpoints provided the physical clues necessary to define several candidate genes that were screened for mutations in patients with *NF1* (Fig. 8-7).

The nucleotide sequence of the *NF1* gene provided an early clue to function when its predicted amino acid sequence was compared with amino acid sequences of known gene products found in computerized databases. Extended similarities were observed with the mammalian GTPase-activating protein (GAP). This was an important finding, because at least one function of GAP is to decrease

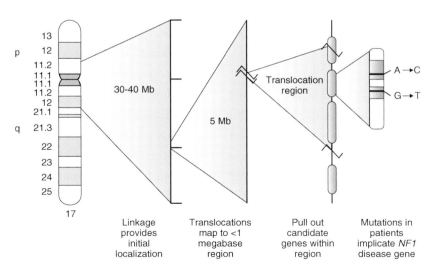

FIG 8-7 Localization of the *NF1* gene on chromosome 17q involved linkage analysis and identification of two translocation breakpoints that interrupted the disease gene. Candidate genes were isolated from this region and tested for mutations in patients with NF1 and in normal controls.

the amount of active GTP-bound RAS. The RAS protein is a key component of the signal transduction pathway, transmitting positive growth signals in its active form. The *NF1* gene product, neurofibromin, also plays a role in signal transduction by down-regulating RAS.

With the identification of the *NF1* gene product as a component in signal transduction, a picture began to form of how the inheritance of a mutation in one *NF1* allele might contribute to the development of neurofibromas and *café-au-lait* spots. Reduced expression of the *NF1* gene permits increased RAS activity and allows the cell to escape from differentiation and continue its growth. Loss of the remaining normal allele in some cells (e.g., Schwann cells) further encourages unchecked growth. Discovery of the *NF1* gene has led to the identification of a key tumor suppressor that helps to regulate the fundamental process of signal transduction.

▶ The gene responsible for *NF1* was mapped to chromosome 17q by linkage in families and was identified through translocations and point mutations in patients. DNA sequencing of the gene predicted a protein product with a domain related to GAP, and a similar role in down-regulating the RAS signal transduction protein was confirmed by biochemical experiments.

The *TP53* Gene

Somatic mutations in the *TP53* gene are found in more than half of all human tumors, making this the most commonly altered cancer-causing gene. Somatic *TP53* mutations are seen, for example, in approximately 70% of colorectal tumors, as well as 40% of breast tumors and 60% of lung tumors. Approximately 80% to 90% of *TP53* mutations are concentrated in the portion of the gene that encodes a DNA-binding domain, typically preventing the p53 protein from binding to DNA of other genes.

Like *RB1* and *NF1*, *TP53* functions as a tumor suppressor gene. Its protein product, p53, increases in quantity in response to cell damage (e.g., double-stranded DNA breaks caused by ionizing radiation). Acting as a transcription factor, p53 helps to regulate dozens of genes that affect cell growth, proliferation, and survival. For example, p53 binds to the promoter of *CDKN1A*, whose protein product, p21, is a CDK inhibitor that blocks CDK4's inactivation of pRb (see Fig. 8-5). This halts the cell cycle in the G1 phase, before DNA replication occurs in S phase. Arrest of the cell cycle before S phase provides time for repair of the damaged DNA. If the cell's DNA is severely damaged, p53 may instead induce programmed cell death (apoptosis). This response is more likely if the pRb pathway for cell cycle arrest is not intact. Lacking the possibility of cell cycle arrest to repair damage, the p53 protein "chooses" cell death by interacting with genes involved in apoptotic pathways (e.g., *PTEN*, *BAX*). In this way, p53 prevents the proliferation of an abnormal, potentially carcinogenic cell.

When *TP53* is mutated, cells with damaged DNA can evade both repair and destruction, and continued replication of the damaged DNA can lead to tumor formation. For this to happen, other components of cell cycle control must also be compromised. For example, several DNA tumor viruses, such as the human papilloma virus that is responsible for most cases of cervical cancer, inactivate both pRb and p53. This produces cells that can neither repair their DNA nor undergo apoptosis in response to damage, leading in some cases to cancer.

Carcinogenic substances can induce specific *TP53* mutations. Dietary ingestion of aflatoxin B_1, which can produce liver cancer, is associated with a mutation that produces an arginine-to-serine substitution at position 249 of the p53 protein. Exposure to benzopyrene, a powerful mutagen and carcinogen found in cigarette smoke, leads to alterations of specific *TP53* base pairs in lung tumors. This demonstrates a direct molecular link between cigarette smoking and lung cancer. Thus, examination of the type of *TP53* mutation seen in a tumor can provide clues to the identity of the causative carcinogenic agent.

Although tumor-causing *TP53* mutations have

been observed mostly in somatic cells, germline mutations of *TP53* are responsible for an inherited cancer condition known as the Li-Fraumeni syndrome (LFS). This rare syndrome is transmitted in autosomal dominant fashion and involves breast and colon carcinomas, soft-tissue sarcomas, osteosarcomas, brain tumors, leukemia, and adrenocortical carcinomas. These tumors usually develop at early ages in members of LFS families, and multiple primary tumors are commonly seen in an affected person. The demonstration of consistent *TP53* mutations in the constitutional DNA of patients with LFS confirmed the causative role of this gene. As in retinoblastoma, the inheritance of a mutated *TP53* gene greatly increases the person's susceptibility to subsequent cell transformation and tumor development when a cell loses the other, normal copy of *TP53* (two-hit model). Among LFS family members who inherit an abnormal *TP53* gene, approximately 50% develop invasive cancer by 30 years of age, and more than 90% develop invasive cancer by age 70 years.

TP53 mutations account for only about 75% of LFS cases. Some of the remaining cases are the result of mutations in another tumor suppressor gene, *CHEK2*. This gene encodes a kinase that normally phosphorylates p53 in response to ionizing radiation, resulting in the accumulation and activation of p53. Loss-of-function mutations in *CHEK2* result in a lack of p53 activation, causing LFS via the p53 pathway.

TP53 is medically important in at least two ways. First, the presence of *TP53* mutations in tumors, particularly those of the breast and colon, often signals a more-aggressive cancer with relatively poor survival prospects. It is thus a useful prognostic indicator. Second, *TP53* might ultimately prove important in tumor prevention. Laboratory experiments show that the insertion of a normal *TP53* gene into tumor cells can induce tumor regression by inducing abnormal cancer cells to undergo apoptosis. This has led to gene therapy protocols (see Chapter 10) in which normal *TP53* copies are inserted into tumors in an effort to eliminate cancerous cells.

Somatic mutations of the *TP53* gene are found in the majority of tumors. This gene encodes a protein that can induce either cell cycle arrest or apoptosis in response to damaged DNA. Inherited *TP53* mutations can cause Li-Fraumeni syndrome.

The Familial Adenomatous Polyposis Gene, *APC*

Colon cancer (CRC) affects approximately 1 in 20 Americans, and, like most common cancers, it is more likely to occur in persons with a positive family history. One's risk of developing CRC is elevated two- to threefold if a first-degree relative is affected; it increases to three- to sixfold if two first-degree relatives are affected. Approximately 2% to 5% of colon cancer cases are inherited as autosomal dominant syndromes, the two most important of which are discussed here.

Familial adenomatous polyposis (FAP) is characterized by the appearance of large numbers adenomas, or polyps, of the colon in the second or third decade of life. Colonic adenomas are now understood to be the immediate precursors to colorectal cancer. The multiple adenomas of the patient with FAP therefore present a grave risk of early malignancy. Because early detection and removal of adenomatous polyps can significantly reduce the occurrence of cancer, it is important to understand the causative gene and its role in the development of polyps (Clinical Commentary 8-1).

The gene responsible for FAP was localized to the long arm of chromosome 5 by linkage analysis in families. Discovery of small, overlapping deletions in two unrelated patients provided the key to isolation of the disease-causing gene, termed *APC* (adenomatous polyposis coli). Among the genes that lay within the 100-kb region that was deleted in both patients, one showed apparent mutations in other patients. This mutation was seen in one patient but not in his unaffected parents (i.e., a de novo mutation; see Chapter 4), which help to confirm the identification of the *APC* gene.

Like *RB1* and *NF1*, *APC* is a tumor suppressor gene, and both copies of *APC* must be inactivated in a cell for tumor progression to begin. Persons who inherit an *APC* mutation typically experience somatic loss-of-function mutations in hundreds of their colonic epithelial cells, giving rise to multiple adenomas. In some cases, loss of function of *APC* occurs because of hypermethylation of *APC*'s promoter region, which results in reduced transcription (see Chapter 4). Hypermethylation, as well as other changes in gene regulation (Box 8-1) has been observed in the inactivation of a number of tumor suppressor and DNA repair genes, including those associated with retinoblastoma (*RB1*), breast cancer (*BRCA1*), hereditary nonpolyposis colorectal cancer (*MLH1*), malignant melanoma (*CDKN2A*), and von Hippel-Lindau disease (*VHL*).

Identification of the *APC* gene has been important in diagnosing and managing colon cancer in families with FAP (see Clinical Commentary 8-1). In addition, and perhaps even more importantly, *APC* mutations are found in 85% of all sporadic, noninherited cases of colon cancer. These somatic *APC* mutations (i.e., those that disable both copies of the gene in a colonic cell) are among the earliest alterations that give rise to colon cancer. But *APC* mutations are not sufficient by themselves to complete the progression to metastatic disease. As shown in Figure 8-8, other genes may also be altered. For example, **gain-of-function mutations** are seen in the *KRAS* gene in approximately 50% of colon tumors. This gene encodes a signal transduction molecule, and a gain-of-function mutation increases signaling and thus cellular proliferation. **Loss-of-function mutations** in the *TP53* gene are also seen in more than 50% of colon tumors and usually occur relatively late in the pathway to cancer. Ordinarily, p53 would be activated in response to mutations like those of *APC* and *KRAS*, leading to DNA repair or apoptosis. Cells that lack p53 activity are free to continue along the path to malignancy in spite of their damaged DNA. Still another tumor suppressor gene, *SMAD4*, is also frequently mutated in the CRC pathway. Thus, multiple mutations are required in tumor suppressor genes and oncogenes to produce a colorectal tumor.

Extensive studies have revealed at least three ways the APC protein acts as a tumor suppressor. Perhaps most importantly, it participates in the phosphorylation and degradation of β-catenin, a key molecule in

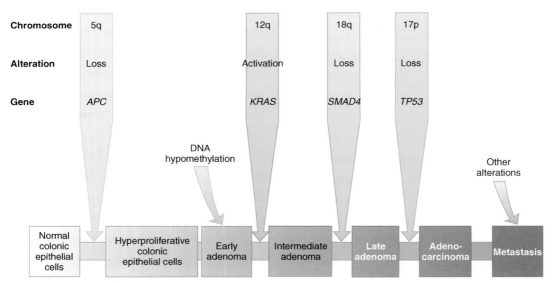

FIG 8-8   The pathway to colon cancer. Loss of the *APC* gene transforms normal epithelial tissue lining the gut to hyperproliferating tissue. Hypomethylation of DNA (which can cause genomic instability and up-regulate proto-oncogenes), activation of the *KRAS* proto-oncogene, and loss of the *SMAD4* gene are involved in the progression to a benign adenoma. Loss of the *TP53* gene and other alterations are involved in the progression to malignant carcinoma and metastasis. Note that these alterations are present in varying frequencies in colon tumor cells. (Modified from Vogelstein B. Cancer genome landscapes. *Science.* 2013;339:1546-1558.)

BOX 8-1   Epigenetics and Cancer

Epigenetics is defined as the study of changes in gene expression or phenotype caused by mechanisms other than variation in DNA sequences. Examples of epigenetic changes include methylation, histone modification, and mRNA-binding by microRNAs. As discussed in Chapter 2, methylation of a gene's promoter region, along with histone hypoacetylation, are associated with chromatin condensation, which inhibits the binding of transcription factors to a gene's promoter. Consequently, expression of the gene (i.e., transcription to mRNA) is reduced. Methylation and histone modification are involved in the processes of genomic imprinting (see Chapter 4) and X inactivation (see Chapter 6). Epigenetic alterations can cause persons with the same DNA sequences (i.e., identical twins) to have quite different disease profiles.

Epigenetic alterations are important in cancer because they can alter the expression of many cancer-associated genes. Tumor cells typically exhibit widespread hypomethylation (decreased methylation), which can increase the activity of oncogenes. Hypomethylation increases as tumors progress from benign neoplasms to malignancy.

In addition, the promoter regions of tumor-suppressor genes (e.g., *RB1* and *BRCA1*) are often hypermethylated, which decreases their rate of transcription and their ability to inhibit tumor formation. Hypermethylation also is seen in specific subgroups of microRNA genes. When these microRNA genes are methylated, their mRNA targets are over-expressed, and this overexpression has been associated with tumorigenesis.

Except through gene therapy (see Chapter 10), mutations in DNA sequences cannot be altered. Epigenetic modifications, however, can be reversed through the administration of therapeutic drugs. For example, 5-azacytidine, a demethylating agent, has been used to treat leukemia and myelodysplastic syndrome. Another class of drugs, histone deacetylase (HDAC) inhibitors, counteracts the histone hypoacetylation that can silence the activity of tumor-suppressor genes. HDAC inhibitors have been used in the treatment of T-cell lymphomas. A challenge in developing drugs that modulate epigenetic alterations is to target only the genes responsible for a specific cancer.

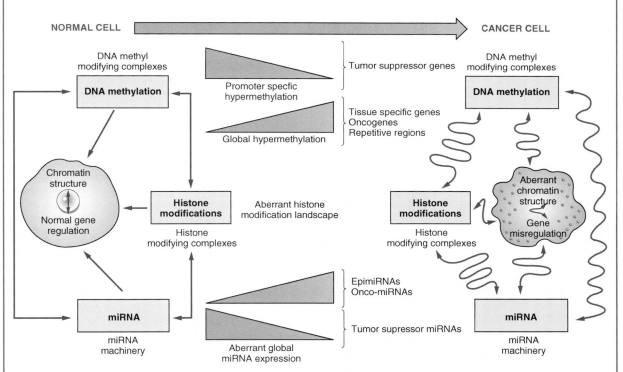

Global epigenomic alterations and cancer. Oncogenesis involves accumulated genetic alterations combined with the epigenetic changes: DNA methylation, histone modifications, and miRNAs. In cancer cells, tumor-suppressor genes become hypermethylated and with histone modifications cause abnormal gene silencing. The gene silencing of tumor-suppressor genes results in tumor progression. Global hypomethylation leads to chromosomal instability and fragility. Additionally, these modifications create abnormal mRNA and miRNA expression, which leads to activation of oncogenes and silencing of tumor-suppressor genes. (From McCance KL, Huether SE, Brashers VL, Rote NS. *Pathophysiology: The Biologic Basis for Disease in Adults and Children.* 7th ed. St Louis: Elsevier; 2014. Adapted from Sandoval J, Esteller M. Cancer epigenomics: beyond genomics. *Curr Opin Genet Dev.* 2012;22:50-55.)

the Wnt signal transduction pathway. Among other things, this pathway is involved in activation of the MYC transcription factor. By reducing β-catenin levels, APC dampens signals that lead to cellular proliferation. Examination of colon carcinomas that do not carry mutations in the *APC* gene revealed that some of them have gain-of-function mutations in the β-catenin gene, thus confirming the potential etiological role of this gene in CRC. *APC* mutations are also thought to affect cell-to-cell and cell-to-matrix adhesion properties (this is important because alteration of cell adhesion control permits cells to invade

---

CLINICAL COMMENTARY 8-1
The APC Gene and Colorectal Cancer

Colorectal cancer (CRC) will be diagnosed in about 1 in 20 Americans. Currently, the mortality rate for this cancer is approximately one third. Genetic and environmental factors, such as dietary fat and fiber, are known to influence the probability of occurrence of colorectal cancer.

As indicated in the text, familial adenomatous polyposis (FAP) is an autosomal dominant subtype of colon cancer that is characterized by a large number of adenomatous polyps (Fig. 8-9). These polyps typically develop during the second decade of life and number in the hundreds or more (polyposis itself is defined as the presence of >100 polyps). The average age of CRC diagnosis in untreated FAP patients is 39 years; 95% of untreated FAP patients will develop CRC by age 50. Germline mutations in the *APC* gene are consistently identified in family members affected with FAP, and approximately one third of cases are the result of new mutations in *APC*. More than 700 different mutations of the *APC* gene have been reported, most of which are nonsense or frameshift mutations. Because these mutations produce a truncated protein product, a **protein truncation test** can be used to help determine whether the at-risk person has inherited an *APC* mutation. (As discussed in Chapter 3, this test involves the in vitro manufacture and analysis of a protein product from the gene of interest.) It is now more common to rely on DNA-based tests, including direct sequencing, to identify *APC* mutations. These diagnostic tests, which identify mutations in about 80% of FAP cases, are important for family members because a positive result alerts them to the need for frequent surveillance and possible colectomy.

FAP is relatively rare, affecting only about 1 in 10,000 to 1 in 20,000 persons and accounting for less than 1% of all cases of colon cancer. The broader significance of the *APC* gene derives from the fact that somatic mutations in this gene are seen in approximately 85% of all colon cancers. Furthermore, *APC* mutations typically occur early in the development of colorectal malignancies. A better understanding of the *APC* gene product, how it interacts with other proteins, and how it interacts with environmental factors such as diet, can provide important clues for the prevention and treatment of common colon cancer. In this way, the mapping and cloning of a gene responsible for a relatively rare cancer syndrome can have widespread clinical implications.

Treatment for FAP usually involves surgical resection of the colon and chemotherapy. However, because CRC is usually preceded by the appearance of benign polyps, it is one of the most preventable of cancers. The National Polyp Study Workgroup estimates that colonoscopic removal of polyps could reduce the nationwide incidence of colon cancer by as much as 90%. The importance of early intervention and treatment further underscores the need to understand early events in colorectal cancer, such as somatic mutations in the *APC* gene.

Because polyps usually begin to appear in the second decade of life in those who inherit an *APC* mutation, an annual colonoscopy is recommended in these persons starting at 10-12 years of age. Upper gastrointestinal polyps are seen in 90% of FAP patients by age 70. Thus, endoscopy of the upper gastrointestinal tract is recommended every 1 to 2 years, starting at ages 20 to 25 years. Because classic FAP results in hundreds to thousands of polyps, colectomy is often necessary by age 20 years. There is evidence that the use of nonsteroidal anti-inflammatory drugs causes some degree of polyp regression. Persons with FAP have increased risks of other cancers, including gastric cancer (<1% lifetime risk), duodenal adenocarcinoma (5%-10% lifetime risk), hepatoblastoma (1% risk), and thyroid cancer.

Mutations in the *APC* gene can also produce a related syndrome, termed attenuated familial adenomatous polyposis. This syndrome differs from FAP in that patients have fewer than 100 polyps (typically 10-20). Most of the mutations that produce this form of FAP are located in the 5' or 3' regions of *APC*.

FAP can also result from recessive mutations in *MUTYH*, a gene that encodes a DNA repair protein. These mutations are estimated to account for about 30% of cases of attenuated FAP and approximately 10% to 20% of classic FAP cases in which an *APC* mutation is not detected.

FIG 8-9   A portion of a colon removed from a patient with familial adenomatous polyposis (FAP), illustrating a large number of adenomatous polyps covering the colon. Each of these benign neoplasms has the potential to become a malignant tumor.

other tissues and to metastasize to other sites). Again, this activity is mediated through β-catenin, which interacts with a cell-surface molecule (E-cadherin) whose loss of function leads to abnormal cell adhesion properties. Finally, APC is expressed in the microtubules that pull chromosomes apart during meiosis (see Chapter 2). Alterations in APC result in altered microtubule activity, such that aneuploidies and chromosome breaks arise during mitosis. Thus, *APC* mutations also promote cancer by increasing genomic instability.

▶ The adenomatous polyposis coli gene (*APC*), which strikingly predisposes to colon cancer, was ultimately identified from mutations in patients. *APC* is also involved in the great majority of sporadic cases of colon cancer and is in fact one of the earliest alterations leading to colon tumorigenesis. This tumor suppressor gene has been shown to function as a major regulator of the Wnt signal transduction pathway via its interaction with β-catenin. It is also involved in cell adhesion control and in maintaining chromosome stability during mitosis.

The Hereditary Nonpolyposis Colon Cancer Genes

Hereditary nonpolyposis colon cancer (HNPCC, or Lynch syndrome), a second form of inherited colon cancer, accounts for approximately 1% to 5% of all colorectal cancer cases. Like FAP, HNPCC is an autosomal dominant, high-penetrance cancer syndrome, with a lifetime colorectal cancer risk of 50% to 80% in heterozygotes. In addition, the risk of endometrial cancer among females with HNPCC is approximately 40% to 60%, and the risk of ovarian cancer is 5% to 10%. Cancers of the small bowel, stomach, brain, pancreas, renal pelvis, and ureter are seen in a smaller percentage of mutation carriers. In contrast to FAP, HNPCC patients do not have polyposis; they typically have a relatively small number of polyps. Also, polyps in HNPCC patients are more likely to occur in the proximal colon, whereas those of FAP patients are more likely to be concentrated in the distal colon.

Approximately 40% to 60% of HNPCC cases are caused by mutations in a gene called *MSH2*, and another 25% to 30% of cases are caused by mutations in the *MLH1* gene. Mutations in two other genes, *PMS2* and *MSH6*, help to account for a small percentage of additional cases. Each of these genes is known to play an important role in DNA mismatch repair in many different organisms (in fact, a critical clue in their identification was the existence of highly similar DNA repair genes in yeast and bacteria). Inactivation of both alleles of any one of these genes increases the genome-wide mutation rate in an affected cell by as much as 1000-fold. This increased rate of mutation results in the alteration of a number of cellular regulatory genes, thus leading to an increased incidence of cancer. A characteristic feature of tumors from HNPCC patients is a high degree of instability of microsatellite loci (see Chapter 3), which generates many new microsatellite alleles. Such **microsatellite instability** is also seen in about 15% of sporadic colorectal carcinomas, but somatic loss-of-function mutations in the HNPCC genes seem to occur only infrequently in these tumors. Instead, the most common alteration seen in these **sporadic tumors** is hypermethylation of the *MLH1* gene, resulting in its inactivation.

A comparison of FAP and HNPCC reveals interesting differences in the way each syndrome leads to colon cancer. In FAP, an inherited *APC* mutation results in hundreds of polyps, each of which has a relatively low probability of incurring all of the other genetic alterations required for progression to metastatic cancer. But, because the number of polyps is large, there is a high probability (almost 100%) that at least one of them will produce a cancerous tumor. In HNPCC, the number of polyps is much smaller (hence the term *nonpolyposis*), but, because of a relative lack of DNA repair, each polyp has a high probability of experiencing the multiple alterations necessary for tumor development. Consequently, the average age of onset of colorectal cancer in HNPCC is only about 10 years later than that of FAP.

HNPCC (Lynch syndrome) is an inherited form of colorectal cancer that is caused by mutations in any of six genes involved in DNA mismatch repair. It represents an example of a cancer syndrome associated with microsatellite instability.

Inherited Breast Cancer

The lifetime prevalence of breast cancer in women is 1 in 8, and a woman's risk of developing breast cancer doubles if a first-degree relative is affected. Two genes, *BRCA1* and *BRCA2*, have been identified as major contributors to inherited breast cancer. This section addresses three critical questions regarding these genes: What percentage of breast cancer cases are the result of *BRCA1* and *BRCA2* mutations? Among those who inherit a mutation, what is the risk of developing cancer? How do mutations in these genes contribute to cancer susceptibility?

Population-based studies show that only a small percentage of all breast cancers—approximately 1% to 3%—can be attributed to inherited mutations in *BRCA1* or *BRCA2*. Among women with breast cancer who also have a positive family history of the disease, the percentage with inherited mutations in either of these genes increases to approximately 20% to 30%. Among affected women who have a positive family history of breast and ovarian cancer, 60% to 80% have inherited a *BRCA1* or *BRCA2* mutation. Inherited mutations in these genes are also more common among women with early-onset breast cancer and among those with bilateral breast cancer.

Women who inherit a mutation in *BRCA1* experience a 50% to 80% lifetime risk of developing breast cancer; the lifetime risk for those who inherit a *BRCA2* mutation is slightly slower, averaging approximately 50%. *BRCA1* mutations also increase the risk of ovarian cancer among women (40%-50% lifetime risk, which is substantially higher than the lifetime risk of 1/70 in the general female population). These mutations also confer a modestly increased risk of prostate and colon cancers. *BRCA2* mutations confer an increased risk of ovarian cancer (20% lifetime risk). Approximately 6% of males who inherit a *BRCA2* mutation develop breast cancer, which represents a 70-fold increase over the risk in the general male population (see Chapter 5 for further discussion of breast cancer risk factors).

BRCA1 and *BRCA2* were both identified by linkage analysis in families, followed by positional cloning. Most *BRCA1* and *BRCA2* mutations result in truncated protein products and a consequent loss of function. As for the *RB1* and *APC* genes, affected persons inherit one copy of a *BRCA1* or *BRCA2* mutation and then experience a somatic loss of the remaining normal allele in one or more cells (following the two-hit model for tumor suppressor genes). In contrast to *RB1* and *APC*, somatic mutations affecting these genes are seldom seen in sporadic (noninherited) breast tumors. *BRCA1* and *BRCA2* are both large genes, and they exhibit extensive allelic heterogeneity (approximately 2000 distinct mutations, most of which are deletions or nonsense or frameshift mutations, have been reported for each gene). This poses challenges for genetic diagnosis (see Chapter 10), which is done primarily by direct DNA sequencing of the coding and regulatory regions of both genes. Typically, a panel of approximately one dozen breast cancer-associated risk genes are now tested for disease causing mutations (see Chapter 10).

Although *BRCA1* and *BRCA2* share no significant DNA sequence similarity, they both participate in the DNA repair process. The protein product of *BRCA1* is phosphorylated (and thus activated) by the ATM and CHEK2 kinases in response to DNA damage (Fig. 8-10). The *BRCA1* protein product binds to the *BRCA2* product, which in turn binds to RAD51, a protein involved in the repair of double-stranded DNA breaks (as with the *HNPCC* genes, yeast and bacteria both have DNA-repair genes similar to RAD51). BRCA1 and BRCA2 thus participate in an important DNA repair pathway, and their inactivation results in incorrect DNA repair and genomic instability. In addition to their roles in the RAD51 pathway, *BRCA1* and *BRCA2* help to suppress tumor formation through their interactions with previously discussed proteins such as p53, pRb, and Myc, and by helping to maintain genomic stability.

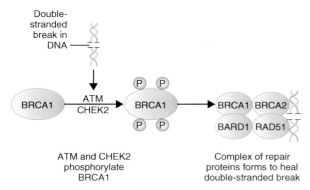

FIG 8-10   The roles of BRCA1 and BRCA2 in DNA repair. BRCA1 is phosphorylated by ATM and CHEK2 in response to double-stranded DNA breaks (produced, for example, by ionizing radiation). BRCA1 binds to BRCA2, which interacts with RAD51 to form a complex involved in DNA repair.

Because all of the genes illustrated in Figure 8-10 are involved in a DNA repair pathway, it might be anticipated that mutations in genes other than *BRCA1* or *BRCA2* could lead to DNA repair defects and possibly cancer. This is indeed the case. As already discussed, mutations in *CHEK2* can cause LFS. Mutations in the *ATM* gene can cause ataxia telangiectasia (see Chapter 3), an autosomal recessive disease that involves extensive genomic instability, cerebellar ataxia, dilated vessels in the eyes and skin (telangiectasia), and cancers of mainly lymphoid origin. Another autosomal recessive chromosome instability syndrome, Fanconi anemia, can be caused by the inheritance of two copies of a *BRCA2* mutation.

Although *BRCA1* and *BRCA2* mutations are the most common known causes of familial breast cancer, this disease can also be caused by inherited mutations in several other tumor suppressor genes (e.g., the previously discussed *CHEK2* and *TP53* genes). Germline mutations in a tumor suppressor gene called *PTEN* are responsible for Cowden disease, which is characterized by multiple benign tumors and an increased susceptibility to breast cancer. The risk of breast cancer among heterozygous carriers of mutations in the *ATM* gene is approximately double that of the general population. Mutations in the *PALB2* gene, which forms a complex with *BRCA1* and *BRCA2* in repairing double-stranded DNA breaks, also double the risk of breast cancer.

It is estimated that the major breast cancer genes, such as *BRCA1*, *BRCA2*, *PTEN*, and *CHEK2*, account for less than 25% of the overall inherited predisposition to breast cancer. Other breast cancer-causing genes are likely to exist, but their individual effects on cancer risk are thought to be relatively small. Large-scale genome-wide association studies have now identified multiple additional inherited genetic variants that contribute small increases in breast cancer risk (Fig. 8-11). For example, a variant in the gene that encodes fibroblast growth factor receptor 2 (FGFR2) increases breast cancer risk by about 25%.

Most studies indicate that the clinical course of breast cancer among patients with *BRCA1* or *BRCA2* mutations is not substantially different from that of other breast cancer patients. However, the substantial increase in risk of ovarian cancer (which has a high mortality rate and is difficult to detect early), has led to the recommendation that women who have a causal *BRCA1* or *BRCA2* mutation should undergo a prophylactic oophorectomy after they have completed their child-bearing years. This reduces ovarian cancer risk by about 90%, and because it reduces breast cancer risk by about 50%. Bilateral prophylactic mastectomy, an option chosen by some *BRCA1* and *BRCA2* carriers, reduces the risk of breast cancer by approximately 90%.

 Mutations in *BRCA1* and *BRCA2* are responsible for a significant fraction of inherited breast cancer cases, especially those of early onset. These mutations usually result in a truncated protein product and loss of function. The protein products of these genes play important roles in DNA repair.

Familial Melanoma

Largely as a result of increased exposure to ultraviolet radiation, the incidence of melanoma has increased about 20-fold in the United States during the past 70 years. It is now one of the most common cancers, with 76,000 new cases per year. The risk of developing melanoma increases by a factor of 2 when a first-degree relative is affected. The risk increases further,

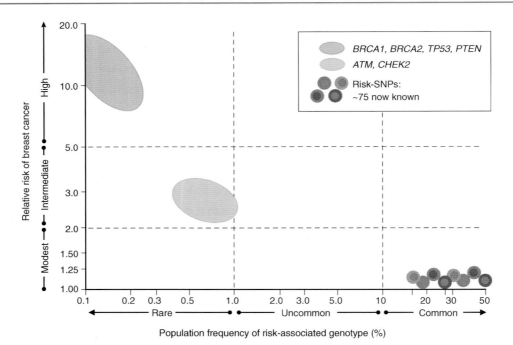

Population frequency of risk-associated genotype (%)

FIG 8-11   The relationship between the relative risk of breast cancer due to a cancer-associated variant (*y*-axis) and the frequency of the variant in the population (*x*-axis). Inherited disease-causing variants in *BRCA1* and *BRCA2* are collectively rare in the population, but they confer a large increase in risk among those who have the variants. Risk alleles in *ATM* and *CHEK2* have higher frequencies, but they confer only a two- to threefold increase in risk. Dozens of common SNP alleles are associated with an increase in breast cancer risk, but they each confer an additional risk of only 5% to 20%. (Courtesy Sean Tavtigian, PhD, Huntsman Cancer Institute, University of Utah Health Sciences Center.)

to approximately six fold, when the first-degree relative is affected before 50 years of age. It is estimated that approximately 5% to 10% of melanoma cases occur in inherited, familial forms.

Germline mutations in the *CDKN2A* gene are estimated to be involved in 20% to 40% of familial melanoma cases. *CDKN2A* encodes two different proteins, both of which are important components of the cell cycle. The first protein, p16, is cyclin-dependent kinase inhibitor which interacts negatively with a cyclin-dependent kinase (CDK4) that phosphorylates and down-regulates the pRb protein (see Fig. 8-5). Because pRb acts as a brake on the cell cycle, its down-regulation by CDK4 promotes progression through the cell cycle and can lead to cell proliferation. By negatively regulating CDK4, p16 acts as an upstream brake on the cell cycle. When p16 activity is lost through loss-of-function mutations in *CDKN2A*, CDK4 activity is increased and cell proliferation can ensue. This can lead to melanomas. The second protein encoded by *CDKN2A* is produced by alternative splic-

ing of the gene's transcript. This protein, termed p14, binds to and inhibits MDM2. The MDM2 protein, as shown in Figure 8-5, binds to and degrades p53. Thus, by inhibiting MDM2, p14 increases p53 expression. As discussed earlier, p53 expression is needed to arrest the cell cycle for DNA repair in response to cell damage, and it can cause damaged cells to undergo apoptosis. A loss of p14 activity leads to a loss of p53 activity, and this can also produce melanomas.

Inherited mutations in the gene that encodes CDK4 can also result in familial melanoma. These gain-of-function mutations convert the cyclin-dependent kinase from a proto-oncogene to an activated oncogene. The activated CDK4 down-regulates pRb, resulting again in a lack of cell cycle control and tumor formation. Melanoma provides an example in which the same tumor type can result from either the activation of a proto-oncogene (*CDK4*) or the loss of a tumor suppressor gene (*CDKN2A*).

CDKN2A plays a role not only in familial melanoma but also in most sporadic melanomas, in which somatic loss-of-function mutations of this gene lead to inactivation of the p16 tumor suppressor protein. About 50% of sporadic melanomas contain somatic deletions of *CDKN2A*, and loss-of-function point mutations are seen in another 5% to 10% of melanomas. Hypermethylation of the promoter region of *CDKN2A*, which down-regulates the gene, is seen in 1/4 to 3/4 of all melanomas. As might be expected, somatic mutations in other genes are also seen in sporadic melanomas. Approximately half of these tumors contain somatic gain-of-function mutations in *BRAF*, a gene that encodes a kinase involved in the RAS signal-transduction pathway (drugs that inhibit BRAF are now being used to treat melanoma). In addition, one of the *RAS* genes, *NRAS*, is mutated in 15% to 30% of sporadic melanomas. Approximately 10% of melanomas have somatic *TP53* mutations, and about 6% have somatic *RB1* mutations (persons who inherit an *RB1* mutation also have an increased risk of melanoma).

Genome-wide association studies using microarrays, as well as exome and whole-genome sequencing, have identified a number of additional genes that influence the risk of melanoma. Many of these genes are involved in producing eumelanin, a skin pigment that helps to protect skin cells from harmful ultraviolet radiation. An example is the *MC1R* gene, in which inherited loss-of-function variants are associated with low levels of eumelanin and high risk of sunburn (red hair and freckling are also associated with these variants). Inheritance of one of these variants increases the risk of melanoma by approximately 50%, and inheritance of multiple *MC1R* variants can more than double the risk of melanoma.

▶ Familial melanoma can be caused by loss-of-function mutations in the *CDKN2A* tumor suppressor gene or by gain-of-function mutations in the *CDK4* proto-oncogene. Both mutations result in a loss of cell cycle control via the pRb and p53 pathways. Somatic mutations of *CDKN2A*, *BRAF*, or *NRAS* are seen in most sporadic melanomas.

The *RET* Proto-Oncogene and Multiple Endocrine Neoplasia

The *RET* proto-oncogene, initially identified by a transfection assay (rearranged during transfection; see previous discussion), encodes a receptor tyrosine kinase that includes an extracellular receptor domain, a transmembrane domain, and an intracellular tyrosine kinase domain. RET is involved in embryonic neural crest cell migration, and it is normally activated by a complex consisting of glial-derived neurotrophic factor (GDNF) and a coreceptor termed GFRα. The RET protein interacts with several signal transduction pathways, including the well-known RAS pathway.

Inherited loss-of-function mutations in *RET* can produce Hirschsprung disease (a lack of enteric nerve cells, resulting in severe, chronic constipation and bowel distention). Gain-of-function mutations in the same gene result in excess tyrosine kinase activity and increased signal transduction, leading ultimately to cellular proliferation and, depending on the type and location of the mutation, any of three forms of autosomal dominant multiple endocrine neoplasia type 2 (MEN2): (1) MEN2A, which accounts for 80% of MEN2 cases, is characterized by medullary thyroid carcinomas (MTC) in nearly 100% of patients, parathyroid hyperplasia in 30% of patients, and pheochromocytoma (an adrenal tumor) in 50% of patients. More than 98% of MEN2A cases are caused by missense mutations that affect cysteine residues in RET's extracellular domain. (2) MEN2B is similar to MEN2A but lacks parathyroid hyperplasia and includes multiple mucosal neuromas and a marfanoid appearance. Nearly all MEN2B alterations are missense mutations that affect RET's tyrosine kinase domain. MEN2B accounts for about 5% of MEN2 cases and is the most aggressive form of MEN2. (3) A syndrome consisting only of familial MTC can be caused by mutations in both the extracellular and tyrosine kinase domains of RET.

RET is one of only a few proto-oncogenes in which mutations can cause inherited cancer syndromes (see Table 8-3 for other examples). (Another inherited form of multiple endocrine neoplasia, MEN1, is characterized by tumors of the parathyroids, anterior pituitary, and pancreas. MEN1 is caused by germline mutations in a gene that encodes the menin tumor suppressor.) Identification of the mutations responsible for each of these inherited cancer syndromes has provided an accurate means of early diagnosis. Patients with apparently sporadic MTC are advised to undergo genetic testing for *RET* mutations because 1% to 7% of these patients have germline *RET* mutations and thus familial, rather than sporadic, MTC. Prophylactic thyroidectomy before 6 years of age is recommended for children who inherit a disease-causing mutation (thyroidectomy before age 3 years may be indicated for the more aggressive MEN2B tumors).

Somatic alterations of RET can produce papillary thyroid carcinomas, the most common type of thyroid tumor. The prevalence of this tumor increased substantially among persons who were exposed to radioactive fallout from the Chernobyl nuclear reactor accident. Sixty percent of the papillary thyroid carcinomas in these persons have contained somatic *RET* alterations.

The *RET* gene provides an example of extraordinary allelic heterogeneity. Loss-of-function mutations in this gene produce defects in the embryonic development of the bowel, and gain-of-function mutations result in increased signal transduction and various forms of endocrine neoplasia. This example illustrates the critical connection between normal development and cancer: Both involve a finely tuned genetic regulation of cell growth and differentiation.

▶ Loss-of-function mutations in the *RET* proto-oncogene can produce Hirschsprung disease, a disorder of embryonic development. Germline gain-of-function mutations in the same gene can lead to any of three different types of inherited multiple endocrine neoplasia. Somatic alterations in *RET* can produce noninherited papillary thyroid carcinoma.

Many additional genes responsible for various inherited cancer syndromes have been identified. These include, for example, the genes that cause neurofibromatosis type 2, von Hippel-Lindau syndrome, and Beckwith-Wiedemann syndrome (see Table 8-1). With the current generation of genomic resources, including the complete human DNA sequence, it is reasonable to expect the identification of more such genes.

IS GENETIC INHERITANCE IMPORTANT IN COMMON CANCERS?

The term "common cancers" is often used to designate those cancers, such as carcinomas of the breast, colon, or prostate, that are not usually part of an inherited cancer syndrome (e.g., Li-Fraumeni syndrome or familial adenomatous polyposis). Recall that germline mutations in genes such as *BRCA1* or *APC*, although very important in aiding our understanding of the basis of carcinogenesis, are responsible for only a small proportion of breast or colon cancer cases. Yet these cancers do cluster in families. Typically, the presence of one affected first-degree relative increases one's risk of developing a common cancer by a factor of two or more. It is likely that additional genes, as well as nongenetic factors that are shared in families, contribute to this increased familial risk (see Chapter 5 for further discussion of these genetic and nongenetic factors in common cancers).

Genome-wide association studies, as well as exome and whole-genome sequencing studies, have revealed many common cancer-predisposing alleles, each with a relatively small effect on overall cancer risk (an example was given by an allele of the *FGFR2* gene in breast cancer). It is critical to determine how these alleles contribute functionally to carcinogenesis. The continuing identification of these alleles, and characterization of the genes in which they occur, can be expected to create new diagnostic and therapeutic tools that ultimately will reduce the cancer burden.

CANCER CYTOGENETICS

Most of the chromosome abnormality syndromes discussed thus far are caused by errors that occur in the meiotic process leading to gamete formation. Chromosome rearrangements can also take place in somatic cells; these are responsible for a number of important cancers in humans. The first of these to be recognized was a chromosome alteration seen consistently in patients with chronic myelogenous leukemia (CML). Initially, it was suggested that the chromosome alteration was a deletion of the long arm of either chromosome 21 or chromosome 22. With the subsequent development of chromosome banding techniques, the abnormality was identified as a reciprocal translocation between chromosomes 9 and 22. The **Philadelphia chromosome**, as this translocation is commonly known, consists of a translocation of most of chromosome 22 onto the long arm of chromosome 9. A small distal portion of 9q in turn is translocated to chromosome 22. The net effect is a smaller chromosome 22, which explains why the Philadelphia chromosome was initially thought to be a deletion. This translocation (Fig. 8-12) is seen in most cases of CML.

Much has been learned about the effects of this translocation by isolating the genes that are located near the translocation **breakpoints** (i.e., the locations on the chromosomes at which the breaks occur preceding translocation). A proto-oncogene called *ABL* is moved from its normal position on 9q to 22q. This alters the *ABL* gene product, causing increased tyrosine kinase activity, which leads to malignancy in hematopoietic cells (i.e., cells that form blood cells such as lymphocytes). Drugs have now been developed to inhibit the tyrosine kinase encoded by this gene, offering much more effective treatment for CML.

A second example of a translocation that produces cancer is given by Burkitt lymphoma, a childhood jaw tumor. In this case, a reciprocal translocation involving chromosomes 8 and 14 moves the *MYC* proto-oncogene from 8q24 to 14q32, near the immunoglobulin heavy chain loci (see Chapter 9). Transcription regulation sequences near the immu-noglobulin genes then activate *MYC*, causing malignancies to form.

More than 100 different rearrangements, involving nearly every chromosome, have been observed in more than 40 different types of cancer. Some of these are summarized in Table 8-4. Increasingly, these translocations are identified using spectral

Normal 9   der(9)

Normal 22   der(22)

FIG 8-12 Reciprocal translocation between chromosome 22 and the long arm of chromosome 9 (the Philadelphia chromosome). The occurrence of this translocation in hematopoietic cells can produce chronic myelogenous leukemia.

TABLE 8-4   Specific Cytogenetic Changes Observed in Selected Leukemias and Solid Tumors

TYPE	MOST COMMON CHROMOSOME ABERRATION
Leukemias	
Chronic myelogenous leukemia	t(9;22)(q34;q11)
Acute myeloblastic leukemia	t(8;21)(q22;q22)
Acute promyelocytic leukemia	t(15;17)(q22;q11-12)
Acute lymphocytic leukemia	t(12;21)(p13;q22)
Solid Tumors	
Burkitt lymphoma	t(8;14)(q24;q32)
Ewing sarcoma	t(11;22)(q24;q12)
Meningioma	Monosomy 22
Retinoblastoma	del(13)(q14)
Wilms tumor	del(11)(p13)
Neuroblastoma	*N-MYC* amplification
Breast cancer	*HER2/NEU* amplification

karyotypes. In many cases, identification of the chromosome rearrangement leads to a more accurate prognosis and better therapy. Hence, the cytogenetic evaluation of bone marrow cells from leukemia patients is a routine part of diagnosis. Furthermore, identification and characterization of the genes that are altered in translocation syndromes are leading to a better understanding of carcinogenesis in general.

 Balanced translocations in somatic cells can sometimes cause malignancies by interrupting or altering genes or their regulatory sequences.

CHROMOSOME INSTABILITY SYNDROMES

Several autosomal recessive disease conditions exhibit an increased incidence of chromosome breaks under specific laboratory conditions. These conditions, which are termed **chromosome instability syndromes**, include ataxia-telangiectasia, Bloom syndrome, Fanconi anemia, and xeroderma pigmentosum (see Chapter 2). Among patients with Fanconi anemia, the frequency of breaks can be increased further if the chromosomes are exposed to certain alkylating agents. Patients with Bloom syndrome also have a high incidence of somatic cell sister chromatid exchange (exchange of chromosome material between sister chromatids; see Chapter 2). Each of these syndromes is associated with a significant increase in cancer risk. All are thought to be the result of faulty DNA replication or repair, as discussed in Chapter 2.

 The chromosome instability syndromes all involve increased frequencies of chromosome breakage and an increased risk of malignancy. All are associated with defects in DNA replication or repair.

SUMMARY

Tumors are categorized as benign or malignant and are identified as neoplasms formed by a group of cells with uncontrollable proliferating ability. A malignant tumor results from a genetic occurrence within somatic cells and is triggered by structural and constitutional alterations of tumor-related genes (including oncogenes and tumor suppressor genes), which are frequently accompanied by genome instability or telomerase activation. The cell integrates and interprets the host of signals it receives from its environment and determines whether to grow or to stop growing and differentiate. Tumor-related genes are normally involved in the regulation of cell growth and repair of DNA damage. However, 5% of cancers are caused by germline mutations and can be passed on to the next generation.

Despite the many scientific discoveries of the 21st century, our understanding of tumor etiology remains insufficient. In addition, cancer incidence and mortality rates continue to increase, even as promising gains against infectious diseases and increases in longevity are made. Increases in cancer incidence and mortality are closely associated with environmental pollution, stress, and unhealthy habits such as smoking. Thus far, however, no apparent determining factor has been identified in the pathogenesis of most malignant tumors, in which a genetic basis is believed to play a critical role. It would be relatively easy to understand the initiation and promotion of cancer if cancer was a disease involving a single gene mutation. Unfortunately, this is not the case. Current theories assume that cancer develops via the accumulation of a series of genetic alterations and that missteps in the induction of proliferation or the regulation of the cell cycle and/or programmed cell death (apoptosis) inevitably lead to the development of a tumor.

IMPORTANT TERMINOLOGY

cancer-predisposing mutation   肿瘤易感基因突变
multi-hit concept of carcinogenesis   肿瘤多步骤起源学说
retinoblastoma   视网膜母细胞瘤
two-hit model of carcinogenesis; two-hit hypothesis   肿瘤起源二次打击学说

somatic mutation　体细胞突变
cancer-causing genes　肿瘤致病基因
gene amplification　基因扩增
germline mutation　生殖细胞突变
chromosomal rearrangement　染色体重排
inherited tumor　遗传型肿瘤

familial adenomatous polyposis　家族性腺瘤样息肉
gain-of-function mutation　功能获得性突变
loss-of-function mutation　功能缺失性突变
microsatellite instability　微卫星不稳定
sporadic tumor　散发型肿瘤
familial melanoma　家族性黑色素瘤

REVIEW QUESTIONS

1. The *G6PD* locus is located on the X chromosome. Studies of *G6PD* alleles in tumor cells from women show that all tumor cells usually express the same single *G6PD* allele, even though the women are heterozygous at the *G6PD* locus. What does this finding imply about the origin of the tumor cells?

2. If we assume that the somatic mutation rate at the *RB1* locus is three mutations per million cells and that there is a population of 2 million retinoblasts per individual, what is the expected frequency of *sporadic* retinoblastoma in the population? What is the expected number of tumors per individual among those who *inherit* a mutated copy of the *RB1* gene?

3. Compare and contrast oncogenes and tumor suppressor genes. How have the characteristics of these classes of cancer-causing genes affected our ability to detect them?

4. Members of Li-Fraumeni syndrome families nearly always develop tumors by 65 to 70 years of age, but mutation carriers do not necessarily develop the same type of tumor (e.g., one has breast cancer, and another has colon cancer). Explain this.

SUGGESTED READINGS AND WEBSITES

1. Couch FJ, Nathanson KL, Offit K. Two decades after BRCA: setting paradigms in personalized cancer care and prevention. *Science*. 2014; 343: 1466-1470.

2. Deng Y, Chan SS, Chang S. Telomere dysfunction and tumour suppression: the senescence connection. *Nat Rev Cancer*. 2008; 8(6): 450-458.

3. Foulkes WD. Inherited susceptibility to common cancers. *N Engl J Med*. 2008; 359(20): 2143-2153.

4. Garraway LA, Lander ES. Lessons from the Cancer Genome. *Cell*. 2013; 153: 17-37.

5. Ghoussaini M, Pharoah PD, Easton DF. Inherited genetic susceptibility to breast cancer: the beginning of the end or the end of the beginning? *Am J Pathol*. 2013; 183: 1038-1051.

6. Hill VK, Gartner JJ, Samuels Y, Goldstein AM. The genetics of melanoma: recent advances. *Annu Rev Genomics Hum Genet*. 2013; 14: 257-279.

7. Jasperson KW, Tuohy TM, Neklason DW, Burt RW. Hereditary and familial colon cancer. *Gastroenterology*. 2010; 138: 2044-2058.

8. Kamihara J, Rana HQ, Garber JE. Germline TP53 mutations and the changing landscape of Li-Fraumeni syndrome. *Hum Mutat*. 2014; 35: 654-662.

9. Kilpivaara O, Aaltonen LA. Diagnostic cancer genome sequencing and the contribution of germline variants. *Science*. 2013; 339: 1559-1562.

10. Knudson AG. Two genetic hits (more or less) to cancer. *Nat Rev Cancer*. 2001; 1(2): 157-162.

11. Lakhani VT, You YN, Wells SA. The multiple endocrine neoplasia syndromes. *Ann Rev Med*. 2007; 58(1): 253-265.

12. Lawrence MS, Stojanov P, Mermel CH, et al. Discovery and saturation analysis of cancer genes across 21 tumour types. *Nature*. 2014; 505: 495-501.

13. Lo JA, Fisher DE. The melanoma revolution: from UV carcinogenesis to a new era in therapeutics. *Science*. 2014; 346: 945-949.

14. McDermott U, Downing JR, Stratton MR. Genomics and the continuum of cancer care. *N Engl J Med*. 2011; 364: 340-350.

15. Muller PA, Vousden KH. Mutant p53 in cancer: new func-

tions and therapeutic opportunities. *Cancer Cell.* 2014; 25: 304-317.

16. Roy HK, Khandekar JD. APC gene testing for familial adenomatosis polyposis. *JAMA.* 2012; 308: 514-515.

17. Sandoval J, Esteller M. Cancer epigenomics: beyond genomics. *Curr Opin Genet Dev.* 2012; 22: 50-55.

18. Venkitaraman AR. Cancer suppression by the chromosome custodians, BRCA1 and BRCA2. *Science.* 2014; 343: 1470-1475.

19. Vogelstein B, Kinzler KW, eds. *The Genetic Basis of Human Cancer.* 2nd ed. New York: McGraw-Hill; 2002.

20. Vogelstein B, Papadopoulos N, Velculescu VE, et al. Cancer genome landscapes. *Science.* 2013; 339: 1546-1558.

21. National Cancer Institute Information site (general information on cancer and cancer genetics, as well as links to other useful websites): http://cancer.gov/cancerinformation

（Xiaobo Cui）

Chapter 9

Immunogenetics

Each day, our bodies are confronted with a formidable series of invaders: viruses, bacteria, and many other disease-causing organisms whose goal is to overcome our natural defenses. These defenses, known collectively as the immune system, consist of a diverse collection of trillions of cells. The immune system must be able to cope with a multitude of invading microorganisms, and it must be able to distinguish "self" from "nonself" with a high degree of accuracy.

As one might expect, the genetic basis of the immune system is complex. The study of the genetics of the immune system, known as **immunogenetics,** has benefited enormously from new developments in gene identification and characterization. Most of the techniques discussed in earlier chapters (e.g., linkage analysis, genome-wide association studies, and high-throughput DNA sequencing) have been used to study genes responsible for the immune response. Many new genes have been discovered, and their functions and interactions have been studied intensely. This chapter provides a brief review of basic immunology and discusses the genes underlying the body's capacity to defend against a highly diverse array of pathogens. Aspects of autoimmune disease are examined, and some of the major immunodeficiency disorders are discussed.

THE IMMUNE RESPONSE: BASIC CONCEPTS

The Innate Immune System

When a pathogenic microorganism is encountered, the body's first line of defense includes **phagocytes** (a type of cell that engulfs and destroys the microorganism) and the **complement system.** The complement proteins can destroy microbes directly by perforating their cell membranes, and they can also attract phagocytes and other immune system agents to microbes by coating the microbial surface (it is because of this assisting role that the term *complement* originated). **Natural killer cells,** a specific type of lymphocyte, can respond to certain viral infections and some tumor cells. Phagocytes complement, and natural killer cells are all part of the **innate immune system,** which is capable of responding very rapidly to pathogens.

The innate immune system is activated by general features that are detected in pathogens but are not found in the host. For example, gram-negative bacteria produce lipopolysaccharides, and gram-positive bacteria produce peptidoglycans. Some bacteria have a high percentage of unmethylated CG sequences, and some viruses produce double-stranded RNA. These distinctive features of pathogenic organisms can be detected by **receptor** molecules located on the surfaces of innate immune system cells. An important example is the Toll-like family of receptors, named after a cell-surface receptor, Toll, that was first described in fruit flies. The genes that encode the human and fruit-fly versions of Toll-like receptors have a remarkable similarity to one another, attesting to their importance in maintaining an innate immune response in a wide variety of organisms. Indeed, all multicellular organisms are thought to possess innate immune systems.

▶ The innate immune system, which includes some phagocytes, natural killer cells, and the complement system, is an early part of the immune response and recognizes general features of invading microorganisms.

The Adaptive Immune System

Although the innate immune system typically helps to hold an infection in check in its early phases, it is sometimes incapable of overcoming the infection. This becomes the task of a more specialized component of the immune response, the **adaptive immune system.** As its name suggests, this part of the immune system is capable of changing, or adapting to features of the invading microorganism in order to mount a more specific and more effective immune response. The adaptive immune system is a more recent evolu-tionary development than the innate immune system and is found only in vertebrates.

Key components of the adaptive immune response (Fig. 9-1) include **T lymphocyte** (or **T cells**) and **B lymphocytes** (or **B cells**). These cells develop in the body's primary lymphoid organs (bone marrow for B cells and the thymus for T cells). In the thymus, developing T cells are exposed to a wide variety of the body's peptides. Those that can recognize and tolerate the body's own peptides are selected, and those that would attack the body's peptides are elimi-nated. The B and T cells progress to secondary lym-

FIG 9-1   Overview of the adaptive immune response. Lymphoid stem cells from the bone marrow migrate to the central lymphoid organs, where they undergo cellular division and differentiation, producing either T cells (thymus) or B cells (bone marrow). At this stage, the B and T cells have not yet encountered antigens, but they have developed considerable diversity in their cell-surface receptors as a result of VDJ recombina-tion and junctional diversity (see text). The cells enter the circulation and migrate to the secondary lymphoid organs (e.g., the spleen and lymph nodes), where they will encounter foreign antigens that are usually processed by antigen-presenting cells (APCs) for presentation to helper T (T$_H$) cells. Only a small subset of T and B cells has receptors capable of binding to a specific foreign antigen, and this subset is selected for further development and differentiation. Somatic hypermutation (see text) occurs in B cells at this stage and results in further receptor diversity and the ability to bind the foreign antigen with greater affinity. The end result of this process is a humoral (B cell) and/or cellular (T cell) response to a foreign antigen. The T-cell response includes cytotoxic T cells that can kill infected cells, regulatory T cells that help to control the immune response, and memory T cells that enable a rapid response if the antigen is encountered later in life. Humoral immunity results in a population of mature B cells (plasma cells) that secrete antibodies into the circulation and a population of memory B cells.

phoid tissues, such as the lymph nodes, spleen, and tonsils, where they encounter disease-causing microorganisms. Mature B lymphocytes secrete circulating **antibodies,** which combat infections. The B lymphocyte component of the immune system is sometimes called the **humoral immune system** because it produces antibodies that circulate in the blood stream. **Helper T lymphocytes** stimulate B lymphocytes and other types of T lymphocytes to respond to infections more effectively, and **cytotoxic T lymphocytes** can directly kill infected cells. Because of this direct interaction with infected cells, the T-cell component of the immune system is sometimes called the **cellular immune system.** It is estimated that the body contains several trillion B and T cells.

> ▶ B lymphocytes are a component of the adaptive immune system; they produce circulating antibodies in response to infection. T lymphocytes, another component of the adaptive immune system, interact directly with infected cells to kill these cells, and they aid in the B-cell response.

The B-Cell Response: Humoral Immune System

A major element of the adaptive immune response begins when specialized types of phagocytes, which are part of the innate immune system, engulf invading microbes and then present peptides derived from these microbes on their cell surfaces. These cells, which include **macrophages** and **dendritic cells,** are termed **antigen-presenting cells (APCs).** B cells are also capable of engulfing microbes and presenting foreign peptides on their cell surfaces. The APCs alert the adaptive immune system to the presence of pathogens in two ways. First, the foreign peptide is transported to the surface of the APC by a **class II major histocompatibility complex (MHC)** molecule, which carries the foreign peptide in a specialized groove (Fig. 9-2). This complex, which projects into the extracellular environment, is recognized by T lymphocytes, which have receptors on their sur-

faces that are capable of binding to the MHC-peptide complex. In addition, the APCs, upon encountering a pathogen, display **costimulatory molecules** on their cell surfaces as a signal that foreign pathogens have been encountered (Fig. 9-3). Binding to the MHC-peptide complex stimulates the helper T lymphocyte to secrete **cytokines,** which are signaling proteins that mediate communication between cells. In particular, these cytokines help to stimulate the subset of B lymphocytes whose cell surface receptors, termed **immunoglobulins,** can bind to the invading microorganism's peptides (see Fig. 9-3). The immunoglobulin's capacity to bind a specific foreign peptide (i.e., its **affinity** for the peptide) is determined by its shape and other characteristics.

> ▶ In the humoral immune response, foreign particles are displayed in conjunction with class II MHC molecules by antigen-presenting cells. These displayed molecules are recognized by helper T cells, which then stimulate proliferation of B cells whose receptors (immunoglobulins) can bind to the foreign pathogen.

It is estimated that upon initial exposure to a foreign microbe, as few as 1 in every 1 million B lymphocytes happens to produce cell-surface receptors capable of binding to the microbe. This number is too small to fight an infection effectively. Furthermore, the receptor's binding affinity is likely to be relatively poor. However, once this relatively small population of B lymphocytes is stimulated, they begin an adaptive process in which additional DNA sequence variation is generated via the process of **somatic hypermutation** (see later discussion). These DNA mutations, which are confined to the genes that encode the cell-surface receptors, in turn produce alterations in the receptors' binding characteristics (e.g., the shape of the protein). Some of these variant receptors possess a higher level of binding affinity for the microorganism. The B cells that produce these receptors are favorably selected because they bind the pathogen for a longer period of time. They thus proliferate rapidly. These B cells then become **plasma cells,** which secrete their cell-surface receptors, or immunoglobulins, into the blood stream. The secreted molecules, which are structurally identical to the receptors on the B cell's surface, are antibodies. It can now be seen how the adaptive immune system gets its name: it involves the initial selection of B cells and T cells whose receptors can bind with the pathogen, followed by subsequent fine-tuning (adaptation) of these cells to achieve higher binding affinity.

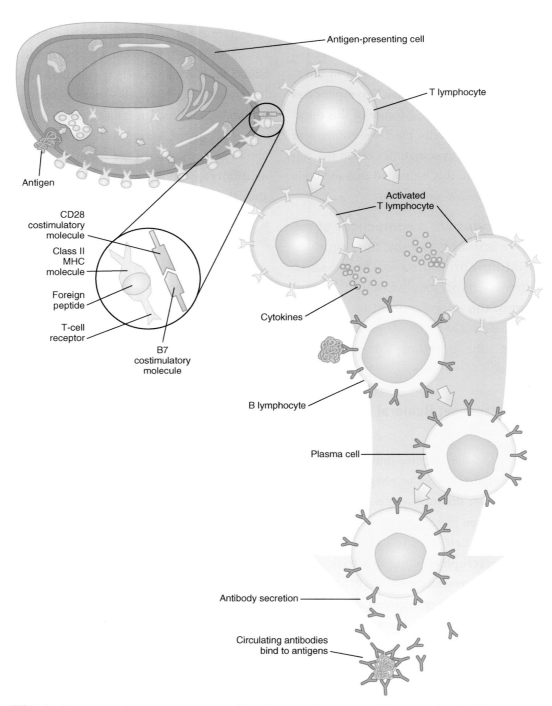

FIG 9-2 The humoral immune response. Class II major histocompatibility complex (MHC) molecules in antigen-presenting cells carry foreign peptides to the surface of the cell, where the foreign peptide is recognized by a helper T cell. The T cell secretes cytokines, which stimulate B cells whose immunoglobulins will bind to the foreign peptide. These B cells become plasma cells, which secrete antibodies into the circulation to bind with the microbe, helping to combat the infection. (Modified from Nossal GJ. Life, death and the immune system. *Sci Am*. 1993; 269: 53-62.)

FIG 9-3   A detailed view of the binding between a helper T cell and a B cell. In addition to the binding of the T-cell receptor to the MHC-peptide complex, a number of other molecules interact with one another, such as the co stimulatory B7-CD28 complex. MHC, major histocompatibility complex. (Modified from Roitt I, Brostoff J, Male D. *Immunology.* 6th ed. St. Louis: Mosby; 2001.)

▶ During the B-cell response to a foreign peptide, the binding affinity of immunoglobulins for the invading pathogen increases. When mature, the B cell becomes an antibody-secreting plasma cell.

After initial stimulation by the disease pathogen, the process of B-cell differentiation and maturation into antibody-producing plasma cells requires about 5 to 7 days for completion. Each plasma cell is capable of secreting approximately 10 million antibody molecules per hour. Antibodies bind to the pathogen's surface **antigens** (a term derived from "*anti*body *gen*erating") and may neutralize the microorganism directly. More often, the antibody tags the pathogen for destruction by other components of the immune system, such as complement proteins and phagocytes.

Another important activity of the humoral immune response is the creation of **memory B cells,** a subset of high affinity-binding B cells that persist in the body after the infection has subsided. These cells, which

have already been highly selected for response to the pathogen, provide a more rapid response should the pathogen be encountered again later in the individual's life. Vaccinations are effective because they induce the formation of memory cells that can respond to a specific pathogen.

The Cellular Immune System

Some microorganisms, such as viruses, are very adept at quickly inserting themselves into the body's cells. Here, they are inaccessible to antibodies, which are water-soluble proteins that cannot pass through the cell's lipid membrane. A second component of the adaptive immune system, the cellular immune system, has evolved to combat such infections. A key member of the cellular immune response is the **class I MHC molecule,** which is found on the surfaces of nearly all of the body's cells. In a normal cell, the class I MHC molecule binds with small peptides (8 to 10 amino acids long) derived from the interior of the cell. It migrates to the cell's surface, carrying the peptide with it and displaying it outside the cell. Because this is one of the body's own peptides, no immune response is elicited. In an infected cell, however, the class I MHC molecule can bind to small peptides that are derived from the infecting organism. Cell-surface presentation of foreign peptides by the class I MHC molecule alerts the immune system, T cells in particular. Recall that T lymphocytes learn to recognize and tolerate self peptides (in conjunction with MHC molecules) while developing in the thymus, but they are highly intolerant of foreign peptides. The MHC-peptide complex binds to receptors on the appropriate T cell's surface, which prompts the T cell to emit a chemical that destroys the infected cell (Fig. 9-4). Because of their ability to destroy cells in this way, these T lymphocytes are termed **cytotoxic T lymphocytes** or **killer T lymphocytes.** (They are also known as CD8+ T cells because of the presence of CD8 [cluster of differentiation antigen 8] coreceptors on their surfaces, which bind to the class I MHC molecule [see Fig. 9-4]. Mature T_H cells have CD4 coreceptors on their cell surfaces, which bind to class II MHC molecules [see Fig. 9-3] and are thus known as CD4+ T cells.) Each cytotoxic T lymphocyte can destroy one infected cell every 1 to 5 minutes.

T cells are often alerted to the presence of an infection when circulating dendritic cells present the foreign peptides on their cell surfaces and migrate to secondary lymphoid tissues, where most of the T cells reside. As with B lymphocytes, only a small fraction of the body's T cells has receptors with binding affinity for the infecting pathogens.

FIG 9-4 In a cell infected by a virus, the viral peptides (*1, 2*) are carried to the cell surface by class I MHC molecules (*3*). The T-cell receptor of a CD8+ cytotoxic T cell binds to the peptide-MHC complex (*4*). Recognizing the peptide as foreign, the cytotoxic T cell secretes chemicals that either kill the infected cell directly or induce it to undergo programmed cell death (apoptosis; see Chapter 8) (*5*). *MHC*, major histocompatibility complex. (Modified from Janeway CA Jr. How the immune system recognizes invaders. *Sci Am*. 1996; 269: 73-79.)

The immune system is capable of destroying the body's cells once they are infected. Peptides from the pathogen are displayed on cell surfaces by class I MHC molecules. These are recognized by cytotoxic (killer) T lymphocytes, which destroy the infected cell.

In contrast to cytotoxic T cells, which destroy infected cells directly, helper T (T_H) cells respond to the presence of pathogens by secreting cytokines. These molecules in turn stimulate the development of other components of the immune system, such as B cells and cytotoxic T cells. T_H cells are classified into subsets, depending on which cytokines they secrete. For example, T_H1 cells, which are involved primarily in combating intracellular pathogens, secrete interleukin-2 (IL-2), interferon-γ, and tumor necrosis factor β. T_H2 cells, which secrete IL-4, IL-5, IL-6, and IL-13, help to fight multicellular parasites and are involved in allergic responses. Other helper T-cell subsets include T_H17 cells, which secrete IL-17, and T_H22 cells, which secrete IL-22.

As in the B-cell component of the adaptive immune system, a subset of long-lived T cells is retained (**memory T cells**) to quickly respond to a foreign pathogen should it be encountered again in the future. Yet another type of T cell, the **regulatory T cell,** helps to regulate the immune system so that self peptides are not inadvertently attacked.

Helper T cells stimulate development of other components of the immune system, such as cytotoxic T cells and B cells, by secreting cytokines. Various subsets of helper T cells have been described, depending on which cytokines they secrete. Memory T cells remain long after an infection and ensure rapid response to a subsequent infection by the same pathogen. Regulatory T cells help to prevent the immune system from attacking the body's own cells.

The Innate, Humoral, and Cellular Immune Systems: A Comparison

Although the innate and adaptive immune systems are described separately, a great deal of interaction takes place between them, and the two systems fulfill complementary functions. The innate system, because it recognizes general features of pathogens, can react very quickly to foreign elements. While doing so, it signals the adaptive immune system to initiate a fine-tuned response to the pathogen. Without this signal, the adaptive immune system is incapable of responding to an infection. After several days during which the adaptive system "learns" the characteristics of the pathogen, it can launch a massive, specialized response. Through the creation of memory B and T cells, the adaptive immune system allows the organism to respond quickly and effectively to a pathogen should it be encountered again. No such memory cells exist for the innate immune system.

The humoral immune system is specialized to combat extracellular infections, such as circulating bacteria and viruses. The cellular immune system combats intracellular infections, such as parasites and viruses within cells. However, this division of labor is not strict, and there is again a great deal of interaction between the humoral and cellular components of the immune system.

IMMUNE RESPONSE PROTEINS: GENETIC BASIS OF STRUCTURE AND DIVERSITY

Immunoglobulin Molecules and Genes

As illustrated in Figure 9-5, each antibody (or immunoglobulin) molecule is composed of four chains: an identical pair of longer **heavy chains** and an identical pair of shorter **light chains,** which are linked together by disulfide bonds. There are five different types of heavy chains (termed γ, μ, α, δ, and ε) and two types of light chains (κ and λ). The five types of heavy chains determine the major **class** (or **isotype**) to which an immunoglobulin (Ig) molecule belongs:

γ, μ, α, δ, and ε correspond to the immunoglobulin isotypes IgG, IgM, IgA, IgD, and IgE, respectively. Immature B lymphocytes produce only IgM, but as they mature, a rearrangement of heavy chain genes called **class switching** occurs. This produces the other four major classes of immunoglobulins, each of which differs in amino acid composition, charge, size, and carbohydrate content. Each class tends to be localized in certain parts of the body, and each tends to respond to a different type of infection. The two types of light chains can be found in association with any of the five types of heavy chains.

The heavy and light chains both contain a **constant** and a **variable** region, which are located at the carboxyl (C)-terminal and amino (N)-terminal ends of the chains, respectively. The arrangement of genes encoding the constant region determines the major class of the Ig molecule (e.g., IgA, IgE). The variable region is responsible for antigen recognition and binding and thus varies within immunoglobulin classes. Three distinct gene segments encode the light chains: C for the constant region, V for the variable region, and J for the region that joins the constant and variable regions. Four gene segments encode the heavy chains, with C, V, and J coding again for the constant, variable, and joining regions, respectively, and a "diversity" (D) region located between the joining and variable regions.

 Immunoglobulin molecules consist of two identical heavy chains and two identical light chains. The heavy chain constant region determines the major class to which an immunoglobulin belongs. The variable regions of the light and heavy chains recognize and bind antigens.

FIG 9-5   An antibody molecule consists of two identical light chains and two identical heavy chains. The light chain includes variable, joining, and constant regions; the heavy chain includes these regions as well as a diversity region located between its variable and joining regions. The *upper portion* of the figure depicts a molecular model of antibody structure.

The Genetic Basis of Antibody Diversity

Because the immune system cannot "know" in advance which types of microbes it will encounter, the system must contain a huge reservoir of structurally diverse immune cells so that at least a few cells can respond (i.e., bind) to any invading microbe. Indeed, the humoral immune system is capable of generating approximately 100 billion structurally distinct antibodies. At one time, it was thought that because each antibody has a unique amino acid sequence, each must be encoded by a different gene. However, this one gene-one antibody hypothesis could not possibly be correct, because the human genome has only 20,000 to 25,000 protein-coding genes. Further study has shown that several mechanisms are responsible for generating **antibody diversity** in somatic cells:

1. Multiple Germline Immunoglobulin Genes

Molecular genetic studies (cloning and DNA sequencing) have shown that for each heavy and light chain, an individual has more than 80 different V segments located contiguously in his or her germline and six different J segments. There are at least 30 D segments in the heavy chain region.

2. Somatic Recombination (VDJ Recombination)

As immunoglobulin molecules are formed during B lymphocyte maturation, a specific combination of single V and J segments is selected for the light chain, and another combination of V, D, and J segments is selected for the heavy chain. This is accomplished by deleting the DNA sequences separating the single V, J, and D segments before they are transcribed into mRNA (Fig. 9-6). The deletion process is carried out in part by **recombinases** (encoded by the *RAG1* and *RAG2* genes), which initiate double-strand DNA breaks at specific DNA sequences that flank the V and D gene segments. After the deletion of all but one V, D, and J segment, the nondeleted segments are joined by ligases. This cutting-and-pasting process is known as **somatic recombination** (in contrast to the germline recombination that takes place during meiosis). Somatic recombination produces a distinc-

tive result: unlike most other cells of the body, whose DNA sequences are identical to one another, mature B lymphocytes vary in terms of their rearranged immunoglobulin DNA sequences. Because there are many possible combinations of single V, J, and D segments, somatic recombination can generate approximately 100,000 to 1,000,000 different types of antibody molecules.

FIG 9-6 **A,** Somatic VDJ recombination in the formation of a heavy chain of an antibody molecule. The functional heavy chain is encoded by only one segment each from the multiple V, D, and J segments. This produces a subset of B cells whose receptors have low-affinity binding for a foreign antigen. Once the antigen is encountered in the secondary lymphoid tissue, somatic hypermutation **(B** and **C)** is initiated. Most of the mutated receptors have little binding affinity **(B),** but eventually somatic hypermutation produces a subset of receptors with high-affinity binding **(C).** The cells that contain these receptors become antibody-secreting plasma cells.

3. Junctional Diversity

As the V, D, and J regions are assembled, slight variations occur in the position at which they are joined, and small numbers of nucleotides may be deleted or inserted at the junctions joining the regions. This creates even more variation in antibody amino acid sequence.

4. Somatic Hypermutation

Typically, only a small subset of B cells has cell-surface receptors (immunoglobulins) that can bind to a specific foreign antigen, and their binding affinity is usually low. Once this subset of B cells is stimulated by a foreign antigen, they undergo an affinity maturation process characterized by somatic hypermutation of the V segments of immunoglobulin genes, as mentioned previously. An enzyme termed *activation-induced deaminase* causes cytosine bases to be replaced by uracil. Error-prone DNA polymerases are recruited, and DNA repair processes are modified so that mutations can persist in the DNA sequence. Consequently, the mutation rate of these gene segments is approximately 10^{-3} per base pair per generation (recall that the mutation rate in the human genome is normally only 10^{-8} per base pair per generation). This causes much additional variation inimmunoglobulin-encoding DNA sequences and thus in the antigen-binding properties of the encoded immunoglobulins. Because mutation is a random process, most of the new receptors have poor binding affinity and are thus not selected. Eventually, however, somatic hypermutation produces a subset of immunoglobulins that have high-affinity binding to the foreign antigen, and the B cells that harbor these immunoglobulins are selected to proliferate extensively. The end result is a population of mature plasma cells that secrete antibodies that are highly specific to the invading pathogen.

5. Multiple Combinations of Heavy and Light Chains

Further diversity is created by the random combination of different heavy and light chains in assembling the immunoglobulin molecule. Each of these mechanisms contributes to antibody diversity. Considering all of them together, it has been estimated that as many as 1011 distinct antibodies can potentially be produced.

 Mechanisms that produce antibody diversity include multiple germline immunoglobulin gene segments, somatic recombination of the immunoglobulin gene segments, junctional diversity, somatic hypermutation, and the potential for multiple combinations of heavy and light chains.

T-Cell Receptors

The T-cell receptors are similar in many ways to the immunoglobulins, or B-cell receptors. Like the immunoglobulins, T-cell receptors must be able to bind to a large variety of peptides derived from invading organisms. Unlike immunoglobulins, however, T-cell receptors are never secreted from the cell, and T-cell activation requires the presentation of foreign peptide along with an MHC molecule. Approximately 90% of T-cell receptors are heterodimers composed of an α and a β chain, and approximately 10% are heterodimers composed of a γ and a δ chain (Fig. 9-7). A given T cell has a population of either α-β receptors or γ-δ receptors.

Most of the mechanisms involved in generating immunoglobulin diversity—multiple germline gene segments, VDJ somatic recombination, and junctional diversity—are also important in generating T-cell receptor diversity. However, somatic hypermutation does not occur in the genes that encode the T-cell receptors. This is thought to help avoid the generation of T cells that would react against the body's own cells (an autoimmune response, which is discussed later in the chapter).

 T-cell receptors are similar in function to B-cell receptors (immunoglobulins). Unlike immunoglobulins, however, they can bind to a foreign peptide only when it is presented by an MHC molecule. Their diversity is created by the same mechanisms that produce immunoglobulin diversity, with the exception of somatic hypermutation.

α chain —| |— β chain

☐ Variable region
☐ Constant region
☐ Joining region
☐ Diversity region

FIG 9-7   The T-cell receptor is a heterodimer that consists of either an α and a β chain or a γ and a δ chain. The complex of MHC molecule and antigen molecule is bound by the variable regions of the α and β chains. (Modified from Raven PH, Johnson GB. *Biology.* 3rd ed. St. Louis: Mosby; 1992.)

Plasma membrane

THE MAJOR HISTOCOMPATIBILITY COMPLEX

Class I, II, and III Genes

The MHC, which includes a series of more than 200 genes that lie in a 4-Mb region on the short arm of chromosome 6 (Fig. 9-8), is commonly classified into three groups: class I, class II, and class III. The class I MHC molecule forms a complex with foreign peptides that is recognized by receptors on the surfaces of cytotoxic T lymphocytes. Class I presentation is thus essential for the cytotoxic T-cell response. Some viruses evade cytotoxic T-cell detection by down-regulating the expression of MHC class I genes in the cells they infect. Class I MHC molecules are composed of a single heavy glycoprotein chain and a single light chain called β2-microglobulin (Fig. 9-9A). The most important of the class I loci are labeled **human leukocyte antigens** A, B, and C (**HLA-A, -B, and -C).** (These molecules were named "human leukocyte antigens" because they were seen in early studies on leukocyte [white cell] surfaces. However,

as mentioned previously, they are found on the surfaces of nearly all cells). Each of these loci has dozens or hundreds of alleles, resulting in a high degree of class I MHC variability among individuals. The class I region spans 1.8 Mb and includes a number of additional genes and **pseudogenes** (genes that are similar in DNA sequence to coding genes but that have been altered so that they cannot be transcribed or translated).

The class I molecules were first discovered in the 1940s by scientists who were experimenting with tissue grafts in mice. When the class I alleles in donor and recipient mice differed, the grafts were rejected. This is the historical basis for the term *major histocompatibility complex.* In humans, matching of the donor's and recipient's class I alleles increases the probability of graft or transplant tolerance. Because grafts and transplants are a relatively new phenomenon in human history, the MHC obviously did not evolve to effect transplant rejection. Instead, T cells, when confronted with foreign MHC molecules on donor cells, interpret these as foreign peptides and attack the cells.

FIG 9-8   A map of the human major histocompatibility complex. The 4-Mb complex is divided into three regions: classes I, II, and III.

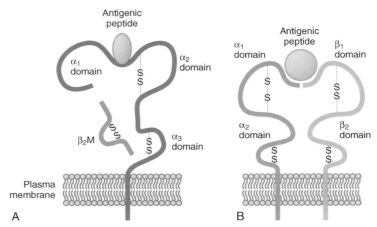

FIG 9-9   A, A class I major histocompatibility complex (MHC) molecule, showing the structure of the heavy chain, which consists of three extracellular domains (α_1, α_2, and α_3), a membrane-spanning domain, and a cytoplasmic domain. A groove formed by the α_1 and α_2 domains carries peptide for presentation to T-cell receptors. The α_3 domain associates closely with the β_2-microglobulin (β_2M) chain. **B,** A class II MHC molecule, showing the structure of the α and β chains. Each has two globular extracellular domains, a membrane-spanning domain, and a cytoplasmic domain. The α_1 and β_1 domains form a groove into which peptide nestles for presentation to T-cell receptors. (Modified from McCance KL, Huether SE. *Pathophysiology: the Biologic Basis for Disease in Adults and Children.* 7th ed. St. Louis: Elsevier; 2014: 234.)

▶ The class I MHC molecules are encoded by the highly polymorphic *HLA-A, -B,* and *-C* loci on chromosome 6. In addition to presenting foreign peptides on the surfaces of infected cells, they can also bring about transplant rejection when non-self MHC molecules stimulate cytotoxic T cells.

Whereas the class I MHC molecules are found on the surfaces of nearly all cells and can bind with cytotoxic T-cell receptors, the class II MHC molecules ordinarily are found only on the surfaces of the immune system's APCs (e.g., phagocytes and B lymphocytes). When associated with foreign peptides, they stimulate helper T cell activity after binding to the T cells' receptors, as described previously. The class II molecules are heterodimers consisting of an α and a β chain, each of which is encoded by a different gene located on chromosome6 (see Fig. 9-9B). In addition to the genes in the major class II groups (*HLA-DP, -DQ,* and *-DR*), this region includes genes that encode peptide transporter proteins (*TAP1* and *TAP2*) that help to transport peptides into the endo-

plasmic reticulum, where they initially form complexes with class I molecules before migrating to the cell surface.

▶ Class II MHC molecules are heterodimers encoded by genes on chromosome 6. They present peptides on the surfaces of antigen-presenting cells. These peptides, in conjunction with class II MHC molecules, are bound by receptors on helper T cells.

Like the major class I MHC loci, the major class II loci are highly polymorphic, expressing hundreds of different alleles. Indeed, the MHC loci are, as a class, the most polymorphic loci known in humans. Each MHC allele encodes a molecule with slightly different binding properties: some variants bind peptide from a given pathogen more effectively than others do. (Because of the relatively limited repertoire of different MHC molecules, the peptide-binding affinity of MHC molecules is usually much lower than the binding affinity of finely tuned T-cell receptors.) Consequently, a person who expresses a greater variety of MHC molecules has a better chance of dealing effectively with infectious organisms. For example, someone who is homozygous for each of the major class I loci (*A*, *B*, and *C*) expresses only three different class I MHC molecules in each cell, whereas someone who is heterozygous for each of these loci expresses six different class I MHC molecules in each cell and can cope more successfully with pathogenic diversity (many thousands of MHC molecules are expressed on a typical cell's surface). A higher degree of polymorphism in the general population increases the chance that any individual in the population is heterozygous. For example, HIV infected persons who are heterozygous for the *HLA-A*, *HLA-B*, and/or *HLA-C* loci have longer survival times than those who are homozygous at these loci. In addition, greater MHC polymorphism in a population decreases the chance that an infectious pathogen can spread easily through the population. Thus, the high degree of polymorphism in MHC genes is thought to be the result of natural selection for allelic variation.

In some cases, specific MHC alleles are known to produce proteins that are effective against specific pathogens. For example, the *HLA-B53* allele was shown to have a strong protective effect against severe malaria in the population of Gambia, and the *HLA-DRB1*13:02* allele protects against hepatitis B infection in the same population. These alleles produce MHC molecules that have higher-affinity binding of the infectious agents.

▶ Like the class I MHC genes, class II genes are highly polymorphic. This increases the ability of individuals and populations to respond to a wide variety of pathogens.

Both class I and class II MHC molecules guide T-cell receptors (cytotoxic and helper, respectively) to specific cells. T-cell receptors recognize peptides only in combination with MHC molecules on cell surfaces, a phenomenon known as **MHC restriction.** Not all components of the immune system are MHC restricted. The complement system, for example, does not require direct interaction with MHC molecules.

Some virus-infected cells and tumor cells take advantage of MHC restriction: they suppress the expression of MHC molecules on their surfaces in an attempt to evade detection by T cells (Clinical Commentary 9-1). Fortunately, natural killer cells are activated by the absence, rather than the presence of MHC molecules on cell surfaces. This activation is mediated by an important and diverse family of receptors found on the surfaces of natural killer cells, **killer cell immunoglobulin-like receptors (KIR).** These receptors inhibit natural killer cells when they bind to MHC class I molecules on the surfaces of normal cells but activate them when MHC class I molecules are absent.

The class III MHC region spans 680 kb and contains at least 36 genes, only some of which are involved in the immune response. Among the most important of these are the genes encoding the complement proteins.

The genes encoding the immunoglobulins, the T-cell receptors, KIR, and the class I and class II MHC proteins all share similar DNA sequences and structural features. Thus, they are members of a gene family, like the globin genes, the color vision genes, and the collagen genes described in earlier Chapters. Table 9-1 provides a summary of the major genes of the immune system and their chromosome locations.

It is important to emphasize that the class I and class II MHC molecules differ greatly *among* individuals, but each cell within an individual has the same class I and class II molecules (this uniformity is necessary for recognition by T cells). In contrast, after VDJ recombination the T-cell receptors and immunoglobulins differ from cell to cell *within* individuals, allowing the body to respond to a large variety of different infectious agents.

 The immunoglobulin, T-cell receptor, KIR, and MHC genes are members of a gene family. Whereas immunoglobulins and T-cell receptors vary between cells within an individual, MHC molecules vary between individuals.

TABLE 9-1 Chromosome Location and Function of Major Immune Response Genes

GENE SYSTEM	CHROMOSOME LOCATION	GENE PRODUCT FUNCTION
Immunoglobulin heavy chain (C, V, D, and J genes)	14q32	Heavy chain, the first part of antibody molecule, which binds foreign antigens
Immunoglobulin κ light chain (C, V, and J genes)	2p13	Light chain, the second part of antibody molecule
Immunoglobulin λ light chain (C, V, and J genes)	22q11	Light chain, the second part of antibody molecule (either κ or λ may be used)
T-cell receptor α	14q11	One chain of the α-β T-cell receptor, which recognizes antigen with MHC molecule
T-cell receptor β	7q35	The second chain of the α-β T-cell receptor
T-cell receptor γ	7p15	One chain of the γ-δ T-cell receptor
T-cell receptor δ	14q11	The second chain of the γ-δ T-cell receptor
MHC (classes I, II, and III); includes TAP1 and TAP2	6p21	Cell-surface molecules that present peptides to T-cell receptors. TAP1 and TAP2 are transporter molecules that process foreign peptides and carry them to the endoplasmic reticulum.
β_2-microglobulin	15q21-22	Forms second chain of the class I MHC molecule
RAG1, RAG2	11p13	Recombinases that participate in VDJ somatic recombination

MHC and Disease Associations

A number of diseases show significant associations with specific MHC alleles: persons who have the allele are much more likely to develop the disease than are those who lack it. Some examples, mentioned in earlier chapters, include the association of HLA-B27 (i.e., allele 27 of the HLA-B locus) with ankylosing spondylitis and of HLA-DQB1 with type 1 diabetes. An especially strong association is seen between several HLA-DR and -DQ alleles and narcolepsy, a disorder characterized by sudden and uncontrollable episodes of sleep. As Table 9-2 shows, most of the HLA-disease associations involve the class II MHC genes.

In some cases the association between MHC alleles and a disease is caused by linkage disequilibrium. For example, the hemochromatosis locus is linked to HLA-A, and significant associations occur between HLA-A3 and the most common hemochromatosis-causing allele. There is no known causal link between HLA-A3 and this disorder, however. More likely, the association represents a past event in which the primary hemochromatosis mutation arose on a copy of chromosome 6 that had the HLA-A3 allele. Similarly, the association between HLA-DQB1 and HLA-DQA1 and narcolepsy is due to linkage disequi-

TABLE 9-2 Examples of Major Histocompatibility Complex and Disease Associations

DISEASE	MHC (HLA) ASSOCIATED LOCUS (LOCI)[*]	APPROXIMATE RELATIVE RISK[†]
Type 1 diabetes	DQB1, DQA1	10
Ankylosing spondylitis	B27	90
Narcolepsy	DR2 and DQA1, DQB1	>100
Celiac disease	DQA1, DQB1	10
Rheumatoid arthritis	DRB1, DQA1	5
Myasthenia gravis	C, DR3, DR7	2.5
Multiple sclerosis	DRB1	4
Systemic lupus erythematosus	DRB1	6
Hemochromatosis	A3	20
Malaria	B53	0.6059
Graves disease	DR3	5
Psoriasis	C	13
Abacavir (anti-HIV drug) hypersensitivity	B57	≈1000

[*]For simplicity, specific alleles are not shown here. For example, the HLA-B57 allele associated with abacavir sensitivity is labeled HLA-B*57:01, and the allele associated with psoriasis is HLA-C*06:02.

[†]Relative risk can be interpreted loosely as the odds that a person who has a risk factor (in this case, an MHC antigen) will develop the disease, compared with a person who lacks the risk factor. Thus, a relative risk of 4 for DRB1 and multiple sclerosis means that persons with a specific DRB1 allele are four times more likely to develop multiple sclerosis than are those without it. A relative risk <1 (as seen for malaria and B53) indicates that the factor is protective against the disease. These relative risks can vary among different human population groups.

librium between the *HLADQ* region and a nearby locus that causes narcolepsy (the hypocretin type 2 receptor gene).

In other cases a causal association may exist. Some MHC-disease associations involve **autoimmunity,** in which the body's immune system attacks its own normal cells. For example, type 1 diabetes is characterized by T-cell infiltration of the pancreas and subsequent T-cell destruction of the insulin-producing beta cells. In some cases, autoimmunity involves "molecular mimicry". Here, a peptide that stimulates an immune response is so similar to the body's own peptides that the immune system begins to attack the body's own cells. This phenomenon helps to explain the onset of ankylosing spondylitis, another autoimmune disease. Infections of *HLAB27*-positive persons with specific microbes, such as *Klebsiella*, can lead to a **cross-reaction** in which the immune system mistakes peptides from some of the body's normal cells for microbial peptides. Another

---

CLINICAL COMMENTARY 9-1

The Immune Response as a Molecular Arms Race

The vast majority of the pathogens that assault the human body are destroyed by our immune system. Consequently, there is strong natural selection for pathogens that can evade immune surveillance and destruction. These microorganisms often have high mutation rates, and their numbers are huge. Thus, despite their biological simplicity, viruses and other pathogens have evolved some very clever ways of overcoming the immune response. Our immune systems, in turn, are constantly creating new ways to deal with pathogenic ingenuity. Three examples of this molecular "arms race" are discussed here.

Cytomegalovirus (CMV) is a common infectious agent that can produce mononucleosis, hemolytic anemia, pneumonitis, congenital infections, and thrombocytopenia (a decrease in the number of platelets). Cells infected with CMV are the targets of destruction by cytotoxic T cells. However, some CMV strains (as well as other viruses and tumor cells) can evade T-cell detection by down-regulating the expression of class I molecules on the surfaces of infected cells. Without viral peptide presentation by class I molecules, the cytotoxic T cells are blind to the presence of CMV, and they do not destroy the infected cell. At this point, the cell would normally become the target of natural killer cells, which attack cells that lack MHC class I molecules on their surfaces. But CMV has devised a way to outwit natural killer cells, too. The virus encodes a cell-surface protein that resembles class I molecules closely enough so that the natural killer cells mistake the viral protein for a true class I molecule. The viral protein is also sufficiently *different* from a true class I MHC molecule that it does not trigger destruction by the more finely tuned cytotoxic T cell. In this way, CMV can often avoid destruction by both T cells and natural killer cells.

An important immunological challenge for placental mammals is pregnancy, in which placental cells express foreign class IMHC molecules derived from the father. Ordinarily, such cells would be quickly destroyed by the mother's cytotoxic T cells. To avoid this, placental cells down-regulate the expression of class I MHC molecules on their surfaces. As with viral down regulation of class I molecules, this lack of MHC class I expression leaves the placental cells liable to destruction by the mother's natural killer cells. In this case, the cells are saved from destruction by presenting HLA-G molecules on their surface. This relatively nonvariant MHC molecule does not stimulate a T-cell response, which is limited to presentation of HLA-A, -B, and -C molecules. It does inhibit the natural killer cell, which has HLA-G receptors on its surface. The fetus, like CMV, has thus devised ways of avoiding destruction by both T cells and natural killer cells.

A third example of the molecular arms race is given by one of the most feared infectious agents of modern times, the human immunodeficiency virus (HIV). Some strains of this virus gain entry into macrophages and helper T cells via a cell-surface receptor, CC chemokine receptor 5 (*CCR5*). Once inside the cell, HIV inserts its genetic material into the nucleus and takes advantage of the cell's machinery to replicate itself (HIV is a retrovirus, a type of virus that is discussed further in Chapter 10. Helper T cells are a critical component of the body's immune system, and their destruction by HIV leads to severe secondary immunodeficiency. Persons who are homozygous for a 32-bp deletion of the *CCR5* gene lack the CCR5 receptor and are thus remarkably resistant to HIV infection. Among those who are heterozygous for this deletion, progression to AIDS symptoms after seroconversion is slowed by 2 to 4 years. This deletion is especially common in northeastern European populations, where the gene frequency reaches 0.20. It is virtually absent in Asian and African populations.

Analysis of linkage disequilibrium in the chromosomal region that contains CCR5 indicates that the deletion arose in European populations only 700 to 2000 years ago. Because HIV appeared in humans only a few decades ago, the high gene frequency in northeastern Europe cannot be due to HIV and must be due to another selective force or perhaps to genetic drift. Considering the age of the deletion, it is possible that it underwent positive selection because it provided resistance to pathogens, such as smallpox, that ravaged European populations in the past. Clearly, there would be strong selection in favor of this mutation in populations now heavily exposed to HIV, and the deletion would eventually rise in frequency in these populations. Even now, knowledge of the consequences of this deletion may help accelerate the medical arms race against HIV, where genetic modification of CCR5 is being tested in HIV clinical trials (see Chapter 10).

such example is given by rheumatic fever, in which a streptococcal infection initiates cross reactivity between streptococcus and cardiac myosin. In each of these scenarios, the body already has a small population of self-reactive T cells, but they remain inactive and quite harmless until they are stimulated to proliferate by a foreign peptide that closely resembles a self peptide.

Autoimmunity can also be caused by specific defects in the regulation of immune system components. For example, regulatory T cells help to prevent the formation of self reactive immune cells and require a transcription factor, encoded by *FOXP3*, for their normal development. Mutations in *FOXP3* result in a deficiency of regulatory T cells and an autoimmune disease called *IPEX* (*i*mmune dysregulation, *p*olyendocrinopathy, *e*nteropathy, *X* linked).

Other common diseases that involve autoimmunity include rheumatoid arthritis, systemic lupus erythematosus, psoriasis, and multiple sclerosis. It is estimated that approximately 5% of the population suffers from some type of autoimmune disease.

 A significant number of diseases are associated with specific MHC alleles. Some of these associations are the result of linkage disequilibrium, but most are likely to result from causal associations involving autoimmunity.

The ABO and Rh Blood Groups

Another component of the immune system involves red blood cell surface molecules that can cause an immune reaction during blood transfusions. The ABO and Rh red cell antigen systems were discussed in Chapter 3 as early examples of polymorphic marker loci. They are also the most important systems that determine blood transfusion compatibility.

The ABO System

There are four major ABO blood types: A, B, AB, and O. The first three groups respectively represent persons who carry the A, B, or A and B antigens on their erythrocyte surfaces. Those with type O have neither the A nor the B antigen. Persons who have one of these antigens on their erythrocyte surfaces possess antibodies against all other ABO antigens in their blood stream. (These antibodies are formed early in life as a result of exposure to antigens that are identical to the A and B antigens but are present in various microorganisms.) Thus, if a type B person received type A or AB blood, his or her anti-A antibodies would produce a severe and possibly fatal reaction. Type O persons, who have neither the A nor the B antigen and thus both anti-A and anti-B antibodies, would react strongly to blood of the other three types (A, B, and AB). It was once thought that type O persons, because they lack both types of antigens, could be "universal donors" (anyone could accept their blood). Similarly, type AB persons were termed "universal recipients" because they lacked both anti-A and anti-B antibodies. However, when patients are given transfusions of whole blood containing large volumes of serum, the donor's antibodies can react against the recipient's erythrocyte antigens. Hence, complete ABO matching is nearly always done for blood transfusions.

 The ABO locus encodes red cell antigens that can cause a transfusion reaction if donors and recipients are not properly matched.

The Rh System

The Rh blood group is encoded by two tightly linked loci, one of which is labeled *D*. The other locus produces Rh antigens labeled *C* and *E* through alternative splicing of the messenger RNA. The *D* locus is of primary interest because it is responsible for Rh maternal-fetal incompatibility and the resulting disease, hemolytic disease of the newborn (HDN). Persons with the *DD* or *Dd* genotype have the Rh antigen on their erythrocytes and are Rh-positive. The recessive homozygotes, with genotype *dd*, are Rh-negative and do not have the Rh antigen. About 85% of persons of European ancestry are Rh-positive and about 15% are Rh-negative.

Unlike the ABO system, in which antibodies normally are formed in response to antigens presented by other organisms, anti-Rh antibody production requires a stimulus by the human Rh antigen itself. An Rh-negative person does not begin to produce anti-Rh antibodies unless he or she is exposed to the Rh antigen, usually through a blood transfusion or during pregnancy. Maternal-fetal incompatibility results when an Rh-positive man and an Rh-negative woman produce children. If the man's genotype is *DD*, all of their offspring will be Rh-positive and will have Rh antigens on their erythrocytes. If the man is a heterozygote, with genotype *Dd*, half of their children will be Rh-positive, on average.

There are usually no difficulties with the first Rh incompatible child, because very few of the fetus's red blood cells cross the placental barrier during gestation. When the placenta detaches at birth, a large number of fetal red blood cells typically enter the mother's blood stream. These cells, carrying the Rh antigens, stimulate production of anti-Rh antibodies by the mother. These antibodies persist in the blood stream for a long time, and if the next offspring is again Rh-positive, the mother's anti-Rh antibodies enter the fetus's bloodstream and destroy its red blood cells. As this destruction proceeds, the fetus becomes anemic and begins to release many erythroblasts (immature nucleated red cells) into its blood stream. This phenomenon is responsible for the descriptive term *erythroblastosis fetalis*. The anemia can lead to a spontaneous abortion or stillbirth. Because the maternal antibodies remain in the newborn's circulatory system, destruction of red cells can continue in the neonate. This causes a buildup of bilirubin and a jaundiced appearance shortly after birth. Without replacement transfusions, in which the child receives Rh-negative red cells, the bilirubin is deposited in the brain, producing cerebral damage and usually death. Infants who do not die can develop intellectual disability, cerebral palsy, and/or high-frequency deafness.

Among persons of European descent, approximately 13% of all matings are Rh-incompatible. Fortunately, a simple therapy now exists to avoid Rh sensitization of the mother. During and after preg-

nancy, an Rh-negative mother is given injections of Rh immune globulin, which consists of anti-Rh antibodies. These antibodies destroy the fetal erythrocytes in the mother's blood stream before they stimulate production of maternal anti-Rh antibodies. Because the injected antibodies do not remain in the mother's blood stream for long, they do not affect subsequent offspring. To avoid sensitization, these injections must be administered with each pregnancy. The Rh-negative mother must also be careful not to receive a transfusion containing Rh-positive blood, because this would also stimulate production of anti-Rh antibodies.

 Maternal-fetal Rh incompatibility (Rh-negative mother and Rh-positive fetus) can produce hemolytic disease of the newborn if the mother's Rh antibodies attack the fetus. Administration of Rh immune globulin to the mother prevents this reaction.

A rarer form of maternal-fetal incompatibility can result when a mother with type O blood carries a fetus with type A or B blood. The hemolytic disease produced by this combination is usually so mild that it does not require treatment. Interestingly, if the mother is also Rh-negative and the child is Rh-positive, the ABO incompatibility *protects* against the more severe Rh incompatibility. This is because any fetal red blood cells entering the mother's circulatory system are quickly destroyed by her anti-A or anti-B antibodies before she can form anti-Rh antibodies.

IMMUNODEFICIENCY DISEASES

Immunodeficiency disease results when one or more components of the immune system (e.g., T cells, B cells, MHC, complement proteins) are missing or fail to function normally. **Primary immunodeficiency diseases** are caused by abnormalities in cells of the immune system and are usually produced by genetic alterations. To date, more than 100 different primary immunodeficiency syndromes have been described, and it is estimated that these diseases affect at least 1 in 10,000 persons. **Secondary**

immunodeficiency occurs when components of the immune system are altered or destroyed by other factors, such as radiation, infection, or drugs. For example, the human immunodeficiency virus (HIV), which causes acquired immunodeficiency syndrome (AIDS), attacks macrophages and helper T lymphocytes, central components of the immune system. The result is increased susceptibility to a multitude of opportunistic infections.

B-cell immunodeficiency diseases render the patient especially susceptible to recurrent bacterial infections, such as *Streptococcus pneumoniae*. An important example of a B-cell immunodeficiency is X-linked **agammaglobulinemia** (XLA). Patients with this disorder, the overwhelming majority of whom are male, lack B cells completely and have no IgA, IgE, IgM, or IgD in their serum. Because IgG crosses the placenta during pregnancy, infants with XLA have some degree of humoral immunity for the first several months of life. However, the IgG supply is soon depleted, and the infants develop recurrent bacterial infections. They are treated with large amounts of γ-globulin. XLA is caused by mutations in a gene (*BTK*) that encodes a B-cell tyrosine kinase necessary for normal B-cell maturation. Mutations in the genes that encode the immunoglobulin heavy and light chains can cause a form of autosomal recessive B-cell immunodeficiency.

T-cell immunodeficiency diseases directly affect T cells, but they also affect the humoral immune response, because B-cell proliferation largely depends on helper T cells. Thus, in the most severe T-cell defects, affected patients develop severe combined immune deficiency (SCID) and are susceptible to many opportunistic infections, including *Pneumocystis jiroveci* (a protozoan that commonly infects AIDS patients). Without bone marrow transplants, these patients usually die within the first several years of life. About half of SCID cases are caused by X-linked recessive mutations in a gene that encodes the γ chain found in six different cytokine receptors (those of interleukins 2, 4, 7, 9, 15, and 21). Lacking these receptors, T cells and natural killer cells cannot receive the signals they need for normal maturation.

These receptors all interact with an intracellular signaling molecule called Jak3. As might be expected, persons who lack Jak3 as a result of autosomal recessive mutations in the *JAK3* gene experience a form of SCID that is very similar to the X-linked form just described.

About 15% of SCID cases are caused by adenosine deaminase (ADA) deficiency, an autosomal recessive disorder of purine metabolism that results in a buildup of metabolites that are toxic to B and T cells. This type of SCID, as well as the X-linked form, can be treated by bone marrow transplantation, and some cases are being treated successfully with gene therapy (see Chapter 10).

SCID can also arise from mutations in *RAG1* or *RAG2*, two of the genes involved in VDJ recombination and the proper formation of T-cell and B-cell receptors. These mutations produce a combined B-cell and T-cell immunodeficiency, although normal natural killer cells are produced. Other examples of SCID are given in Table 9-3.

Several immune system defects result in lymphocytes that lack MHC molecules on their surfaces. These are collectively termed *bare lymphocyte syndrome*, one form of which is caused by mutations in the *TAP2* gene. *TAP2* encodes a protein that helps to transport peptides to the endoplasmic reticulum, where they are bound by class I MHC molecules. A defect in the TAP2 protein destabilizes the class I MHC molecules so that they are not expressed on the cell surface. Because exposure to MHC molecules is necessary for normal T-cell development in the thymus, bare lymphocyte syndrome results in a severe reduction in the number of functional T and B cells. Bare lymphocyte syndrome can also be caused by defects in several different transcription factors that bind to promoters in the class II MHC region. The result is a lack of class II MHC molecules on APCs, a deficiency of helper T cells, and a consequent lack of antibody production.

Chronic granulomatous disease (CGD) is a primary immunodeficiency disorder in which phagocytes can ingest bacteria and fungi but are then unable to kill them. This brings about a persistent cellular immune

TABLE 9-3   Examples of Primary Immunodeficiency Diseases

CONDITION	MODE OF INHERITANCE	BRIEF DESCRIPTION
X-linked agammaglobulinemia	XR	Absence of B cells leads to recurrent bacterial infections
SCID (γ chain cytokine receptor defect or ADA deficiency)	XR, AR	T-cell deficiency leading also to impairment of humoral immune response; fatal unless treated by bone marrow transplantation or gene therapy
SCID due to Jak3 deficiency	AR	Protein kinase deficiency leading to T-cell deficiency, NK cell deficiency, and impaired humoral immune response.
SCID (also Omenn syndrome) due to *RAG1* or *RAG2* deficiency	AR	Lack of recombinase activity impairs VDJ recombination, which leads to B-cell and T-cell deficiency
SCID due to interleukin-7 α chain deficiency	AR	T-cell deficiency leading to impaired B-cell response
Zap70 kinase deficiency	AR	Lack of cytotoxic T cells; defective helper T cells; impaired antibody response
Purine nucleoside phosphorylase deficiency	AR	Purine metabolism disorder leading to T-cell deficiency
Bare lymphocyte syndrome (BLS)	AR	Deficient MHC class I expression (*TAP2* mutation) leads to T-cell and B-cell deficiency in type 1 BLS; mutations in transcription factors for MHC class II genes lead to a relative lack of helper T cells in type 2 BLS
Complement system defects	Mostly AR	Increased susceptibility to bacterial and other infections
DiGeorge anomaly	AD, sporadic	Congenital malformations include abnormal facial features, congenital heart disease, and thymus abnormality leading to T-cell deficiency
Ataxia telangiectasia	AR	DNA repair defect characterized by unsteady gait (ataxia), telangiectasia (dilated capillaries), and thymus abnormality producing T-cell deficiency
Wiskott-Aldrich syndrome	XR	Abnormal, small platelets, eczema, and abnormal T cells causing susceptibility to opportunistic infections
Chediak-Higashi syndrome	AR	Partial albinism, defective lysosomal assembly, giant cytoplasmic granules, abnormal natural killer cells, and neutrophils leading to recurrent bacterial infections
Leukocyte adhesion deficiency	AR	Mutations in integrin receptor genes produce phagocytes that cannot recognize and ingest microorganisms, which results in severe bacterial infections
Chronic granulomatous disease	XR, AR	Phagocytes ingest microbes but cannot kill them; leads to formation of granulomas and recurrent infections
Hyper IgE syndrome	AD, AR	Recurrent staphylococcal infections, markedly elevated serum IgE levels, progressively coarse facial features
IRAK-4 deficiency		Toll-like receptor defect caused by deficiency of interleukin-1 receptor associated kinase-4 (IRAK-4), resulting in extracellular bacterial (especially *Streptococcus pneumoniae*) infections.

AD, Autosomal dominant; *AR*, autosomal recessive; *SCID*, severe combined immune deficiency; *XR*, X-linked recessive.

response to the ingested microbes, resulting in the formation of the granulomas (nodular inflammatory lesions containing macrophages) for which the disease is named. These patients develop pneumonia, lymph node infections, and abscesses in the skin, liver, and other sites. The most common cause of CGD is an X-linked mutation, but there are also at least three autosomal recessive genes that can cause CGD. The gene that causes X-linked CGD was the first disease-causing gene to be isolated through posi-

tional cloning. It encodes a subunit of cytochrome b, a protein that the phagocyte requires for a burst of microbe-killing oxygen metabolism.

Multiple defects in the various proteins that make up the complement system have been identified. Most of these are inherited as autosomal recessive disorders, and most result in increased susceptibility to bacterial infections.

Systemic lupus erythematosus (SLE) is a serious autoimmune disease, in which the body's immune system mistakenly attacks healthy tissue. The reported worldwide prevalence of SLE in the population is 20 to 150 cases per 100,000, the estimated incidence of SLE is higher among Asians and Africans, and SLE is much more common in women than men. In China, SLE affects about 5 million people. In SLE, the body's immune system produces antibodies against itself, particularly against proteins in the cell nucleus. The Symptoms of SLE vary from person to person, most often harms the heart, joints, skin, lungs, blood vessels, liver, kidneys, and nervous system. The causes of SLE are believed to be a combination of environmental and genetic factors, whereas the underlying genetic reason is not fully known. SLE does run in families, HLA class I and class II genes appear to influence a person's chance of developing lupus when triggered by environmental factors.

Finally, a number of syndromes include immunodeficiency as one of their features. One example is the DiGeorge sequence (see Chapter 6), in which a lack of thymic development leads to T-cell deficiency. Wiskott-Aldrich syndrome is an X-linked recessive disorder that involves deficiencies of platelets and progressive T-cell dysfunction. It is caused by loss-of-function mutations in a gene (*WAS*) whose protein product is expressed in hematopoietic cells, where it relays signals from the cell surface to the cytoskeleton. Wiskott-Aldrich syndrome, like SCID, has been successfully treated with gene therapy (see Chapter10). Immunodeficiency is also seen in several syndromes that involve DNA instability (e.g., ataxi-atelangiectasia, Bloom syndrome, Fanconi anemia; see Chapter 3).

▶ Primary immunodeficiency diseases involve intrinsic defects of immune response cells (e.g., B cells, T cells, MHC, complement system, or phagocytes) and are usually caused by genetic alterations. Secondary immunodeficiency disorders, of which AIDS is an example, are caused by external factors. Immunodeficiency is also seen in a number of genetic syndromes, including several DNA instability disorders.

SUMMARY

Immunogenetics is the branch of medical genetics that explores the immune response and its genetic basis. This chapter begins with a brief description of the human immune system, which is composed of the innate and adaptive systems. The innate immune system is designed for the immediate response to pathogen invasion by an evolutionarily conserved set of pattern-recognition receptors, such as the Toll-like receptors, coupled with a prompt defensive response by cells such as macrophages. The adaptive immune system includes the cellular immune system and the humoral immune system, which are characterized by greater degrees of antigen specificity determined by the T- and B-cell receptor repertoires and by the formation of memory T and B cells.

The cellular immune system is regulated by the major histocompatibility complex (MHC), which is encoded by a series of more than 200 genes. The major role of the MHC is to bind small peptides and present them to the cell surface, where the antigen can be recognized by T-cell receptors. Individuals identical for this region can exchange grafts more successfully than those with different MHC combinations. The humoral immune system is capable of generating approximately 100 billion structurally distinct antibodies. Mechanisms are responsible for such diversity including multiple germline immunoglobulin genes, somatic recombination (VDJ recombination), junctional diversity, and somatic hypermutation. Knowledge of the genetics of the ABO and Rh blood systems has provided a solid foundation for modern transfusion medicine.

This chapter also lists a number of genetically based immunodeficiency diseases that may result from genetic alteration of one or more components of the immune system (eg, T cells, B cells, MHC complement proteins). Gene mutations caused by B-cell or T-cell immunodeficiency (eg, X-linked agammaglobulinemia, severe combined immunodeficiency) could render an individual especially susceptible to opportunistic infections. In addition, autoimmune diseases, which are caused by an extreme reaction of the immune system to the body's own tissues, may be due in part to genetic variation (eg, systemic lupus erythematosus and narcolepsy show familial aggregation). Therefore, advances in human genomics will likely contribute to the diagnosis and treatment of immunodeficiency diseases.

IMPORTANT TERMINOLOGY

immunogenetics　免疫遗传学
innate immune system　天然免疫系统
adaptive immune system　适应性免疫系统
humoral immune system　体液免疫系统
cellular immune system　细胞免疫系统
antibody diversity　抗体多样性
major histocompatibility complex　主要组织相容性复合体
human leukocyte antigens　人白细胞抗原
autoimmunity　自身免疫性
immunodeficiency　免疫缺陷
agammaglobulinemia　丙种球蛋白缺乏血症
chronic granulomatous disease　慢性肉芽肿性疾病
systemic lupus erythematosus (SLE)　系统性红斑狼疮

REVIEW QUESTIONS

1. Compare the functions of class I and class II MHC molecules.

2. MHC molecules and immunoglobulins both display a great deal of diversity but in different ways. How and why do these types of diversity differ?

3. In what ways are T-cell receptors and immunoglobulins similar? In what ways are they different?

4. If there are 80 V segments, 6 J segments, and 30 D segments that can encode an immunoglobulin heavy chain of one particular class, how many different immunoglobulins can be formed on the basis of somatic recombination alone?

5. When matching donors and recipients for organ transplants, siblings are often desirable donors because they are more likely to be HLA-compatible with the recipient. If we assume no crossing over within the HLA loci and assume four distinct HLA haplotypes among the parents, what is the probability that a transplant recipient will be HLA identical with a sibling donor?

6. What types of matings will produce Rh maternal-fetal incompatibility?

SUGGESTED READINGS AND WEBSITES

1. Bonilla FA, Oettgen HC. Adaptive immunity. *J Allergy ClinImmunol*. 2010; 125: S33-S40.

2. Cho JH, Gregersen PK. Genomics and the multifactorial nature of human autoimmune disease. *N Engl J Med*. 2011; 365: 1612-1623.

3. Conley ME, Casanova J-L. Discovery of single-gene inborn errors of immunity by next generation sequencing. *CurrOpinImmunol*. 2014; 30: 17-23.

4. Durandy A, Kracker S, Fischer A. Primary antibody deficiencies. *Nat Rev Immunol*. 2013; 13: 519-533.

5. Finn JA Jr, Crowe JE. Impact of new sequencing technologies on studies of the human B cell repertoire. *CurrOpinImmunol*. 2013; 25: 613-618.

6. Howell WM. HLA and disease: guilt by association. *Int J Immunogenet*. 2014; 41: 1-12.

7. Kumar V, Wijmenga C, Xavier RJ. Genetics of immune-mediated disorders: from genome-wide association to molecular mechanism. *Curr Opin Immunol*. 2014; 31: 51-57.

8. Male D, Brostoff J, Roth D, Roitt I. *Immunology*. 8th ed. St. Louis: Elsevier; 2013.

9. Milner JD, Holland SM. The cup runneth over: lessons from the ever-expanding pool of primary immunodeficiency diseases. *Nat Rev Immunol*. 2013; 13: 635-648.

10. Netea MG, van der Meer JWM. Immunodeficiency and genetic defects of pattern-recognition receptors. *N Engl J Med*. 2011; 364: 60-70.

11. Parvaneh N, Casanova J-L, Notarangelo LD, Conley ME. Primary immunodeficiencies: a rapidly evolving story. *J Allergy Clin Immunol*. 2013; 131: 314-323.

12. Peled JU, Kuang FL, Iglesias-Ussel MD, et al. The biochemistry of somatic hypermutation. *Annu Rev Immunol.* 2008; 26: 481-511.

13. Schroeder HW Jr, Cavacini L. Structure and function of immunoglobulins. *J Allergy Clin Immunol.* 2010; 125: S41-S52.

14. Sollid LM, Pos W, Wucherpfennig KW. Molecular mechanisms for contribution of MHC molecules to autoimmune diseases. *Curr Opin Immunol.* 2014; 31: 24-30.

15. Trowsdale J, Knight JC. Major histocompatibility complex genomics and human disease. *Annu Rev Genomics Hum Genet.* 2013; 14: 301-323.

16. Turvey SE, Broide DH. Innate immunity. *J Allergy Clinimmunol.* 2010; 125: S24-S32.

17. Immunogenetics Database: http://www.ebi.ac.uk/imgt/

18. Molecular Immunology Tutorial: http://www.mi.interhealth.info/

(Feng Li)

Chapter 10

Genetic Testing and Gene Therapy

As we have seen in previous chapters, significant advances have occurred in many areas of medical genetics, including DNA sequencing technology, disease-gene identification, and cytogenetics. These developments have paved the way for more accurate and efficient testing of genetic disorders. **Genetic testing** can be defined as the analysis of chromosomes, DNA, RNA, proteins, or other analytes to detect abnormalities that can cause a genetic disease (An analyte is any substance that is subject to analysis). Indications for genetic testing include prenatal diagnosis, heterozygote carrier detection, and presymptomatic diagnosis of genetic disease. The principles and applications of genetic testing in these contexts are one focus of this chapter.

The other focus is the treatment of genetic disease. Many aspects of disease management involve areas of medicine, such as surgery and drug treatment, that are beyond the scope of this book. However, gene therapy, in which patients' cells are genetically altered to combat specific diseases, is being used increasingly to treat disease and is discussed in the second part of this chapter.

POPULATION SCREENING FOR GENETIC DISEASE

Screening tests represent an important component of routine health care. These tests are usually designed to detect treatable human diseases in their presymptomatic stage. Papanicolaou (Pap) tests for detecting cervical dysplasia and population screening for hypercholesterolemia are well-known examples of this public health strategy. **Population screening** is large-scale testing of populations for disease in an effort to identify persons who probably have the disease and those who probably do not. Screening tests are not intended to provide definitive diagnoses; rather, they are aimed at identifying a subset of the population on whom further, more exact, diagnostic tests should be carried out. This important distinction is commonly misunderstood by the lay public and seldom clarified by the popular media.

Genetic screening is population screening for genetic variants that can cause the disease in the person carrying the variant or in the descendants of the carrier. Newborn screening for inherited metabolic diseases (see Chapter 7) is a good example of the first type of genetic screening, and heterozygote detection for Tay-Sachs disease (discussed later) exemplifies the second. These two examples involve screening of populations, but genetic screening can also be applied to members of families with a positive history of a genetic condition. An example is testing for a balanced reciprocal translocation in families in which one or more members have had a chromosome disorder (see Chapter 6). Box 10-1 lists the various types of genetic screening, including several forms of prenatal diagnosis, that are discussed in this chapter.

 The goal of screening is early recognition of a disorder so that intervention will prevent or reverse the disease process (as in newborn screening for inborn errors of metabolism) or so that informed reproductive decisions can be made (as in screening for heterozygous carriers of an autosomal recessive mutation). A positive result from a genetic screening test is typically followed by a more precise diagnostic test.

BOX 10-1   Types of Genetic Screening and Prenatal Diagnosis

Population Screening for Genetic Disorders
Newborn Screening
Blood
- Phenylketonuria, all 50 states in the United States
- Galactosemia, all 50 states in the United States
- Hypothyroidism, all 50 states in the United States
- Hemoglobinopathies, nearly all states
- Other: cystic fibrosis, congenital adrenal hyperplasia, maple syrup urine disease, homocystinuria, tyrosinemia, and several other diseases or inborn errors of metabolism are screened in the US and Europe
  Universal newborn hearing screening (>60% of congenital hearing loss is due to genetic factors)

Heterozygote Screening
Tay-Sachs disease, Ashkenazi Jewish population
Sickle cell disease, African-American population
Thalassemias in at-risk ethnic groups
Cystic fibrosis in some populations (persons of European descent, Ashkenazi Jews)

Prenatal Diagnosis of Genetic Disorders
Diagnostic Testing (Invasive Prenatal Diagnosis)
Amniocentesis
Chorionic villus sampling
Percutaneous umbilical blood sampling (PUBS)
Preimplantation genetic diagnosis

Fetal Visualization Techniques
Ultrasonography
Radiography
Magnetic resonance imaging

Population Screening
Maternal age >35 years
Family history of condition diagnosable by prenatal techniques
Quadruple screen: maternal serum α-fetoprotein, estriol, human chorionic gonadotropin, inhibin-A
First trimester screening: ultrasonography, PAPP-A, and free β subunit of human chorionic gonadotropin
Noninvasive prenatal screening using cell-free DNA from maternal plasma

Family Screening for Genetic Disorders
Family history of chromosomal rearrangement (e.g., translocation)
Screening female relatives in an X-linked pedigree (e.g., Duchenne muscular dystrophy, fragile X syndrome)
Heterozygote screening within at-risk families (e.g., cystic fibrosis)
Presymptomatic screening (e.g., Huntington disease, breast cancer, colon cancer)

Principles of Screening

The basic principles of screening were developed in the 1960s and are still widely recognized. Characteristics of the disease, the test, and the health-care system should be considered when deciding whether population screening is appropriate.

First, the condition should be serious and relatively common. This ensures that the benefits to be derived from the screening program will justify its costs. The natural history of the disease should be clearly understood. There should be an acceptable and effective treatment, or, in the case of some genetic conditions, prenatal diagnosis should be available. As for the screening test itself, it should be acceptable to the population, easy to perform, and relatively inexpensive. The screening test should be valid and reliable. Finally, the resources for diagnosis and treatment of the disorder must be accessible. A strategy for communicating results efficiently and effectively must be in place.

Screening programs typically use tests that are widely applicable and inexpensive to identify an at-risk population (e.g., the phenylketonuria [PKU] screening program, discussed in Clinical Commentary 10-1). Members of this population are then targeted for subsequent tests that are more accurate but also more expensive and time consuming. In this context, the screening test should be able to effectively separate persons who have the disease from those who do not. This attribute, which defines the test's **validity**, involves two components: **sensitivity** and **specificity**. Sensitivity reflects the ability of the test to correctly identify those *with* the disease. It is measured as the fraction of affected persons in whom the test is positive (i.e., **true positives**). Specificity is the ability of the test to correctly identify those *without* the disease. It is measured as the fraction of unaffected persons in whom the test is negative (i.e., **true negatives**). Sensitivity and specificity are determined by comparing the screening results with those of a definitive diagnostic test (Table 10-1).

Screening tests are seldom, if ever, 100% sensitive and 100% specific. This is because the range of test values in the disease population overlaps that of the unaffected population (Fig. 10-1). Thus, results

CLINICAL COMMENTARY 10-1
Neonatal Screening for Phenylketonuria
Disease Characteristics
Population screening of newborns for PKU represents an excellent example of the application of the screening model to genetic disease. As discussed in Chapter 4, the prevalence of this autosomal recessive disorder of phenylalanine metabolism is about 1 in 10,000 to 15,000 white births in the United States. The natural history of PKU is well understood. More than 95% of untreated PKU patients develop moderate to severe intellectual disability. The condition is difficult to diagnose clinically in the first year of life because the physical signs are subtle and PKU usually manifests only as developmental delay. Dietary restriction of phenylalanine, when begun before 4 weeks of age, is highly effective in altering the course of the disease. A low-phenylalanine diet, although not particularly palatable, largely eliminates the IQ loss that would otherwise occur (an important exception is those who have a defect in biopterin metabolism, in whom a different therapy is used).

Test Characteristics
Until recently PKU was typically detected by the measurement of blood phenylalanine using a bacterial inhibition assay, the Guthrie test. Blood is collected in the newborn period, usually by heel stick, and placed on filter paper. The dried blood is placed on an agar plate and incubated with a strain of bacteria (*Bacillus subtilis*) that requires phenylalanine for growth. Measurement of bacterial growth permits quantification of the amount of phenylalanine in the blood sample. Tandem mass spectrometry (see below) is now usually used to screen for PKU and a number of other inborn errors of metabolism. Positive test results are repeated and followed by a quantitative assay of plasma phenylalanine and tyrosine. If the test is performed after 2 days of age and after regular feeding on a protein diet, the detection rate (sensitivity) is about 98%. If it is performed at less than 24 hours of age, the sensitivity is about 84% and for this reason a repeat test is recommended a few weeks after birth. Specificity is close to 100%.

System Characteristics
Because of the requirement of normal protein in the diet, many states request rescreening at 2 to 4 weeks of age. At that point, sensitivity approaches 100%. A high sensitivity level is important because of the severe impact of a missed diagnosis.

Phenylalanine levels in children with classic PKU typically exceed 20 mg/dl. For every 20 positive PKU screening results, only one infant has classic PKU. The others represent either false-positive findings (usually due to a transient reversible tyrosinemia) or infants with a form of hyperphenylalaninemia (elevated phenylalanine) not caused by classic PKU.

The cost of PKU screening is typically less than a few dollars per test. Several studies have shown that the cost of nationwide PKU screening is significantly less than the savings it achieves by avoiding institutionalization costs and lost productivity.

These principles apply to many of the other inborn errors that are now screened for in the expanded newborn screening programs in North America and Europe (see Chapter 7).

of a screening test (as opposed to the definitive follow-up diagnostic test) will be incorrect for some members of the population. Usually a cutoff value is designated to separate the diseased and nondiseased portions of the population. A tradeoff exists between the impact of nondetection or low sensitivity (i.e., an increased **false-negative** rate) and the impact of low specificity (an increased **false-positive** rate). If the penalty for missing affected persons is high (as in untreated PKU), then the cutoff level is lowered so that nearly all disease cases will be detected (higher sensitivity). This also lowers the specificity by increasing the number of unaffected persons with positive test results (false positives) who are targeted for subsequent diagnostic testing. If confirmation of a positive test is expensive or hazardous, then false-positive rates are minimized (i.e., the cutoff level is increased, producing high specificity at the expense of sensitivity).

> The basic elements of a test's validity include its sensitivity (proportion of true positives accurately detected) and specificity (proportion of true negatives accurately detected). When sensitivity is increased, specificity decreases, and vice versa.

A primary concern in the clinical setting is the accuracy of a positive screening test. One needs to

TABLE 10-1 **Definitions of Sensitivity and Specificity**[*]		
RESULT OF SCREENING TEST	**ACTUAL DISEASE STATE**	
	AFFECTED	**UNAFFECTED**
Test positive (+)	a (true positives)	b (false positives)
Test negative (−)	c (false negatives)	d (true negatives)

[*]a, b, c, and d represent the number of individuals in a population who were found to have the disease and test result combinations shown. The test sensitivity = a/(a + c); specificity = d/(b + d); positive predictive value = a/(a + b); and negative predictive value = d/(c + d).

FIG 10-1   The distribution of creatine kinase (CK) in normal women and in women who are heterozygous carriers for a mutation in the Duchenne muscular dystrophy gene. Note the overlap in distribution between the two groups: About two thirds of carriers have CK levels that exceed the 95th percentile in normal women. If the 95th percentile is used as a cutoff to identify carriers, then the sensitivity of the test is 67% (i.e., two thirds of carriers will be detected), and the specificity is 95% (i.e., 95% of normal women will be correctly identified).

know the fraction of persons with a positive test result who truly have the disease in question [i.e., a/(a + b) in Table 10-1]. This quantity is defined as the **positive predictive value**. It is also useful to know the **negative predictive value**, which is the fraction of persons with a negative result who truly do not have the disease [d/(c + d)].

The concepts of sensitivity, specificity, and positive predictive value can be illustrated by an example. Congenital adrenal hyperplasia (CAH) due to a deficiency of 21-hydroxylase is an inborn error of steroid biosynthesis that can produce ambiguous genitalia in females and adrenal crises in both sexes. The screening test, a 17-hydroxyprogesterone assay, has a sensitivity of about 95% and a specificity of 99% (Table 10-2). The prevalence of CAH is about 1/10,000 in most white populations, but it rises to about 1/400 in the Yupik Native Alaskan population.

Let us assume that a screening program for CAH has been developed in both of these populations. In a population of 500,000 whites, the false-positive rate (1—specificity) is 1%. Thus, about 5000 unaffected persons will have a positive test. With 95% sensitivity, 47 of the 50 white persons who have CAH will be detected through a positive test. Note that the great majority of people who have a positive test result would not have CAH: the positive predictive value is 47/(47 + 5000), or less than 1%. Now suppose that 10,000 members of the Yupik population are screened for CAH. As

TABLE 10-2   Hypothetical Results of Screening for Congenital Adrenal Hyperplasia in a Low-Prevalence White Population and in a High-Prevalence Yupik Population*

RESULT OF SCREENING TEST	CAH PRESENT	CAH ABSENT
Positive		
White	47	5000
Yupik	24	100
Negative		
White	3	494,950
Yupik	1	9875

*White positive predictive value = 47/(47 + 5000) ≈ 1%; Yupik positive predictive value = 24/(24 + 100) ≈ 19%. CAH, congenital adrenal hyperplasia.

Table 10-2 shows, 24 of 25 persons with CAH will test positive, and 100 persons without CAH will also test positive. Here, the positive predictive value is much higher than in the white population: 24/ (24 + 100) = 19%. This example illustrates an important principle: *For a given level of sensitivity and specificity, the positive predictive value of a test increases as the prevalence of the disease increases.*

 The positive predictive value of a screening test is defined as the percentage of positive tests that are true positives. It increases as the prevalence of the target disorder increases.

Newborn Screening for Inborn Errors of Metabolism

Newborn screening programs represent an ideal opportunity for presymptomatic detection and prevention of genetic disease. At present, all states in the United States screen newborns for PKU, galactosemia (see Chapter 7), and hypothyroidism. All of these conditions fulfill the previously stated criteria for population screening. Each is a disorder in which the person is at significant risk for intellectual disability, which can be prevented by early detection and effective intervention.

In recent years, most states of the United States and many other nations have instituted screening programs to identify neonates with hemoglobin disorders (e.g., sickle cell disease). These programs are justified by the fact that up to 15% of untreated children with sickle cell disease die from infections before 5 years of age (see Chapter 3). Effective treatment, in the form of prophylactic antibiotics, is available. Some communities have begun screening for Duchenne muscular dystrophy by measuring creatine kinase levels in newborns. The objective is not presymptomatic treatment; rather it is identification of families who should receive genetic counseling in order to make informed reproductive decisions.

Increasingly, **tandem mass spectrometry** is used to screen newborns for protein variants that signal amino acid disorders (e.g., PKU, tyrosinemia, homocystinuria), organic acid disorders, and fatty acid oxidation disorders (e.g., MCAD and LCHAD deficiencies; see Chapter 7). This method begins with a sample of material from a dried blood spot, which is subjected to analysis by two mass spectrometers. The first spectrometer separates ionized molecules according to their mass, and the molecules are fragmented. The second spectrometer assesses the mass and charge of these fragments, which allows a computer to generate a molecular profile of the sample. Tandem mass spectrometry is highly accurate and very rapid: more than 30 disorders can be screened in approximately 2 minutes.

As screening technologies have continued to advance, many countries have established **expanded newborn screening** programs to deal with positive results and to provide rapid treatment of verified disease conditions. The American College of Medical Genetics and Genomics has developed guidelines and action plans for all of the conditions that are currently screened (https://www.acmg.net) and is consistently developing new plans for disorders for which screening is being considered (e.g., Pompe disease). Conditions for which newborn screening is commonly performed are summarized in Table 10-3.

TABLE 10-3	Characteristics of Selected Newborn Screening Programs			
DISEASE	**INHERITANCE**	**PREVALENCE**	**SCREENING TEST**	**TREATMENT**
Phenylketonuria	Autosomal recessive	1/10,000-1/15,000	Tandem mass spectrometry	Dietary restriction of phenylalanine
Galactosemia	Autosomal recessive	1/50,000-1/100,000	Transferase assay	Dietary restriction of galactose
Congenital hypothyroidism	Usually sporadic	1/5000	Measurement of thyroxine (T_4) or thyroid stimulating hormone (TSH)	Hormone replacement
Sickle cell disease	Autosomal recessive	1/400-1/600 blacks	Isoelectric focusing or DNA diagnosis	Prophylactic penicillin
Cystic fibrosis	Autosomal recessive	1/2500	Immunoreactive trypsinogen confirmed by DNA diagnosis	Antibiotics, chest physical therapy, pancreatic enzyme replacement if needed

Data from guidelines of the American College of Medical Genetics, http://www.acmg.net/resources/policies/ACT/condition-analyte-links.htm.

> Newborn screening is an effective public health strategy for treatable disorders such as PKU, hypothyroidism, galactosemia, and sickle cell disease. The use of tandem mass spectrometry has expanded the number of diseases that can be detected by newborn screening.

Heterozygote Screening

The aforementioned principles of population screening can be applied to the detection of unaffected carriers of disease-causing mutations. The target population is a group known to be at risk. The intervention consists of the presentation of risk figures and options such as prenatal diagnosis. Genetic diseases amenable to heterozygote screening are typically autosomal recessive disorders for which **prenatal diagnosis** and genetic counseling are available, feasible, and accurate.

An example of a highly successful heterozygote screening effort is the Tay-Sachs screening program in North America. Infantile Tay-Sachs disease is an autosomal recessive lysosomal storage disorder in which the lysosomal enzyme β-hexosaminidase A (HEX A) is deficient (see Chapter 7), causing a buildup of the substrate, G_{M2} ganglioside, in neuronal lysosomes. The accumulation of this substrate damages the neurons and leads to blindness, seizures, hypotonia, and death by about 5 years of age. Tay-Sachs disease is especially common among Ashkenazi Jews, with a heterozygote frequency of about 1 in 30. Thus, this population is a reasonable candidate for heterozygote screening. Accurate carrier testing is available (assays for HEX A or direct DNA testing for mutations). Because the disease is uniformly fatal, options such as pregnancy termination or artificial insemination by noncarrier donors are acceptable to many couples. A well-planned effort was made to educate members of the target population about risks, testing, and available options. As a result of screening, the number of Tay-Sachs disease births among Ashkenazi Jews in the United States and Canada declined by 90%, from 30 to 40 per year before 1970, to 3 to 5 per year in the 1990s, and to zero by 2003.

β-Thalassemia major, another serious autosomal recessive disorder, is especially common among many Mediterranean and South Asian populations (see Chapter 7). Effective carrier screening programs have produced a 75% decrease in the prevalence of newborns with this disorder in Greece, Cyprus, and Italy. Carrier screening is also possible for cystic fibrosis, another autosomal recessive disorder (Clinical Commentary 10-2). Table 10-4 presents a list of selected conditions for which heterozygote screening programs have been developed in many countries.

In addition to the criteria for establishing a population screening program for genetic disorders, guidelines have been developed regarding the ethical and legal aspects of heterozygote screening programs. These are summarized in Box 10-2.

> Heterozygote screening consists of testing (at the phenotype or genotype level) a target population to identify unaffected carriers of a disease gene. The carriers can then be given information about risks and reproductive options.

			AT-RISK COUPLE	DISEASE INCIDENCE
DISEASE	ETHNIC GROUP	CARRIER FREQUENCY	FREQUENCY	IN NEWBORNS
Sickle cell disease	Blacks	1/12	1/150	1/600
Tay–Sachs disease	Ashkenazi Jews	1/30	1/900	1/3600
β-Thalassemia	Greeks, Italians	1/30	1/900	1/3600
α-Thalassemia	Southeast Asians, Chinese	1/25	1/625	1/2500
Cystic fibrosis	Northern Europeans	1/25	1/625	1/2500
Phenylketonuria	Northern Europeans	1/50	1/2500	1/10,000

TABLE 10-4   Selected Examples of Heterozygote Screening Programs in Specific Ethnic Groups

Modified from McGinniss MJ, Kaback MM. Carrier screening. In: Rimoin DL, Conner JM, Pyeritz RE, Korf BR, eds. *Emery and Rimoin's Principles and Practice of Medical Genetics*, 5th ed. New York: Churchill Livingstone; 2007, pp 752-762.

CLINICAL COMMENTARY 10-2
Population Screening for Cystic Fibrosis

Approximately 2,000 mutations have now been reported in the *CFTR* gene, and, although some are benign variants, most can cause cystic fibrosis. It would be technologically impractical to test for all reported mutations in a population screening program. However, among the mutations that can cause CF in whites, about 70% are the three-base deletion termed F508del (see Chapter 4). In this population, carrier screening using PCR-based detection of F508del would detect approximately 90% of couples in which one or both are heterozygous carriers of this mutation ($1-0.30^2$, where 0.30^2 represents the frequency of carrier couples in whom neither carries the F508del mutation). It is now recommended to test simultaneously for 25 of the most common *CFTR* mutations, which will detect approximately 85% of all *CFTR* mutations in persons of European descent (because mutation frequencies vary among populations, this figure is somewhat lower in other U.S. populations, such as African-Americans and Hispanics). Among whites, 98% of couples in which one or both members carry a CF mutation would be recognized (i.e., $1-0.15^2$), yielding a high level of sensitivity. The American College of Medical Genetics and Genomics and the American College of Obstetricians and Gynecologists recommend that couples who are planning a pregnancy, or who are currently pregnant, should be offered a screen for CF carrier status. Couples in which both parents are heterozygotes would define a subset of the population in which prenatal diagnosis for CF might be offered. CF is now commonly screened in the newborn population (expanded newborn screening, see above), typically using an immunoreactive trypsinogen assay, followed, if indicated, by direct testing for *CFTR* mutations.

BOX 10-2   **Public Policy Guidelines for Heterozygote Screening**

Recommended guidelines:

Screening should be voluntary, and confidentiality must be ensured.

Screening requires informed consent.

Providers of screening services have an obligation to ensure that adequate education and counseling are included in the program.

Quality control of all aspects of the laboratory testing, including systematic proficiency testing, is required and should be implemented as soon as possible.

There should be equal access to testing.

From Elias S, Annas GJ, Simpson JL. Carrier screening for cystic fibrosis: implications for obstetric and gynecologic practice. *Am J Obstet Gynecol*. 1991; 164: 1077-1083.

Presymptomatic Diagnosis

With the development of genetic diagnosis by direct mutation detection, **presymptomatic diagnosis** has become feasible for many genetic diseases. At-risk persons can be tested to determine whether they have inherited a disease-causing mutation before they develop clinical symptoms of the disorder. Presymptomatic diagnosis is available, for example, for Huntington disease, adult polycystic kidney disease, and autosomal dominant breast/ovarian cancer. By informing persons that they do or do not carry a disease-causing mutation, presymptomatic diagnosis can aid in making reproductive decisions. It can provide reassurance to those who learn that they do not carry a disease-causing mutation. In some cases, early diagnosis can improve health supervision. For example, persons who inherit an autosomal dominant breast cancer mutation can undergo mammography at an earlier age to increase the chances of early tumor detection. Persons at risk for the inheritance of *RET* mutations (see Chapter 8), who are highly likely to develop multiple endocrine neoplasia type 2 (MEN2), can undergo a prophylactic thyroidectomy to reduce their chance of developing a malignancy. Those who inherit mutations that cause some forms of familial colon cancer (adenomatous polyposis coli [APC] and hereditary non-polyposis colorectal cancer [HNPCC]; see Chapter 8) can also benefit from early diagnosis and treatment.

Because most genetic diseases are relatively uncommon in the general population, universal presymptomatic screening is currently impractical. It is usually recommended only for persons who are known to be at risk for the disease, generally because of a positive family history.

 Genetic testing can sometimes be performed to identify persons who have inherited a disease-causing gene before they develop symptoms. This is termed *presymptomatic diagnosis*.

Psychosocial Implications of Genetic Screening and Diagnosis

Screening for genetic diseases has many social and psychological implications. The burden of anxiety, cost, and potential stigmatization surrounding a positive test result must be weighed against the need for detection. Often, screening tests are misperceived as diagnostically definitive. The concept that a positive screening test does not necessarily indicate disease presence must be emphasized to those who undergo screening (see Box 10-2).

The initial screening programs for sickle cell carrier status in the 1970s were plagued by misunderstandings about the implications of carrier status. Occasionally, carrier detection led to cancellation of health insurance or employer discrimination. Such experiences underscore the need for effective genetic counseling and public education. Other issues include the right to choose *not* to be tested and the potential for invasion of privacy.

The social, psychological, and ethical aspects of genetic screening will become more complicated as newer techniques of DNA diagnosis become more accessible. For example, even though presymptomatic diagnosis of Huntington disease is available, several studies have shown that fewer than 20% of at-risk persons elected this option. Largely, this reflects the fact that no effective treatment is currently available for this disorder. Presymptomatic diagnosis of *BRCA1* and *BRCA2* (see Chapter 8) carrier status has also met with mixed responses. In part, this has been a reaction to the cost of the test: because of the large number of different mutations in *BRCA1* or *BRCA2* that can cause breast or ovarian cancer, testing typically consists of sequencing all exons and promoters of both genes, as well as some intronic nucleotides near each exon. This has been a costly procedure, although new technologies and increasing competition are now decreasing the cost. Preventive measures such as prophylactic mastectomy and oophorectomy (removal of the breasts and ovaries, respectively) are known to reduce cancer risk by approximately 90%, but they do not completely eliminate it.

For some genetic diseases, such as autosomal dominant colon cancer syndromes, early diagnosis can lead to improved survival because effective preventive treatments are readily available (colectomy or polypectomy for precancerous colon polyps). In addition, many at-risk persons will find that they do not carry a disease-causing allele, allowing them to avoid unpleasant (and possibly hazardous) diagnostic procedures such as colonoscopy or mammography. However, as screening for such diseases becomes more common, the issues of privacy and confidentiality and the need for accurate communication of risk information must also be addressed.

MOLECULAR TOOLS FOR SCREENING AND DIAGNOSIS

In the past, genetic screening usually relied on assays of the disease phenotype, such as a β-hexosaminidase assay for Tay-Sachs disease or a creatine kinase assay for Duchenne muscular dystrophy. Advances in DNA technology have led to diagnosis at the level of the genotype. In most cases direct assays of disease-causing mutations have been developed. Genetic diagnosis at the DNA level is now supplementing, and in many cases supplanting, tests based on phenotypic assays.

Linkage analysis and direct mutation diagnosis have been used for diagnostic testing within families, for prenatal diagnosis of genetic disorders, and, more recently, in population screening. Improved technology and an increased demand for testing have led to the establishment of clinical molecular laboratories in many medical centers throughout the world.

Linkage Analysis

DNA polymorphisms such as SNPs or STRs can be used as markers in **linkage analysis**. Once linkage phase is established in a family, the marker locus can be assayed to determine whether an at-risk person has inherited a chromosome segment that contains a disease-causing mutation or a homologous segment that contains a normal allele (Fig. 10-2). Because this approach uses linked markers but does not involve direct examination of the disease-causing mutations, it is a form of **indirect diagnosis**.

Linkage analysis has been employed successfully in diagnosing many of the genetic diseases discussed in this text. In principle, it can be used to diagnose any mapped genetic disease. It has the advantages that the disease-causing gene and its product need not be known. The marker simply tells us whether or not the at-risk person has inherited the chromosome region that contains a disease-causing mutation.

The disadvantages of this approach are that several family members must be tested in order to establish linkage phase; not all markers are informative (sufficiently heterozygous) in all families; and recombination can occur between the marker and the disease-causing mutation, introducing a source of diagnostic error. With advances in direct mutation detection, indirect diagnosis with linked markers is applied less commonly than in the past, but it is still useful when a disease-causing mutation is being transmitted in a family but cannot be directly identified.

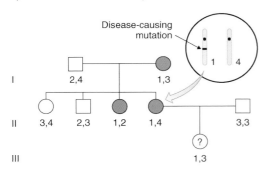

FIG 10-2   In this pedigree for autosomal dominant breast cancer, the analysis of a closely linked marker on chromosome 17 shows that the mutation is on the same chromosome as marker allele 1 in the affected mother in generation II. This indicates that the daughter in generation III has inherited the mutation-bearing chromosome from her mother and is highly likely to develop a breast tumor.

▶ Linkage analysis, a form of indirect genetic diagnosis, uses linked markers to determine whether a person has inherited a chromosome containing a disease gene from his or her parent. The need for typing of numerous family members and the possibilities of recombination and uninformative matings are disadvantages of this approach.

Direct Mutation Analysis

Direct diagnosis, in which the disease-causing mutation itself is detected, has become the approach used most commonly in genetic diagnosis. Compared to indirect diagnosis, it has the advantages that family information is not needed (the mutation is viewed directly in each individual), uninformative matings are not a problem, and there is no error resulting from recombination. (Table 10-5 summarizes the advantages and disadvantages of direct and indirect diagnosis.) Several forms of direct diagnosis (Table 10-6) have been described in preceding chapters. For example, **fluorescence in situ hybridization** (FISH) or **array comparative genomic hybridization** (array CGH) can be used to detect deletions or duplications of chromosome regions (see Chapter 6). Southern blotting or **multiplex ligation-dependent probe amplification** (MLPA) can be used to detect copy number variants or large repeat expansions (see Chapter 3).

If the DNA sequence surrounding a mutation is known, the region containing the sequence can be amplified by PCR (see Chapter 3) and an oligonucleotide probe can be synthesized that will hybridize (undergo complementary base pairing) only to the mutated sequence (such probes are often termed **allele-specific oligonucleotides**, or ASOs). A second probe that will hybridize to the normal DNA sequence is also synthesized. Stringent hybridization conditions are used so that a one-base mismatch will prevent hybridization. DNA from persons who are homozygous for the mutation hybridizes only with

| | TABLE 10-5   **Summary of Attributes of Indirect and Direct Diagnosis** | | |
ATTRIBUTE	INDIRECT DIAGNOSIS	DIRECT DIAGNOSIS
Family information needed	Yes	No
Errors possible because of recombination	Yes	No
Markers may be uninformative	Yes	No
Single test can uncover multiple mutations	Yes	No
Disease-causing mutation must be known	No	Yes

TABLE 10-6   Methods of Direct Genetic Testing[*]

METHOD	SINGLE-GENE MUTATIONS	COPY NUMBER VARIANTS (INCLUDING DELETIONS AND DUPLICATIONS)	UNIPARENTAL DISOMY	REPEAT EXPANSIONS	EXAMPLES OF APPLICATIONS
FISH		X			Prader-Willi syndrome; Williams syndrome; aneuploidy
Array CGH		X	X		Intellectual disability or other conditions of unknown etiology; suspected microdeletions, microduplications, or aneuploidy
SNP microarrays	X	X			Drug sensitivity; intellectual disability; cardiovascular disease risk
Allele-specific oligonucleotide (ASO) hybridization	X			X	Sickle cell disease; α_1-antitrypsin deficiency
Sanger DNA sequencing	X				Familial breast/ovarian cancer
Southern blot or MLPA		X		X	Myotonic dystrophy; fragile X syndrome
Targeted disease-sequencing panels	X				Familial cardiomyopathy; long QT syndrome; familial colorectal cancer
Whole-exome or whole-genome sequencing	X	X			Undiagnosed conditions or diseases of uncertain etiology

[*]Adapted from Katsanis SH, Katsanis N. Molecular genetic testing and the future of clinical genomics. *Nat Rev Genet.* 2013; 14: 415-426.

the ASO containing the mutated sequence, whereas DNA from persons homozygous for the normal sequence hybridizes with the normal ASO. DNA from heterozygotes hybridizes with both probes (Fig. 10-3). The length of the ASO probes, usually about 18 to 20 nucleotides, is critical. Shorter probes would not be unique in the genome and would therefore hybridize to multiple regions. Longer probes are more difficult to synthesize correctly and could hybridize to both the normal and the mutated sequence.

Genetic diagnosis using ASO probes requires that the disease-causing gene has been identified and sequenced. In addition, each disease-causing mutation requires a different oligonucleotide probe. For this reason, this approach, while powerful, can become more challenging if the disease can be caused

by a large number of different mutations that each has low frequency in the population.

> Direct genetic diagnosis is accomplished by assaying the disease-causing mutation itself. It is potentially more accurate than indirect diagnosis and does not require family information. Direct diagnosis can be performed by hybridization of a person's DNA with allele-specific oligonucleotide probes. This approach is feasible if the DNA sequence causing a genetic disease is known and if the number of disease-causing mutations is limited.

Examples of diseases caused by a limited number of mutations include sickle cell disease and α_1-antitrypsin deficiency (Clinical Commentary 10-3). Although

GTG CAC CTG ACT CCT GAG GAG   Normal probe
CAC GTG GAC TGA GGA CTC CTC   Normal β-globin sequence (antisense strand)

GTG CAC CTG ACT CCT GTG GAG   Probe containing mutation
CAC GTG GAC TGA GGA CAC CTC   Missense mutation in β-globin sequence

Missense mutation

A

Probe with normal sequence

Probe with mutated sequence

B   Probe hybridization pattern

FIG 10-3   A, A 21-bp allele-specific oligonucleotide (ASO) probe (*yellow*) is constructed to undergo complementary base pairing only with the normal β-globin sequence, and another ASO probe (*green*) is constructed to undergo complementary base pairing only with a β-globin sequence that contains a missense mutation that produces a substitution of valine for glutamic acid at position 6 of the β-globin polypeptide (see Chapter 3), causing sickle cell disease in homozygotes. **B,** In this family, the parents are both heterozygous carriers of the missense mutation, so their DNA hybridizes to both ASO probes. The first female offspring has a homozygous normal genotype, the second offspring is heterozygous, and third offspring is an affected homozygote. A variety of methods, including microarrays (see Chapter 3), can be used to detect these ASO hybridization patterns.

approximately 2,000 cystic fibrosis mutations have been identified, 25 of the most common ones account for the great majority of mutations in many populations (see Clinical Commentary 10-2). Thus, direct diagnosis can be used to identify most cystic fibrosis homozygotes and heterozygous carriers. Prenatal diagnosis is also possible. Direct diagnosis can also be used to detect deletions or duplications (e.g., those of the dystrophin gene that cause most cases of Duchenne muscular dystrophy). Currently, clinical genetic testing is available for more than 4000 genetic diseases, including almost all of the single-gene conditions discussed in this textbook. Despite this wide availability, it should be kept in mind that genetic

testing, like all testing procedures, has a number of limitations (Box 10-3).

Microarrays, in which large numbers of oligonucleotide probes on a silicon chip are hybridized with labeled patient DNA (see Chapter 3), represent a large-scale extension of the ASO technology just described. Microarrays have many convenient properties, including miniaturization and automated computerized processing. They can be designed to assay large numbers of sequence variants (including disease-causing mutations) in a single rapid analysis (Box 10-4). For example, one microarray contains thousands of oligonucleotide probes that hybridize to large numbers of possible sequence variants in the *CYP2D6* and *CYP2C19* genes. The products of these genes influence the rate of metabolism of about 25% of all prescription drugs, and analysis of their variation might help to predict how individual patients will respond to these drugs.

Although microarray technology is relatively inexpensive and efficient, it allows only the detection of the DNA variants present in the probes included in the microarray platform. This drawback can be overcome with high-throughput DNA sequencing (see Chapters 3), which has become increasingly rapid and affordable. In **disease-targeted sequencing**, only the genes known to be associated with a specific disease are sequenced. For example, an individual with a positive family history of colorectal cancer could be tested for disease-causing variants in any of the dozen or so genes in which mutations have been shown to cause hereditary colorectal cancer (see Chapter 8). This approach has the advantage of detecting all pathogenic variants, including previously undiscovered ones, in the genes included in the testing panel. Disease-targeted sequencing panels have been developed for a number of hereditary conditions, including cardiomyopathies, cardiac arrhythmias (e.g., long QT syndrome), muscular dystrophies, and many hereditary cancers (e.g., cancers of the breast, colon, ovaries, or pancreas).

Disease-targeted sequencing is necessarily limited to the genes included in the sequencing panel. Whole-exome and whole-genome sequencing (see

CLINICAL COMMENTARY 10-3
The Genetic Diagnosis of α₁-Antitrypsin Deficiency

An inherited deficiency of α_1-antitrypsin (AAT) is one of the most common autosomal recessive disorders among whites, affecting approximately 1 in 2000 to 1 in 5000. AAT, synthesized primarily in the liver, is a serine protease inhibitor. As its name suggests, it binds trypsin. However, AAT binds much more strongly to neutrophil elastase, a protease that is produced by neutrophils (a type of leukocyte) in response to infections and irritants. It carries out its binding and inhibitory role primarily in the lower respiratory tract, where it prevents neutrophil elastase from digesting the alveolar septa of the lung.

Persons with less than 10% to 15% of the normal level of AAT activity experience significant lung damage and typically develop emphysema during their 30s, 40s, or 50s. In addition, at least 10% develop liver cirrhosis as a result of the accumulation of variant AAT molecules in the liver. AAT deficiency accounts for almost 20% of all nonalcoholic liver cirrhosis in the United States. Cigarette smokers with AAT deficiency develop emphysema much earlier than do non-smokers because cigarette smoke irritates lung tissue, increasing secretion of neutrophil elastase. At the same time, it inactivates AAT, so there is also less inhibition of elastase. One study showed that the median age of death of nonsmokers with AAT deficiency was 62 years, whereas it was 40 years for smokers with this disease. The combination of cigarette smoking (an environmental factor) and an AAT mutation (a genetic factor) produces more-severe disease than either factor alone; thus, this is an example of a **gene-environment interaction**.

Typically, AAT deficiency is tested first by a straightforward assay for reduced serum AAT concentration. Because a variety of conditions can reduce serum AAT, additional testing, via a type of protein electrophoresis (see Chapter 3) or DNA testing, is carried out to confirm a diagnosis of AAT deficiency. Direct DNA testing became feasible with the identification of *SERPINA1*, the gene that encodes AAT. More than 100 *SERPINA1* mutations have been identified, but only two missense variants, labeled the *S* and *Z* alleles, are common and clinically significant. Approximately ninety-five percent of cases of AAT deficiency are either *ZZ* homozygotes or *SZ* compound heterozygotes. The latter genotype generally produces less severe disease symptoms. Two large studies have indicated that the risk of developing emphysema among *ZZ* homozygotes is 70% for nonsmokers and 90% for smokers. Because the great majority of AAT cases are caused by two alleles, *Z* and *S*, this disease can be diagnosed efficiently and with 95% sensitivity by allele-specific DNA testing. If necessary, rare disease-causing mutations can be detected by sequencing the entire gene.

BOX 10-3   Limitations of Genetic Testing

Although genetic testing offers many advantages, its limitations must also be borne in mind. These limitations can be summarized as follows:
- No genetic test is 100% accurate. Although most genetic tests do achieve a high level of accuracy, factors such as mosaicism can complicate cytogenetic diagnosis, and genotyping errors can occur in the diagnosis of single-gene disorders.
- Genetic tests reveal mutations, not the presence of disease, because many disease-causing mutations have incomplete penetrance. For example, approximately 50% to 80% of women with *BRCA1* or *BRCA2* mutations develop breast cancer, and 70% to 90% of persons with mutations in one of the HNPCC genes develop colorectal cancer. Even when penetrance approaches 100% (as in neurofibromatosis type 1 or Huntington disease), detection of the mutation often reveals little about the severity or age of onset of the disease.
- Genetic testing might not detect all of the mutations that can cause a disease. Even in the absence of genotyping or sequencing errors, many genetic tests lack sensitivity. For example, the panels commonly used to test for cystic fibrosis mutations have typically less than 90% sensitivity to detect homozygotes (see Clinical Commentary 10-2). When a large number of different mutations can produce a genetic disease (e.g., neurofibromatosis, autosomal dominant breast cancer, Marfan syndrome), it might not be practical to test for all possible mutations. In this case, the analysis of linked markers can provide additional diagnostic accuracy if multiple family members are affected. Other factors that can reduce accuracy include locus heterogeneity and the presence of phenocopies.
- Genetic testing can lead to complex ethical and social considerations. The results of a genetic test might lead to stigmatization or to discrimination by employers or insurance companies. (However, a federal law, the Genetic Information Nondiscrimination Act, now prohibits discrimination by employers or health insurance providers based on the results of genetic testing [see Chapter 12].) Effective treatment is not available for some genetic diseases (e.g., Huntington disease, familial Alzheimer disease), decreasing the value of early diagnosis through genetic testing. Because genes are shared in families, the results of a genetic test might affect not only the tested person but also other members of the family (who might not wish to know about their risk for a genetic disease). These and other ethical and social issues are discussed further in Chapter 12.

BOX 10-4   Direct-to-Consumer Genetic Testing

Several private companies now offer microarray-based genetic testing on a direct-to-consumer basis. Typically, the customer collects and submits a cheek swab or mouthwash. DNA is extracted from the sample and hybridized to a microarray that can test simultaneously for a large number of DNA variants, including some of the variants associated, for example, with cystic fibrosis, hemochromatosis, age-related macular degeneration, type 1 diabetes, type 2 diabetes, psoriasis, and breast, prostate, and colorectal cancer. The customer is informed of the results and is given some explanatory information to aid in interpreting them. In some cases, genetic counseling is available. The cost of this procedure typically ranges from one hundred to several thousand dollars.

This type of testing, sometimes termed "recreational genomics," has understandable appeal. Many people want to know more about their genomes and how DNA variation might affect their health. Many will likely present the results of these tests to their primary care physicians, expecting explanations and even predictions. Several important considerations should be kept in mind.

For most disease conditions, these tests have relatively low sensitivity and low specificity. A positive result seldom predicts disease with precision (see Box 10-3), and a negative result should not induce a false sense of security. For common multifactorial diseases, most of the responsible genetic variants have not yet been identified, and, as discussed in Chapter 5, nongenetic factors typically play a large role in causing the disease. The relative increase in disease risk associated with most variants is quite small, on the order of a few percentage points. These risk estimates are usually based on specific populations, typically Europeans or Americans of European descent; they might not apply accurately to members of other populations. There is considerable potential for misunderstanding of these results, and many of the concerns discussed in Box 10-3 (stigmatization, potential for loss of privacy) apply to direct-to-consumer testing. For these reasons, this type of genetic testing should be regarded with considerable caution.

Chapters 3) can overcome this limitation by detecting nearly all disease-causing variants in an individual genome. However, the enormous amount of data generated by exome and whole-genome sequencing presents additional challenges, each human exome contains hundreds of potential disease-causing candidate variants. Many of these are **variants of unknown significance** whose effect on the phenotype is not yet known or understood. Large-scale efforts, involving sophisticated computer algorithms, ever-expanding databases of reported pathogenic variants, and functional studies of model organisms, are improving our ability to discriminate disease-causing variants from harmless ones.

A second challenge is that individuals who undergo exome or whole-genome sequencing for an indicated condition (e.g., a family history of colorectal cancer) are sometimes found to harbor a known pathogenic variant that causes another disease (e.g., an inherited cardiomyopathy). Currently, it is recommended to report these incidental findings to the patient if they are well validated and cause a condition that is considered to be clinically "actionable" (see the American College of Medical Genetics guidelines summarized by Green et al., 2013). As the number of sequenced individuals grows, and as

our understanding of the genetic basis of diseases increases, the list of actionable sequence variants is like to expand.

 New methods of direct mutation detection, including the use of microarrays and high-throughput sequencing, have greatly increased the speed and accuracy of genetic screening and diagnosis. Challenges raised by exome and whole-genome sequencing include large numbers of variants of unknown significance and issues regarding the reporting of incidental findings.

PRENATAL DIAGNOSIS OF GENETIC DISORDERS AND CONGENITAL DEFECTS

Prenatal diagnosis is a major focus of genetic testing, and several important areas of technology have evolved to provide this service. The principal aim of prenatal diagnosis is to supply at-risk families with information so that they can make informed choices during pregnancy. The potential benefits of prenatal testing include providing reassurance to at-risk families when the result is normal; providing risk information to couples who, in the absence of such information, would not choose to begin a pregnancy; allowing a couple to prepare psychologically for the birth of an affected baby; helping the health-care professional to plan delivery, management, and care of the infant when a disease is diagnosed in the fetus; and providing risk information to couples for whom pregnancy termination is an option.

Given the controversy surrounding the issue of pregnancy termination, it should be emphasized that the great majority of prenatal diagnoses yield a normal test result. Thus, most families receive reassurance, and only a small minority face the issue of pregnancy termination.

Both screening and diagnostic tests can be done prenatally. An example of a population screening test is the analysis of maternal serum at 15 weeks' gestation for increased or decreased levels of **α-fetoprotein** (AFP) and several other serum components that can indicate an abnormal pregnancy. A positive test result identifies a subgroup for further testing for aneuploidy syndromes or **neural tube defects** (NTDs). A subsequent **amniocentesis** (the withdrawal of amni-

otic fluid during pregnancy) would represent a more accurate, specific diagnostic test. Prenatal diagnostic methods can be divided into two major types: analysis of fetal tissues (amniocentesis, chorionic villus sampling, cordocentesis, and preimplantation genetic diagnosis) and visualization of the fetus (ultrasonography, magnetic resonance imaging). Amniocentesis is considered an invasive method of prenatal diagnosis, in contrast to noninvasive methods such as maternal serum screening tests and fetal visualization. In this section, each of these procedures is described, and their accuracy, safety, and feasibility are discussed.

Amniocentesis

Amniocentesis is typically performed at 15 to 17 weeks after a pregnant woman's last menstrual period (LMP). After real-time ultrasound imaging localizes the placenta and determines the position of the fetus, a needle is inserted through the abdominal wall into the amniotic sac (Fig. 10-4). Between 20 and 30 ml of amniotic fluid is withdrawn; this fluid contains living cells (**amniocytes**) shed by the fetus. The amniocytes

FIG 10-4   A schematic illustration of an amniocentesis, in which 20 to 30 ml of amniotic fluid is withdrawn transabdominally (with ultrasound guidance), usually at 15 to 17 weeks' gestation.

are cultured to increase their number (a procedure that requires up to 7 days), and standard cytogenetic studies are carried out on the cultured amniocytes. In addition, cells can be grown for biochemical assays or DNA-based diagnosis of any genetic disease for which mutation testing is available. The results of cytogenetic studies are typically available in 10 to 12 days. Because fluorescent in situ hybridization (FISH) can be carried out on a small number of uncultured amniocytes, it can provide an indication of fetal aneuploidy in just 1 to 2 days. If the FISH result is positive, subsequent, confirmatory diagnosis by routine cytogenetic methods is recommended. Indications for prenatal diagnosis by amniocentesis are listed in Box 10-5.

Amniocentesis is also used to measure α-fetoprotein (AFP), a fetal protein that is produced initially by the yolk sac and subsequently by the fetal liver. The AFP level normally increases in amniotic fluid until about 10 to 14 weeks' gestation and then decreases steadily. Amniotic fluid AFP is significantly higher in pregnancies in which the fetus has an NTD. When an amniotic fluid AFP assay is used with ultrasonography (see later) in the second trimester, more than 98% of fetuses with an open spina bifida and virtually all of those with anencephaly can be recognized. Among women who undergo amniocentesis for cytogenetic analysis, it is routine to also measure their amniotic fluid AFP level.

In addition to a fetal NTD, there are several other causes of elevated (or apparently elevated) amniotic fluid AFP. These include underestimation of gestational age, fetal death, presence of twins, blood contamination, and several specific malformations (e.g., omphalocele or gastroschisis, which are abdominal wall defects). Usually, targeted ultrasonography can distinguish among these alternatives.

The safety and accuracy of amniocentesis have been established by several large collaborative studies. The risk of maternal complications is very low. Transient fluid leakage occurs in about 1% of mothers, and maternal infections are extremely rare. The risk of primary concern is fetal loss. Amniocentesis increases the risk of fetal loss by no more than 0.2%

to 0.3% (approximately 1/300 to 1/500) above the background risk at 15 to 17 weeks post-LMP (i.e., if the risk of pregnancy loss after 17 weeks were 3% in mothers who did not have an amniocentesis, the risk would increase to 3.2% to 3.3% in those who had the procedure). One must weigh the risk of fetal loss against the probability that the fetus is affected with a diagnosable condition (Clinical Commentary 10-4).

Although amniocentesis provides highly accurate results, chromosomal mosaicism can lead to misdi-

---

BOX 10-5   Indications for Prenatal Diagnosis by Amniocentesis

Maternal age >35 years
Previous child with chromosome abnormality
History of structural chromosome abnormality in one parent
Family history of genetic defect that is diagnosable by biochemical or DNA analysis
Increased risk of neural tube defect due to positive family history
Abnormal quadruple or integrated screen

CLINICAL COMMENTARY 10-4
The Amniocentesis Decision

When a prenatal screening test (see text) identifies a risk of fetal abnormality greater than 1 in 500, it is common for a pregnant woman to consider the possibility of amniocentesis. Several factors enter into the decision-making process. First is quantitative risk estimate, determined by the screening result, for Down syndrome and other chromosomal disorders. A second factor is the risk of fetal loss from the procedure (about 0.2% to 0.3% above the background risk). A third issue is the expense of an amniocentesis with ultrasound and cytogenetic analysis, which ordinarily costs about $2000. These factors must be weighed in terms of their relative costs and benefits for the woman and her family.

As this decision is explored in greater depth, other considerations often arise. If a woman has had previous miscarriages, the additional risk of fetal loss may be weighed more heavily. In addition, the seriousness of bearing a child with disabilities may be perceived differently from family to family. Some couples are uncomfortable with the amount of time that elapses before test results are available (usually 10-12 days). This discomfort should be acknowledged and validated. The possibility of an ambiguous result (e.g., mosaicism) also deserves discussion. Finally, it is important for the clinician to specify that an amniocentesis typically detects only a specific class of disorders (i.e., chromosome abnormalities and neural tube defects) and not the entire range of birth defects and genetic disorders.

agnosis. Most apparent mosaicism is caused by the generation of an extra chromosome during in vitro cell culture and is labeled as **pseudomosaicism**. This can be distinguished easily from true mosaicism if techniques are used in which all cells in a colony are the descendants of a single fetal cell. If only some cells in the colony have the extra chromosome, it is assumed that pseudomosaicism exists. If, however, consistent aneuploidy is visualized in all cells of multiple colonies, then true fetal mosaicism is diagnosed. Further confirmation of fetal mosaicism (which is generally a rare condition) can be obtained by fetal blood sampling, as described later.

Some centers have evaluated amniocentesis performed earlier in pregnancy, at about 12 to 14 weeks post-LMP. Because less amniotic fluid is present at this time, the risk of fetal loss or injury may be higher. A number of large-scale evaluations have indicated significantly higher rates of fetal loss for **early amniocentesis**, and some studies have shown increased rates of specific congenital anomalies (club foot in particular).

▶ Amniocentesis, the withdrawal of amniotic fluid during pregnancy, is performed at about 16 weeks post-LMP and is used to diagnose many genetic diseases. The amniotic α-fetoprotein level is elevated when the fetus has a neural tube defect and provides a reliable prenatal test for this condition. The rate of fetal loss attributable to this procedure is approximately 1/300 to 1/500 above the background risk level. Amniocentesis can also be performed earlier in the pregnancy; some studies indicate an elevated rate of fetal loss after early amniocentesis.

Chorionic Villus Sampling

Chorionic villus sampling (**CVS**), the other commonly used invasive prenatal diagnostic technique, is performed by aspirating fetal trophoblastic tissue (chorionic villi) by either a transcervical or transabdominal approach (Fig. 10-5). Because it is usually performed at 10 to 11 weeks post-LMP, CVS has the advantage of providing a diagnosis much earlier in pregnancy than second-trimester amniocentesis. This may be important for couples who consider pregnancy termination as an option.

Cell culture (as in amniocentesis) and direct analysis from rapidly dividing trophoblasts can provide material for cytogenetic analysis. When chorionic villi are successfully obtained, CVS provides diagnostic results in more than 99% of cases. **Confined placental mosaicism** (mosaicism in the placenta but not in the fetus itself) is seen in about 1% to 2% of cases in which direct analysis of villus material is performed. This can confuse the diagnosis, because the mosaicism observed in placental (villus) material is not actually present in the fetus. This problem can usually be resolved by a follow-up amniocentesis. A disadvantage of CVS is that amniotic fluid AFP cannot be measured. Women who undergo CVS may have their serum AFP level measured at 15 to 16 weeks after LMP as a screen for NTDs.

CVS, like amniocentesis, is generally a safe procedure. Several collaborative studies revealed a post-CVS fetal loss rate of approximately 1% above the background rate, compared with 0.2% to 0.3% above background for amniocentesis. Factors that increase the risk of fetal loss include a lack of experience with the procedure and an increase in the number of transcervical passages used to obtain the villus sample. In experienced hands, transcervical and transabdominal procedures appear to entail similar risk levels.

Some studies have indicated that CVS can increase the risk of limb deficiencies. Although other investigations have not corroborated this result, the apparent association has been of concern because the proposed mechanism (vascular insult leading to hypoperfusion of the limb) is biologically plausible. The risk is greatest when CVS is performed earlier than 10 weeks post-LMP and decreases to no more than one in several thousand when the procedure is performed at 10 to 11 weeks post-LMP. Accordingly, many professionals now recommend against performing CVS before 10 weeks after LMP.

FIG 10-5   A schematic illustration of a transcervical chorionic villus sampling procedure. With ultrasound guidance, a catheter is inserted, and several milligrams of villus tissue are aspirated.

CVS is performed earlier than amniocentesis (at 10 to 11 weeks post-LMP), using either a transcervical or a transabdominal approach. The risk of fetal loss attributable to CVS is approximately 1% to 1.5%. Confined placental mosaicism can confuse the diagnosis. There is some evidence that CVS can increase the risk of limb deficiencies; this risk is greatest when the procedure is performed before 10 weeks post-LMP.

Inborn errors of metabolism (see Chapter 7), which are usually autosomal or X-linked recessive diseases, can be diagnosed prenatally by amniocentesis or CVS if the specific metabolic defect is expressed in amniocytes or trophoblastic tissue. They can also be diagnosed prenatally by DNA-based methods if the disease-causing mutation can be identified. Table 10-7 lists selected inborn errors of metabolism and single-gene disorders for which amniocentesis or CVS is available.

TABLE 10-7   Selected Inborn Errors of Metabolism That Are Diagnosable through Amniocentesis and/or Chorionic Villus Sampling

DISEASE	MEASURABLE ENZYME
Disorders of Amino Acid or Organic Acid Metabolism	
Maple syrup urine disease	Branched-chain ketoacid decarboxylase
Methylmalonic acidemia	Methylmalonic coenzyme A mutase
Multiple carboxylase deficiency	Biotin responsive carboxylase
Disorders of Carbohydrate Metabolism	
Glycogen storage disease, type 2	α-Glucosidase
Galactosemia	Galactose-1-uridyl transferase
Disorders of Lysosomal Enzymes	
Gangliosidosis (all types)	β-Galactosidase
Mucopolysaccharidosis (all types)	Disease-specific enzyme (see Chapter 7)
Tay-Sachs disease	Hexosaminidase A
Disorders of Purine and Pyrimidine Metabolism	
Lesch-Nyhan syndrome	Hypoxanthine-guanine phosphoribosyl transferase
Disorders of Peroxisomal Metabolism	
Zellweger syndrome	Long-chain fatty acids

Other Methods of Fetal Tissue Sampling

Cordocentesis, or **percutaneous umbilical blood sampling** (**PUBS**), has become the preferred method to access fetal blood. PUBS is usually carried out after the 16th week of gestation and is accomplished by ultrasound-guided puncture of the umbilical cord and withdrawal of fetal blood. The fetal loss rate attributable to PUBS is low, but it is slightly higher than that of amniocentesis or CVS.

There are three primary applications of PUBS. It is used for cytogenetic analysis of fetuses with structural anomalies detected by ultrasound when rapid diagnosis is required. Cytogenetic analysis from fetal blood sampling is completed in 2 to 3 days, whereas diagnosis after amniocentesis can require 10 to 12 days if amniocytes must be cultured. This time difference can be critical in the later stages of a pregnancy. A second application is diagnosis of hematological diseases that are analyzed most effectively in blood samples or diagnosis of immunologic disorders such as chronic granulomatous disease (see Chapter 9). PUBS is also used to make a rapid distinction between true fetal mosaicism and false mosaicism caused by maternal contamination of an amniotic fluid sample.

▶ Percutaneous umbilical blood sampling (PUBS, or cordocentesis) is a method of direct sampling of fetal blood and is used to obtain a sample for rapid cytogenetic or hematological analysis or for confirmation of mosaicism.

Ultrasonography

Technological advances in real-time **ultrasonography** have made this an important tool in prenatal diagnosis. A transducer placed on the mother's abdomen sends pulsed sound waves through the fetus. The fetal tissue reflects the waves in patterns corresponding to tissue density. The reflected waves are displayed on a monitor, which allows real-time visualization of the fetus. Ultrasonography can help to detect many fetal malformations, and it enhances

the effectiveness of amniocentesis, CVS, and PUBS. Box 10-6 lists some of the congenital malformations that are diagnosable by fetal ultrasound.

Ultrasonography is sometimes used to test for a specific condition in an at-risk fetus (e.g., a short-limb skeletal dysplasia). More often, fetal anomalies are detected during the evaluation of obstetrical indicators such as uncertain gestational age, poor fetal growth, or amniotic fluid abnormalities. Second-trimester ultrasound screening has become routine in developed countries. Studies of ultrasound screening suggest that sensitivity for the detection of most major congenital malformations ranges from 30% to 50%. Specificity, however, approaches 99%.

The sensitivity of ultrasonography is higher for some congenital malformations. In particular, ultrasound can detect virtually all fetuses with anencephaly and 85% to 90% of those with spina bifida (Fig. 10-6). It also sometimes identifies a fetus with a chromosome

---

BOX 10-6   Selected Disorders Diagnosed by Ultrasound in the Second Trimester*

Symptom Complex
Hydrops
Oligohydramnios
Polyhydramnios
Intrauterine growth retardation

Central Nervous System
Anencephaly
Encephalocele
Holoprosencephaly
Hydrocephalus

Chest
Congenital heart disease
Diaphragmatic hernia

Abdomen, Pelvis
Gastrointestinal atresias
Gastroschisis
Omphalocele
Renal agenesis
Cystic kidneys
Hydronephrosis

Skeletal System
Limb deficiencies
Many chondrodystrophies, including thanatophoric dysplasia and osteogenesis imperfecta

Craniofacial
Cleft lip

*Detection rate varies by condition

abnormality by detecting a congenital malformation, intrauterine growth retardation, hydrops (abnormal accumulation of fluid in the fetus), or an alteration of the amniotic fluid volume.

FIG 10-6 **A,** Photograph of an ultrasound result, revealing a fetus with a normal spinal column. **B,** Ultrasound result for a fetus with a meningomyelocele, visible as fluid-filled sacs (*arrows*) located toward the base of the spinal column.

Ultrasonography is the technique used most commonly for fetal visualization, but other techniques are also used. Radiography is still used occasionally, for example, to evaluate a fetus for skeletal defects. Magnetic resonance imaging (MRI) offers much greater resolution than ultrasonography and is becoming more widely available for prenatal screening.

Prenatal diagnosis includes invasive techniques designed to analyze fetal tissue (CVS, amniocentesis, PUBS) and noninvasive procedures that visualize the fetus (ultrasonography, MRI).

Maternal Serum Screening in the First and Second Trimesters

Soon after the link between elevated amniotic fluid AFP and NTDs was recognized, an association between increased levels of **maternal serum AFP** (MSAFP) and NTDs was identified. AFP diffuses across the fetal membranes into the mother's serum, so MSAFP levels are correlated with amniotic fluid AFP levels. Thus, it is possible to measure amniotic fluid AFP noninvasively by obtaining a maternal blood sample at 15 to 17 weeks post-LMP.

Because 90% to 95% of NTD births occur in the absence of a family history of the condition, a safe, noninvasive population screening procedure for NTDs is highly desirable. However, there is considerable overlap of MSAFP levels in women carrying a fetus with an NTD and those carrying an unaffected fetus (Fig. 10-7). Thus, the issues of sensitivity and specificity must be considered. Typically, an MSAFP level is considered to be elevated if it is 2 to 2.5 times higher than the normal median level (adjustments for maternal weight, presence of diabetes mellitus, and ancestry are included in these calculations). Approximately 1% to 2% of pregnant women exhibit MSAFP levels above this cutoff level. After adjusting for advanced gestational age, fetal demise, and presence of twins, about 1 in 15 of these women has an elevated amniotic fluid AFP. The positive predictive

FIG 10-7 Maternal serum α-fetoprotein (MSAFP) levels in mothers carrying normal fetuses and in mothers carrying fetuses with Down syndrome and open spina bifida. MSAFP is somewhat lowered when the fetus has Down syndrome, and it is substantially elevated when the fetus has an open spina bifida. (From Milunsky A. *Genetic Disorders and the Fetus: Diagnosis, Prevention, and Treatment,* 4th ed. Baltimore: Johns Hopkins University Press; 1998.)

value of the MSAFP screening test is thus rather low, approximately 6% (1/15). However, the sensitivity of the test is fairly high: MSAFP screening identifies approximately 90% of anencephaly cases and about 80% of open spina bifida cases. Although this sensitivity level is lower than that of amniotic fluid AFP testing, MSAFP measurement poses no risk of fetal loss and serves as an effective screening measure. Women who have an elevated MSAFP may choose to undergo diagnostic amniocentesis to determine whether they are in fact carrying a fetus with an NTD.

An association was found in the 1990s between *low* MSAFP and the presence of a fetus with Down syndrome. Previously, population screening for Down syndrome consisted of amniocentesis for women older than 35 years. Although highly accurate, this screening strategy has a sensitivity of only 20%: because the great majority of births occur in women younger than 35 years, only about 20% of all babies with trisomy 21 are born to mothers older than age 35. MSAFP measurement has expanded the option of population screening for Down syndrome.

MSAFP levels overlap considerably in normal and Down syndrome pregnancies. The risk for Down syndrome in women younger than 35 years increases by a factor of 3 to 4 when the adjusted MSAFP value is lower than 0.5 multiples of the normal population median (see Fig. 10-7). In deriving a risk estimate, complex formulas take into account the mother's weight, age, and MSAFP level. A woman who is 25 years of age ordinarily has a risk of about 1/1250 for producing a fetus with Down syndrome, but if she has a weight-adjusted MSAFP of 0.35 multiples of the median, her risk increases to 1/171. This risk is higher than that of a 35-year-old woman in the general population. Most screening programs use a risk factor of 1/380 (equivalent to the average risk for a 35-year-old woman to produce a newborn with Down syndrome) as an indication for subsequent diagnostic evaluation by amniocentesis.

The accuracy of Down syndrome screening can be increased by measuring the serum levels of unconjugated estriol, human chorionic gonadotropin, and inhibin-A in addition to MSAFP (the **quadruple screen**). Although MSAFP alone identifies only about 40% of Down syndrome pregnancies, the four indicators together can identify approximately 80% (with a false-positive rate of 5%). The quadruple screen can also detect most cases of trisomy 18.

First-trimester maternal serum screening (at 10 to 13 weeks) for Down syndrome is being used increasingly in the United States and Europe. Three of the most useful measurements are the free β subunit of human chorionic gonadotropin (FβhCG), pregnancy-associated plasma protein A (PAPP-A), and an ultrasound assessment of nuchal translucency (NT, the abnormal accumulation of fluid behind the neck of a fetus). Measurement of these three quantities in the first trimester enables detection of 80% to 85% of Down syndrome cases (with a false-positive rate of 5%, or 95% specificity). Combining first- and second-trimester screening, called integrated screening, increases the sensitivity of Down syndrome detection to approximately 90%, with 95% specificity. Measurement of FβhCG and PAPP-A is also useful for detection of trisomy 13 and trisomy 18 in the first trimester. These screening results may be combined with CVS or amniocentesis to provide a more precise diagnostic test.

> MSAFP provides a screening approach that increases the prenatal detection of fetuses with various abnormalities, including NTDs, trisomy 18, and Down syndrome. This non-invasive procedure entails virtually no risk, but its sensitivity and specificity for detecting NTDs are lower than those of amniotic AFP diagnosis. Use of additional markers (e.g., the quadruple screen) in the second trimester increases sensitivity for detecting Down syndrome. Screening of maternal serum for Down syndrome, trisomy 13, and trisomy 18 can be carried out in the first trimester.

Analysis of Fetal DNA in Maternal Circulation

The ability to isolate fetal cells and DNA from maternal blood during pregnancy has opened up new opportunities for prenatal screening and diagnosis. This approach, called **noninvasive prenatal screening** (**NIPS**), has become widely used in recent years, and some authorities think it will replace the current first- and second-trimester screening approaches. During pregnancy, a small number of fetal cells cross the placental barrier to enter the mother's circulation as early as 6 to 8 weeks post-LMP. These cells can be analyzed using techniques such as FISH or PCR, but isolating fetal cells specifically in maternal blood has been a challenge.

Recently, researchers have focused on fragments of **cell-free DNA** (**cfDNA**) released into the maternal circulation from trophoblasts that undergo programmed cell death. This cfDNA represents the fetal genome and composes a significant proportion (5% to 50%) of all cfDNA found in maternal plasma. This proportion tends to increase during pregnancy, and at approximately 9-10 weeks post-LMP a small quantity of maternal blood (10 ml) can be sampled to obtain cfDNA. Fetal cfDNA is differentiated from maternal cfDNA by identifying SNP haplotypes that occur in excess frequency in the maternal circulation. cfDNA has been used to identify the sex of the fetus and its Rh blood type (especially important if the mother is Rh-negative and the fetus may be Rh-positive; see Chapter 9). High-throughput sequencing techniques can be used with fetal cfDNA, and full fetal genome sequences have now been obtained. Sequencing read counts can reveal aneuploidy (e.g., trisomy 21 would produce a 50% excess in reads from chromosome 21). Recent studies indicate that maternal plasma cell-free DNA has at least several-fold higher specificity and positive predictive value for detection of trisomies 13, 18, and 21 than does standard screening. The sensitivity of the test for aneuploidy detection is virtually 100%. It is important to stress that NIPS is a screening test, not a diagnostic test, so positive test results are confirmed by CVS or amniocentesis. By decreasing the number of false positive tests, current NIPS techniques can reduce the need for invasive tests such as amniocentesis and CVS.

 Cell-free DNA (cfDNA) that enters the maternal circulation can be evaluated for mutations or aneuploidy using high-throughput sequencing. This procedure entails no risk of fetal loss and has greater specificity and positive predictive value for aneuploidy detection than other first- and second-trimester screening procedures.

Preimplantation Genetic Diagnosis

The most common type of **preimplantation genetic diagnosis** (**PGD**) is carried out on a blastomere obtained in the course of **in vitro fertilization**. Diagnosis is begun 3 days after fertilization, when the embryo contains six or eight cells. One or two blastomeres can safely be removed from the embryo. FISH analysis of the cell (see Chapter 6) can be used to diagnose aneuploidy. Also, the cell's DNA can be amplified using PCR, permitting the diagnosis of single-gene diseases. If the embryo from which the **blastomere** was obtained is morphologically normal and neither the disease-causing mutation nor aneuploidy is detected, the embryo is implanted into the mother's uterus. Testing protocols have been developed for dozens of genetic diseases (e.g., cystic fibrosis, Tay-Sachs disease, β-thalassemia, myotonic dystrophy, Huntington disease, Duchenne muscular dystrophy), and thousands of normal babies have been born after blastomere diagnosis.

An occasional problem with blastomere PGD is that one of the two alleles of a locus may be undetectable, which could cause a heterozygote to appear as a homozygote. This phenomenon, termed "allelic dropout," occurs because of partial PCR amplification failure when using DNA from only a single cell. This has led to misdiagnosis in a small number of cases, and several methods are used to increase accuracy. For example, highly heterozygous STRs closely linked to the disease-causing locus can be tested as part of the PCR analysis. If only one of the parents' STR alleles can be observed in the blastomere's DNA, it is likely that allelic dropout has also occurred for the disease-causing locus. The testing of two cells, rather than one, helps to avoid allelic dropout.

PGD can also be carried out at the 100-cell blastocyst stage, using cells from the trophoectoderm of the blastocyst. This procedure has the advantage that a larger collection of cells is analyzed, helping to avoid allelic dropout. A disadvantage is that extra-embryonic tissue (the trophoectoderm) is diagnosed, rather than the embryo itself.

Polar body diagnosis involves an examination of the first or second polar body produced along with the ovum (see Chapter 2). The polar body's DNA is tested to determine whether it contains a disease-causing mutation. If it does, it is assumed that the egg does not contain the mutation. This egg is then fertilized and implanted using the usual in vitro techniques. Because only the polar body is examined, paternal mutations cannot be evaluated. Polar body diagnosis is thus most useful when only the mother is at risk for transmitting a disease-causing mutation or when testing for aneuploidy (because most aneuploidies are contributed by the mother [see Chapter 6]).

PGD is most commonly used by couples who have resorted to in vitro fertilization and wish to test for diagnosable genetic conditions. It can also be useful for couples who want prenatal diagnosis but would not consider a pregnancy termination. PGD, however, is costly and technically challenging, and its availability is still limited.

▶ Preimplantation genetic diagnosis can be carried out on polar bodies, blastomeres, or blastocyst cells, on which PCR analysis and/or FISH is performed. Diagnosis of genetic conditions permits implantation of only unaffected embryos and avoids the issue of pregnancy termination.

FETAL TREATMENT

A potential goal of prenatal diagnosis is treatment of the affected fetus. Although this is not currently possible for most conditions, some examples can be cited. Many of these procedures are experimental.

Two of the best-established forms of in utero intervention are treatment for rare inborn errors of metabolism and treatment for hormone deficiencies. An important example of a treatable biochemical disorder is biotin-responsive multiple carboxylase deficiency, an autosomal recessive condition that can be diagnosed by amniocentesis. In one case report, oral administration of biotin to the mother was initiated at 23 weeks of pregnancy and resulted in the birth of a normal baby.

CAH is a second example of a condition for which in utero treatment has been successful after prenatal diagnosis. Because of excessive androgen secretion by the enlarged fetal adrenal glands, female fetuses with CAH become masculinized. Administration of dexamethasone to the mother beginning at 10 weeks post-LMP diminishes or prevents this masculinization.

Surgical treatment of fetuses, primarily for conditions involving urinary tract obstruction, has met with moderate success. Surgical correction of diaphragmatic hernia at 20 weeks' gestation has also been attempted, but results have been discouraging and this approach has been abandoned. Clinical trials have shown that surgical closure of myelomeningocele (spina bifida) at approximately 26 weeks gestation helps to restore the normal flow of cerebrospinal fluid and can reduce hydrocephalus. However, the procedure also increases the likelihood of preterm birth and maternal complications. Some success has been achieved in transplantation of hematopoietic stem cells into fetuses with X-linked severe combined immune deficiency (see Chapter 9).

GENE THERAPY

As we have seen, gene discovery provides opportunities for improved understanding and diagnosis of many diseases. The identification of these genes also leads to the possibility of genetic alteration of the cells of affected persons (**gene therapy**). Although gene therapy is still in its infancy and has only begun to affect the lives of patients, its potential for curing genetic diseases has excited a great deal of interest in both professional and lay circles. Approximately 2000 gene therapy protocols involving more than 100 different genes have been approved for clinical trials (see Table 10-8 for some examples). In this section we review gene therapy techniques and discuss their application in the treatment of disease.

Somatic Cell Therapy

Somatic cell gene therapy, which has been the focus of gene therapy research in humans, consists of the alteration of genes in human somatic cells to treat a specific disorder. The patient's cells are extracted and manipulated outside the body (*ex vivo* therapy), or in some cases the cells are treated while they are in the body (*in vivo* therapy).

Some types of somatic cells are more amenable to gene therapy than others. Good candidates should be easily accessible and should have a long life span in the body. Proliferating cells are preferred for some gene-delivery systems, because the vector carrying the gene can then integrate into the cells' replicating DNA. The bone marrow stem cell meets all of these qualifications and thus has been a prime candidate for somatic therapy. Although these cells are difficult to manipulate and to isolate from bone marrow (the great majority of bone marrow cells are not stem cells), they have now been successfully isolated and genetically altered in many gene therapy treatments. Other cell types have also been investigated as potential targets, including skin fibroblasts, muscle cells, vascular endothelial cells, hepatocytes, and lymphocytes. A disadvantage of using such cells is that their life span may be relatively short. Thus, therapy using them can require repeated treatment and administration of genetically altered cells.

Gene Replacement Therapy

Most current gene therapy techniques involve replacing a missing gene product by inserting a normal gene into somatic cells. This approach is best suited to correcting loss-of-function mutations that result in a nonfunctional or missing gene product; inserting the normal gene supplies the missing product. Even a partially effective gene therapy strategy, producing perhaps 5% to 20% of the normal amount

of the gene product, can provide significant health benefits.

There are many techniques for introducing genes into cells, but viruses, having naturally evolved clever strategies for inserting their genetic material into cells, are the most commonly used gene therapy vectors. In the following paragraphs viral vectors are discussed first, followed by a discussion of some potentially effective non-viral delivery systems.

Retroviral Vectors

Retroviruses, a form of RNA virus, can insert copies of their genomes into the nuclei of host cells after reverse-transcribing their viral RNA into double-stranded DNA (see Chapter 8). The insertion of foreign DNA into a host cell via a viral vector is termed **transduction**. Retroviruses transduce host cells with a high degree of efficiency, and they seldom provoke immune responses, making them a reasonable choice as a gene-delivery vector (Fig. 10-8). Recombinant DNA techniques are used to create replication-defective retroviruses in which the three retroviral protein-coding genes are replaced with a normal copy of a human gene and a promoter element (the "insert," which can be as large as 8-12 kb in a retrovirus). The modified retroviruses are then incubated with the patient's somatic cells (e.g., bone marrow stem cells, lymphocytes) so that the retrovirus transduces the normal human gene into the DNA of the host cells. Ideally, the inserted gene will then encode a normal gene product in the patient's somatic cells. This type of protocol has been used experimentally with many diseases, including forms of severe combined immunodeficiency (Clinical Commentary 10-5).

Although retroviruses offer the advantages of stable and efficient integration into the genome, they also present specific disadvantages. Because retroviruses integrate preferentially near promoter sequences, a retroviral vector can insert near a proto-oncogene, activating it and thus causing tumor formation. Most types of retrovirus can enter the nucleus only when its membrane dissolves during cell division, so they can transduce only dividing cells and are ineffective in nondividing or slowly dividing cells (e.g., neurons).

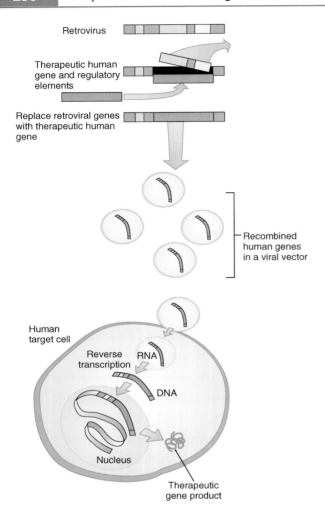

FIG 10-8 Gene therapy using a retroviral vector. The retrovirus is prevented from replicating by removal of most of its genome, and a normal human gene is inserted into the retrovirus. Incubation with human somatic cells allows the retrovirus to insert copies of the normal human gene into the cell. Once integrated into the cell's DNA, the inserted gene produces a normal gene product.

Although this attribute is typically a disadvantage, it can be useful when the goal of therapy is to target only dividing cells and to avoid non-dividing cells (e.g., in the treatment of a brain tumor, where tumor cells are dividing but nearby healthy neurons are not).

Adenoviral Vectors

Because of the inability of most retroviruses to transduce non-dividing cells, other delivery systems have been explored that are not limited in this way. An important example is the **adenovirus**, a double-stranded DNA virus that is often used in vaccine prepa-

rations. In addition to its ability to transduce non-dividing cells, the adenoviral vector can now be designed to accept inserts of approximately 36 kb in size. Adenoviruses do not integrate into the host cell's DNA, which provides the advantage that they will not activate a proto-oncogene or otherwise disturb the genome. However, lack of integration is also a disadvantage because adenoviruses are eventually inactivated. This often results in transient gene expression (though long-term expression is sometimes achieved) and can require readministration of the vector. Because only part of the adenovirus genome is typically removed, the vector often provokes an immune response (e.g., inflammatory responses in the airways of cystic fibrosis patients in whom adenoviruses were used to introduce normal copies of the *CFTR* gene into airway epithelial cells). This problem increases with repeated introduction of the adenovirus, which stimulates further immune response to the foreign protein. Current research is focusing on "gutless" adenoviruses, in which nearly all of the viral genome is removed to reduce the immune response and increase the potential size of the insert.

Adeno-Associated Viral Vectors

Adeno-associated viruses (**AAVs**) are a type of parvovirus that requires the presence of adenoviruses for their normal replication (hence the term *adeno-associated*). Like adenoviruses, AAVs are DNA viruses that can transduce nondividing cells. In addition, they elicit much less immune response than do adenoviruses and have little, if any, pathogenic effect. They are also capable of sustaining protracted therapeutic expression (months to years). These vectors, however, can accept a DNA insert of only about 4.5 kb. (In some cases, this problem can be circumvented by dividing the insert into two parts, placing each part in a vector, and designing the mRNA products to reassemble.) Because of their many useful properties, AAVs have become much more popular as a gene therapy vector during the past several years. They have been tested in clinical trials for the treatment of cystic fibrosis, hemophilia B, α_1-antitrypsin deficiency, Duchenne muscular dystrophy, Parkinson disease, Alzheimer disease, and many other disorders.

CLINICAL COMMENTARY 10-5
Gene Therapy and Severe Combined Immunodeficiency

Gene therapy has been attempted for several forms of **severe combined immunodeficiency (SCID)**, including adenosine deaminase deficiency SCID (ADA-SCID) and X-linked SCID. ADA, which is produced primarily in lymphoid tissues, is an important component of the purine salvage pathway. ADA deficiency, an autosomal recessive disorder that accounts for about 15% of SCID cases, results in the abnormal accumulation of purine metabolites toxic to T lymphocytes. Subsequently, B lymphocytes are also reduced in function and number. The resulting SCID is usually fatal by the age of 2 years if untreated.

The preferred treatment for ADA-SCID is bone marrow transplantation. However, complications of bone marrow transplantation increase patient morbidity and are sometimes fatal. In addition, major histocompatibility complex (MHC)-compatible sibling donors are available for less than 30% of ADA-SCID patients. Patients may be treated with polyethylene glycol (PEG)-conjugated ADA (administered once or twice weekly by intramuscular injection), but the response to this treatment is variable, and some patients develop antibodies against PEG-ADA.

Because it is a systemic disorder caused by an enzyme deficiency, ADA-SCID represents a good candidate for gene replacement therapy. Ideally, proliferating bone marrow stem cells would be modified by retroviral vectors containing the normal ADA gene, resulting in a permanent cure for the disorder. Because of difficulties in dealing with bone marrow stem cells, gene therapy for ADA-SCID was initiated instead in 1990 by retroviral insertion of ADA genes into lymphocytes that were extracted from patients. After retroviral insertion, the lymphocytes were injected back into the patients' peripheral circulation. This was the first application of gene therapy to an inherited human disorder. More recently, ADA-SCID has been treated by retroviral insertion of the ADA gene into bone marrow stem cells, rather than lymphocytes. This treatment has produced long-term increases in B-cell and T-cell counts and normal immune function in treated patients.

X-linked SCID results from mutations in the gene, *SCIDX1*, that encodes subunits of the γ chain found in six different cytokine receptors (those of interleukins 2, 4, 7, 9, 15, and 21; see Chapter 9). Lacking these receptors, T cells and natural killer cells cannot receive the signals they need for normal maturation. The T-cell deficiency in turn produces a deficiency of normal B cells, resulting in SCID. As with ADA deficiency, this disorder can be treated with bone marrow transplantation if an MHC-compatible donor is available. Without a bone marrow transplant, the disease is fatal early in childhood.

In 1999, retroviral therapy was initiated to introduce *SCIDX1* into patients' bone marrow stem cells. Fewer than 1% of bone marrow stem cells were effectively transduced with the therapeutic gene. However, the transduced cells enjoyed a selective growth advantage over other bone marrow stem cells because the inserted gene increased the cytokine signaling needed for normal cell function. In most treated patients, the number of natural killer cells, T cells, and B cells increased to near-normal levels, with sustained resistance to infections continuing for more than a decade after therapy.

These positive outcomes in most ADA and X-linked SCID patients have been widely heralded as the first successful uses of somatic cell gene therapy in the treatment of an inherited disease. However, five X-linked SCID patients developed leukemia-like disease (clonal T-cell proliferation) as a result of random insertion of the retroviral vector in or near *LMO2*, a proto-oncogene that is activated in about half of all cases of acute lymphocytic leukemia. This was fatal in one patient, but the others were treated successfully by chemotherapy and continued to benefit from gene therapy. Leukemia has also occurred in patients with chronic granulomatous disease and Wiskott-Aldrich syndrome (Table 10-8) who have been treated with retroviral therapy. It is likely that the promoter and enhancer sequences in the retroviral vector up-regulate the *LMO2*

TABLE 10-8   Examples of Diseases in Which Somatic Cell Gene Therapy Has Had Significant Therapeutic Effect

DISEASE	TARGET CELL	PRODUCT OF INSERTED OR MODIFIED GENE
Severe combined immunodeficiency (SCID) due to adenosine deaminase deficiency	Circulating lymphocytes, bone marrow stem cells	Adenosine deaminase
X-linked SCID	Bone marrow stem cells	γ subunit of interleukin receptors
Hemophilia B	Hepatocytes, skin fibroblasts	Factor IX
Duchenne muscular dystrophy	Myocytes	Dystrophin (modified by exon skipping)
Wiskott-Aldrich syndrome (primary immunodeficiency)	Hematopoietic stem cells	Wiskott-Aldrich Syndrome Protein (WASP)
X-linked adrenoleukodystrophy	Hematopoietic stem cells	Adenosine triphosphate-binding cassette transporter
Leber congenital amaurosis (childhood blindness)	Rod photoreceptor cells	Retinal pigment epithelium-specific protein 65
β-Thalassemia	Hematopoietic stem cells	β-Globin
Lipoprotein lipase deficiency	Myocytes	Lipoprotein lipase

CLINICAL COMMENTARY 10-5
Gene Therapy and Severe Combined Immunodeficiency (Continued)

gene. Self-inactivating retroviral vectors, in which enhancer sequences are deleted, are now being tested in clinical trials.

These examples illustrate some of the promise, as well as some of the perils, of somatic cell gene therapy.

Clearly, gene therapy poses hazards that must be closely monitored. However, these protocols can lead to effective treatment of otherwise lethal diseases, and they have provided invaluable information for the development of gene therapy protocols for other genetic diseases.

Lentiviral Vectors

Lentiviral viruses are complex RNA retroviruses that, unlike simple retroviruses, can transduce non-dividing cells through pores in the nuclear membrane (human immunodeficiency virus [HIV] is an example of a **lentivirus**). Like other retroviruses, lentiviruses can integrate stably into the genome, and they can accept reasonably large inserts (8 kb). There is no evidence that lentiviruses integrate preferentially near genes, as most retroviruses do. Because they combine the desirable properties of greater safety, stable integration, and the ability to transduce nondividing cells, lentiviruses are currently the focus of much research and development.

Challenges in Viral Gene Therapy

Although viral gene therapy holds considerable promise, there are several important challenges:

- *Transient and low-level expression.* The gene product may be expressed at subtherapeutic levels, often less than 1% of the normal amount. In part, this reflects the fact that only some of the target cells successfully incorporate the normal gene. In addition, random insertion of the virus into the host's genome can affect gene regulation (e.g., some of the regulatory sequences required for normal expression levels are not present). Cells sometimesrespond to foreign inserted DNA by methylating—and thus inactivating—it. For these reasons, transcription of the gene often ceases after a few weeks or months. It should be noted, however, that transient expression is sufficient, and even desirable, for some types of therapy, such as provoking an immune response against a tumor or generating new blood vessels (discussed later).
- *Difficulties in reaching or specifying target tissue.*

Although some systemic disorders are relatively easy to target by modifying lymphocytes or bone marrow stem cells, others present formidable challenges. It may be difficult, for example, to target affected neurons responsible for central nervous system disorders. In addition, vectors must be modified so that they enter only the desired cell type.

- *Necessity for precise regulation of gene activity.* Accurate regulation of gene activity is not a concern for some diseases (e.g., a 50-fold overexpression of adenosine deaminase has no clinically significant effects). However, it is critical for diseases such as thalassemia, in which the number of α-globin and β-globin chains must be closely balanced (see Chapter 7). It is often difficult to achieve such precision using viral gene therapy.
- *Potential for insertional mutagenesis.* The unpredictable integration of a retroviral vector into the host's DNA can have undesired consequences, as discussed earlier. Although insertional mutagenesis appears to be a rare event, it has occurred in several patients (see Clinical Commentary 10-5).

Considerable research is being devoted to overcoming these and other problems. For example, the levels and permanence of gene expression are being increased by incorporating stronger promoter sequences in DNA inserts. Vectors are being modified to reduce immune responses and to increase target-cell specificity. Methods are being developed for targeted insertion of corrected DNA sequences. For example, proteins are engineered to bind to a specific mutated DNA sequence and to induce double-stranded DNA breaks followed by the insertion of a normal DNA sequence. The CRISPR/Cas9 gene editing method uses specific noncoding RNAs to guide the DNA-cutting Cas9 nuclease to a specific location in the genome, where DNA bases are then removed or altered. With targeted insertion, the mutated DNA is corrected in situ, avoiding difficulties with random insertion of DNA and taking advantage of the native promoter and enhancer sequences in the host's genome.

 Viral vectors offer highly efficient transfer of therapeutic genes into somatic cells. However, they have several drawbacks, including low or transient expression of the gene product, limited insert size, generation of immune responses, difficulty in precise regulation, and, for some vectors, a lack of ability to transduce nondividing cells and the potential for oncogenesis.

Nonviral Vectors

Although viral vectors provide the advantage of efficient gene transfer into cells, the disadvantages just listed have prompted researchers to investigate several types of nonviral vectors. One of the most extensively studied is the liposome, a fat body that can accept large DNA inserts. **Liposomes** sometimes fuse with cells, allowing the DNA insert to enter the cell. Because the liposome has no peptides, it does not elicit an immune response. Its primary disadvantage is that it lacks the transfer efficiency of viruses: most of the liposomes are degraded in the cytoplasm, and most of those that are not degraded are unable to enter the nucleus.

Surprisingly, it is possible to insert plasmids containing human DNA directly into cells without using any delivery vector at all. Although most "naked" DNA is repelled by the cell membrane, the DNA occasionally enters the cell, escapes degradation, and temporarily encodes proteins. Attempts are under way to use naked DNA as a vaccine that encodes a pathogenic protein against which the body mounts an immune response.

An intriguing development with potential for somatic cell therapy is the synthesis of **human artificial chromosomes**. Because these synthetically constructed chromosomes contain functional centro-

meres and telomeres, they should be able to integrate and replicate in human cell nuclei. Also, they are capable of accepting inserts as large as the entire 2.4 Mb Duchenne muscular dystrophy gene (*DMD*).

 Gene therapy using nonviral vectors, including liposomes and naked DNA, offers some advantages over viral vectors, but they currently lack the transfer efficiency of viral vectors.

Gene-Blocking Therapies

Gene-replacement techniques are not effective in correcting gain-of-function or dominant negative mutations (e.g., Huntington disease, Marfan syndrome). To correct these conditions, the defective gene product must be blocked or disabled in some way. Although not as well developed as gene-replacement therapy methods, a number of gene-blocking methods are showing considerable therapeutic promise.

Antisense Therapy

The principle behind **antisense therapy** is simple: an oligonucleotide is engineered whose DNA sequence is complementary to that of the messenger RNA (mRNA) sequence produced by a gain-of-function mutation. This antisense oligonucleotide binds to the abnormal mRNA, preventing its translation into a harmful protein (Fig. 10-9A). Antisense oligonucleotides can also be engineered to bind to the double-stranded DNA containing the disease-causing mutation, creating a triple helix that cannot be transcribed into mRNA. A difficulty with antisense therapy is that anti-sense oligonucleotides are often degraded before they can reach their target. Also, because of variation in the shape of the target DNA or RNA molecule, the antisense oligonucleotide might not be able to bind to its complementary sequence. Nevertheless, antisense therapy is being tested in a number of experimental applications, including blocking *KRAS* oncogene (see Chapter 8) expression in pancreatic and colorectal tumor cells.

Antisense oligonucleotides can also be used to induce alternative splice sites in pre-mRNA (mRNA

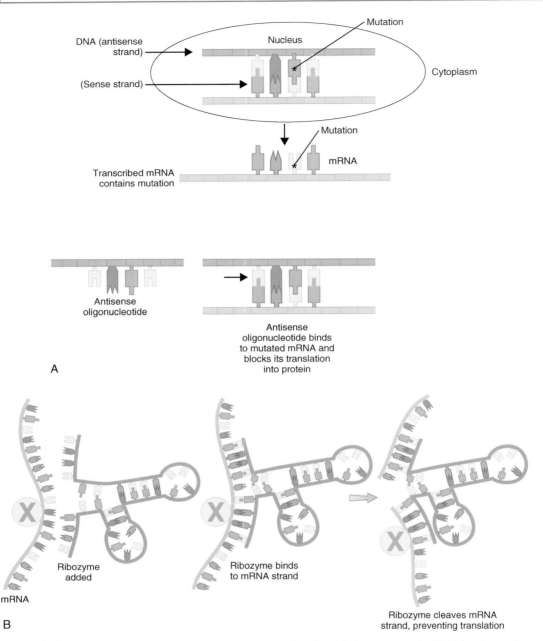

FIG 10-9 A, Gene therapy using an antisense technique. Binding of the abnormal mRNA by the antisense molecule prevents it from being translated into an abnormal protein. **B,** Gene therapy using a hammerhead ribozyme, which binds to a mutated mRNA, cleaving and eliminating it.

from which the introns have not yet been removed; see Chapter 2) to remove an exon that is affected by a frameshift mutation. This **exon skipping** approach has shown considerable promise, for example, in treating patients with Duchenne muscular dystrophy, where a large proportion of cases are caused by frameshift insertions or deletions (see Chapter 4). The result is a *DMD* mRNA transcript in which one exon is missing but the remainder of the transcript has an intact reading frame (the phenotype is expected to be similar to that of the milder Becker muscular dystrophy). In phase Ⅲ clinical trials, treated patients show substantial increases in dystrophin production.

Ribozyme Therapy

Ribozymes are enzymatic RNA molecules, some of which can cleave mRNA. They can be engineered to disrupt specific mRNA sequences that contain a mutation, destroying them before they can be translated into protein (see Fig. 10-9B). Ribozyme therapy is being tested, for example, as a method of countering the overexpression of epidermal growth factor receptor type 2, a feature of many breast tumors.

RNA Interference

A third method of gene blocking involves **RNA interference** (RNAi; Fig. 10-10), a natural phenomenon that evolved to defend cells against viral invasion. Because many viruses produce double-stranded RNA, cells of all multi-cellular organisms recognize this form of RNA and use an enzyme called *dicer* to digest it into small 20-bp pieces. These pieces are then used as a template to direct the destruction of any single-stranded RNA that has the same sequence as the double-stranded viral RNA (e.g., the single-stranded mRNA that the virus would use to encode viral proteins). By artificially synthesizing double-stranded RNA molecules that correspond to a disease-causing DNA sequence, RNAi can be induced to destroy the mRNA produced by the mutated sequence.

RNAi faces challenges similar to those of antisense and ribozyme therapy, such as degradation of the RNA molecule before it reaches the target. This difficulty is being overcome by inserting RNAi molecules into lentiviral and adeno-associated viral vectors. RNAi

has shown some promise in reducing, for example, the number of transcripts produced by oncogenic *KRAS*, and it has also been shown to block transcripts of the *BCR-ABL* fusion gene, which causes chronic myelogenous leukemia (see Chapter 8). It is being tested for the treatment of age-related macular degeneration, asthma, hepatitis C, and Huntington disease.

 Gene-blocking techniques may be used to counter the effects of dominant-negative or gain-of-function mutations. They include the use of antisense molecules, RNA-cleaving ribozymes, and RNA interference.

Gene Therapy for Non-inherited Diseases

Gene therapy is by no means limited to inherited diseases. Indeed, about two thirds of the gene therapy protocols now under way involve non-inherited cancers, and a significant proportion involve acquired immunodeficiency syndrome (AIDS) therapy. For example, the *TP53* tumor suppressor gene, which is inactivated in about half of all cancers (see Chapter 8), has been inserted into lung tumors in an effort to halt tumor progression. As discussed in Chapter 9, some tumors evade immune system detection by discarding cell-surface molecules that are recognized by

FIG 10-10   Gene-blocking therapy using RNA interference (RNAi). A dicer cleaves double-stranded RNA (dsRNA) into 20-bp single-stranded RNA fragments called *short interfering RNAs* (siRNAs). These fragments form a template that is recognized and bound by the RNA-induced silencing complex (RISC), which cleaves and destroys the complementary RNA strand. In RNAi, a dsRNA is engineered to produce siRNA strands that are complementary to a mutated mRNA, causing the RISC complex to destroy the mRNA.

T cells. Liposomes containing DNA that encodes the B7 costimulatory molecule (see Chapter 9) have been introduced into malignant melanoma cells, which results in B7 expression on the cell surface and subsequent cell destruction by cytotoxic T cells. In some cases, this has led to regression of the melanoma.

A variety of gene therapy approaches are being formulated to combat HIV. Most of these efforts are aimed at halting replication of the virus or preventing its spread to healthy cells. For example, a dominant-negative mutation introduced into HIV-infected T cells produces a protein that interferes with proteins produced by HIV, blocking their normal action. Trials are also in progress to reduce expression of CCR5, a chemokine coreceptor used by HIV to enter cells of the immune system (see Chapter 9).

Another example of gene therapy for a noninherited disease involves the treatment of coronary artery disease. Copies of the genes that encode members of the vascular endothelial growth factor (VEGF) and fibroblast growth factor (FGF) families have been injected into ischemic myocardium (using viral vectors or as naked DNA) with the hope of producing new coronary vessels.

Germline Therapy

Somatic cell therapy consists of altering only specific somatic cells and thus differs little in principle from many other types of medical intervention (e.g., bone marrow transplantation). In contrast, **germline gene therapy** involves altering all cells of the body, including those that give rise to the gametes. Thus, this type of gene therapy would affect not only the patient but also his or her descendants.

Germline therapy was first achieved in the mouse in 1983, when copies of a human growth hormone gene were successfully introduced into mouse embryos by microinjection (the gene was inserted directly into the embryo using a very small needle). Among the minority of embryos in which the gene integrated, the gene was expressed and the mice grew to abnormally large size. The gametes were also modified, and the human growth hormone gene was transmitted to future generations.

Although germline therapy is, in principle, possible in humans, it presents significant problems (Box 10-7). First, injected embryos usually die, and some develop tumors and malformations. Second, even in an autosomal dominant disorder, half of the embryos produced by a heterozygous parent are genetically normal. If it were possible to distinguish the genetically normal embryos (e.g., through pre-implantation genetic diagnosis), it would be simpler to implant the normal embryos than to alter the abnormal ones. Finally, numerous ethical questions are associated with the permanent alteration of a human's genetic legacy. For these reasons, it appears unlikely that human germline therapy would be useful or desirable.

Gene Therapy: A Perspective

The majority of gene therapy protocols are still in phase I and phase II trials, but more than 100 are now in phase III clinical trials. (The NIH web site, https://clinicaltrials.gov/, is an excellent resource for reviewing the current and ongoing trials.) The past several years have witnessed the first arguable successes of gene therapy, some of which have been discussed in this chapter (successful therapy for X-linked SCID and ADA deficiency, hemophilia B, and other conditions listed in Table 10-8; evidence of therapeutic effects in various cancers). However, success has been achieved thus far in only a relatively small number of persons.

Gene therapy is not without risk. In addition to the insertional mutagenesis potential already discussed, a young man with ornithine transcarbamylase deficiency (see Chapter 7) died in 1999 as a result of an adverse immune reaction to an adenovirus vector. In addition, retroviral therapy has occasionally resulted in insertional mutagenesis (see Clinical Commentary 10-5). Despite these reservations, gene therapy research is providing many new insights of fundamental biological significance. As with many avenues of biomedical research, the potential of gene therapy research is considerable, and current progress suggests strongly that it may provide efficacious treatment of some important human diseases.

BOX 10-7   Germline Therapy, Genetic Enhancement, Human Cloning, and Embryonic Stem Cells: Controversial Issues in Medical Genetics

For reasons outlined in the text, germline gene therapy is not being undertaken in humans. Nevertheless, germline gene therapy is in many ways technically easier to perform than is somatic cell therapy. Germline therapy also offers (in theory) the possibility of "genetic enhancement," the introduction of favorable genes into the embryo. However, a gene that is favorable in one environment may be unfavorable in another (e.g., the sickle cell mutation, which is advantageous only for heterozygotes in a malarial environment). And, because of pleiotropy, the introduction of advantageous genes can have completely unintended consequences (e.g., a gene thought to enhance one characteristic could negatively affect another). For these reasons, and because germline therapy usually destroys the targeted embryo, neither germline therapy nor genetic enhancement is advocated by the scientific community.

Controversy also surrounds the prospect of cloning humans. Many mammalian species (e.g., sheep, pigs, cattle, goats, mice, cats, dogs) have been successfully cloned by introducing a diploid nucleus from an adult cell into an egg cell from which the original haploid nucleus was removed (a technique termed **somatic cell nuclear transfer**, or SCNT; see the figure that follows). The cell is manipulated so that all of its genes can be expressed (recall that most genes in a typical differentiated adult cell are transcriptionally silent). This procedure, when allowed to proceed through a full-term pregnancy, could likely be used to produce a human being (reproductive cloning).

Some argue that human cloning offers childless couples the opportunity to produce children to whom they are biologically related or even to replace a child who has died. It is important to keep in mind, however, that a clone is only a *genetic* copy. The environment of the individual, which also plays a large role in development, cannot be replicated. Furthermore, the great majority of cloning attempts in mammals fail: in most cases, the embryo either dies or has gross malformations. Because the consequences of human reproductive cloning would almost certainly be similar, reproductive cloning of humans is condemned almost universally by scientists.

It is important to distinguish reproductive cloning from the cloning and cultivation of cells for therapeutic purposes. **Embryonic stem cells** (**ESCs**), which are derived from the inner-cell mass of blastocyst-stage embryos, can be cloned and have the unique potential to differentiate into any type of cell in the human body (**pluripotency**). For example, they can potentially form neurons for the treatment of Parkinson disease or cardiac myocytes for the treatment of ischemic heart disease. However, with current technology, the embryo is destroyed to obtain ESCs, and this is controversial in many circles. Ongoing research efforts are aimed at inducing pluripotency in differentiated adult cells. Research is also under way to extract usable single cells from 3-day blastomere embryos (as in pre-implantation genetic diagnosis) so that embryos are not destroyed. It remains to be seen whether these technologies can produce cells that have the same flexibility and utility as ESCs.

One difficulty in using cells derived from ESCs is that they might induce an immune response in the recipient. This problem could be largely overcome if ESC clones were available from many persons with different MHC types. The recipient would then be immunologically matched to the appropriate ESC. However, only a limited number of ESC lines are currently available to most researchers. Another suggestion is that SCNT could be used with a patient's own cells to create ESCs that would be identical in DNA sequence to the patient.

Although these technologies offer the hope of effective treatment for some recalcitrant diseases, they also present thorny ethical issues. Clearly, decisions regarding their use must be guided by constructive input from scientists, legal scholars, philosophers, and others.

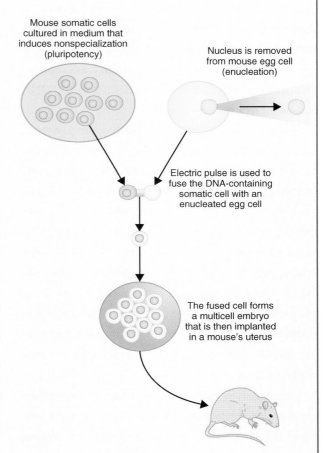

Somatic cell nuclear transfer to create a mouse clone. A mouse diploid somatic cell (e.g., a fibroblast) is cultured and grown in media that cause it to become pluripotent. It is fused with an enucleated egg cell, creating a diploid one-cell embryo. This embryo is allowed to develop to a multicell stage and implanted in a mouse's uterus. The resulting mouse is genetically identical (a clone) to the mouse that provided the somatic cell.

SUMMARY

Numerous genetic disorders can be diagnosed at the chromosome, DNA, RNA, or protein levels by genetic tests using blood, body fluids, and other tissues. Population and prenatal genetic screening are very important for preventing specific genetic diseases in certain areas or countries. Molecular genetic tests can detect mutations in single genes that lead to a genetic disorder. FISH and multiplex ligation-dependent probe amplification (MLPA) can analyze entire chromosomes or long lengths of DNA to determine if there are large genetic changes, such as an extra copy or deletion of a chromosome, or duplication of a large segment of a chromosome, that causes a genetic abnormality, and biochemical genetic tests study the amount or activity of proteins or enzymes, abnormalities of which may indicate changes to the DNA that result in a genetic disease.

With the development of molecular genetics, sequencing technology, and the sequencing of the human genome, much progress has and will be made in this area. Family members of the affected can benefit from genetic diagnosis, which can be carried out with fetal tissues such as the chorionic villus and amniocytes, as well as cell-free DNA. In the near future, additional diagnostic technologies, including detection methods that can analyze at large scale, will be developed, and the information provided will offer improvements in genetic testing and counseling. Genetic counseling will play an important role in preventing genetic diseases.

Surgery, drug treatment, and dietary restriction are standard treatments for genetic diseases and other disorders; however, gene therapy, including in vivo and ex vivo cell therapy, offer revolutionary and hopeful therapeutic breakthroughs, and significant progress has been made in the past few years. Gene therapy strategies include gene replacement for monogenic diseases, gene addition for complex disorders and infectious diseases, gene expression alteration targeting RNA, and gene editing to introduce targeted changes into the host genome. Among these, gene replacement is the main therapy.

Advances include improvements in viral as well as nonviral vector gene delivery systems, exon skipping, RNA interference, newly developed gene editing based on CRISPR-Cas 9, and the application of embryonic stem cells. Phase 2 and 3 clinical trials of gene therapy, in clinical trial II and III after obtaining regulatory approvals have surged for many kinds of genetic and nongenetic diseases. There are many disagreements regarding the use of germline cell therapies, given ethical reasons, compared to somatic cell therapies. In addition, a serious issue is the potential mutagenesis of inserted DNA, which may affect the safety of certain gene therapies. Consideration should be given to genetic intervention to clinical application. Current progress in gene therapy will likely lead to efficacious treatments for important human diseases in the near future.

IMPORTANT TERMINOLOGY

genetic testing   遗传检测
population screening   群体筛查
genetic screening   遗传筛查
newborn screening   新生儿筛查
heterozygote screening   杂合子筛查
presymptomatic diagnosis   症状前诊断
linkage analysis   连锁分析
fluorescence in situ hybridization (FISH)   荧光原位杂交
array comparative genomic hybridization (array CGH)   微阵列比较基因组杂交
multiplex ligation-dependent probe amplification (MLPA)   多重连接依赖探针扩增
allele-specific oligonucleotide (ASO)   等位基因特异的寡核苷酸
prenatal diagnosis   产前诊断
α-fetoprotein (AFP)   甲胎蛋白
neural tube defect   神经管缺陷
amniocentesis   羊膜穿刺术
pseudomosaicism   假嵌合体
chorionic villus sampling (CVS)   绒毛膜绒毛取样
percutaneous umbilical blood sampling (PUBS)   脐静脉血取样
ultrasonography   超声波检查法

noninvasive prenatal screening　非侵袭性产前筛查
cell-free DNA (cfDNA)　游离 DNA
preimplantation genetic diagnosis　植入前遗传学
　诊断
in vitro fertilization　体外受精
blastomere　卵裂球
gene therapy　基因治疗
gene replacement therapy　基因替代治疗

retrovirus　逆转录病毒
transduction　转导
adenovirus　腺病毒
severe combined immunodeficiency (SCID)　严重
　联合免疫缺陷
lentivirus　慢病毒
RNA interference　RNA 干扰
embryonic stem cell (ESC)　胚胎干细胞

REVIEW QUESTIONS

1. A newborn-screening program for a metabolic disease has just been initiated. Of 100,000 newborns, 100 were shown by a definitive test to have been affected with the disease. The screening test identified 93 of these neonates as affected and 7 as unaffected. It also identified 1000 neonates as affected who were later shown to be unaffected. Calculate the sensitivity, specificity, and positive predictive value of the screening test, and specify the rate of false positives and false negatives.

2. Study the family shown in the pedigree in Figure 10-11. Individual 3 has PKU, an autosomal recessive disease. A two-allele SNP closely linked to the PKU locus has been assayed for each family member, and the figure shows the genotypes of each individual. Based on the genotypes of the linked marker, is individual 6 affected, a heterozygous carrier, or a normal homozygote?

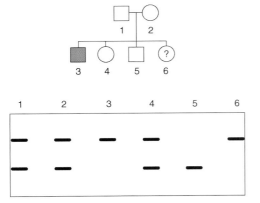

FIG 10-11　Pedigree to accompany Study Question 2.

3. Study the family shown in the pedigree in Figure 10-12. The affected individuals have neurofibromatosis type 1 (NF1), an autosomal dominant condition. A four-allele STR locus closely linked to the NF1 locus has been typed for each family member. Based on the genotypes shown in the accompanying figure, will individual 6 develop NF1?

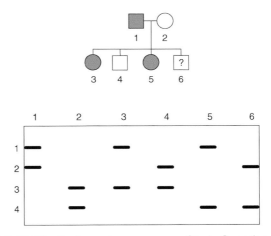

FIG 10-12　Pedigree to accompany Study Question 3.

4. In the pedigree for an autosomal dominant disorder shown in Figure 10-13, a tightly linked two-allele SNP has been typed in each family member. Based on this information, what can you tell the family about the risk that the offspring in generation III will develop the disorder? How might diagnostic accuracy be improved in this case?

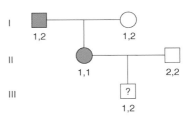

FIG 10-13　Pedigree to accompany Study Question 4.

5. Compare the advantages and disadvantages of amniocentesis and chorionic villus sampling (CVS).

6. What type of gene therapy would be most appropriate for Huntington disease? Why?

SUGGESTED READINGS AND WEBSITES

1. Alldred SK, Deeks JJ, Guo B, et al. Second trimester serum tests for Down's syndrome screening. *Cochrane Database Syst Rev*. 2012; (6): CD009925.

2. Bamshad MJ, Ng SB, Bigham AW, et al. Exome sequencing as a tool for Mendelian disease gene discovery. *Nat Rev Genet*. 2011; 12: 745-755.

3. Bianchi DW, Parker RL, Wentworth J, et al. DNA sequencing versus standard prenatal aneuploidy screening. *N Engl J Med*. 2014; 370(9): 799-808.

4. Biesecker LG, Green RC. Diagnostic clinical genome and exome sequencing. *N Engl J Med*. 2014; 370: 2418-2425.

5. Bodurtha J, Strauss JF. Genomics and perinatal care. *N Engl J Med*. 2012; 366: 64-73.

6. Cavazzana-Calvo M, Fischer A, Hacein-Bey-Abina S, Aiuti A. Gene therapy for primary immunodeficiencies: part 1. *Curr Opin Immunol*. 2012; 24: 580-584.

7. Green RC, Berg JS, Grody WW, et al. ACMG recommendations for reporting of incidental findings in clinical exome and genome sequencing. *Genet Med*. 2013; 15: 565-574.

8. Gregg AR, Gross SJ, Best RG, et al. ACMG statement on noninvasive prenatal screening for fetal aneuploidy. *Genet Med*. 2013; 15(5): 395-398.

9. Griesenbach U, Alton EW. Moving forward: cystic fibrosis gene therapy. *Hum Mol Genet*. 2013; 22: R52-R58.

10. Grody WW, Thompson BH, Gregg AR, et al. ACMG position statement on prenatal /preconception expanded screening. *Genet Med*. 2013; 15(6): 482-483.

11. High KA. The gene therapy journey for hemophilia: are we there yet? *Blood*. 2012; 120: 4482-4487.

12. Harper JC, Sengupta SB. Preimplantation genetic diagnosis: state of the art 2011. *Hum Genet*. 2012; 131: 175-186.

13. Hudson KL. Genomics, health care, and society. *N Engl J Med*. 2011; 365: 1033-1041.

14. Katsanis SH, Katsanis N. Molecular genetic testing and the future of clinical genomics. *Nat Rev Genet*. 2013; 14: 415-426.

15. Korf BR, Rehm HL. New approaches to molecular diagnosis. *JAMA*. 2013; 309: 1511-1521.

16. Milunsky A, Milunsky J. *Genetic Disorders and the Fetus: Diagnosis, Prevention and Treatment*. 6th ed. Hoboken, NJ: Wiley-Blackwell; 2010.

17. Shulman LP, Elias S. Techniques for prenatal diagnosis. In: Rimoin DL, Pyeritz RE, Korf BR, eds. *Emery and Rimoin's Principles and Practice of Medical Genetics*. 6th ed. Philadelphia: Elsevier; 2013.

18. Simpson JL. Preimplantation genetic diagnosis at 20 years. *Prenat Diagn*. 2010; 30: 682-695.

19. Verma IM. Medicine. Gene therapy that works. *Science*. 2013; 341: 853-855.

20. Yang Y, Muzny DM, Reid JG, et al. Clinical whole-exome sequencing for the diagnosis of mendelian disorders. *N Engl J Med*. 2013; 369: 1502-1511.

21. ACMG ACTSHEETS and Algorithms: http://www.ncbi.nlm.nih.gov/books/NBK55832/

22. Comprehensive list of ongoing clinical trials: https://clinicaltrials.gov/

23. Gene Clinics/Gene Tests (reviews of genetic diseases and lists of laboratories that perform diagnostic tests): http://www.geneclinics.org/

24. Gene Therapy Clinical Trials Worldwide (updated list of all gene therapy protocols): http://www.abedia.com/wiley/

25. National Newborn Screening and Global Resource Center: http://genes-r-us.uthscsa.edu/

26. National Organization for Rare Diseases (database of rare disorders that includes brief reviews and information on diagnostic tests and treatment for families and professionals): http://www.rarediseases.org

(Benchang Shen)

Chapter 11

Genetics and Personalized Medicine

Scientific, technological, and medical advances have made it possible to detect, diagnose, and treat most common diseases (e.g., asthma, diabetes, hypertension) early in their course and more effectively than ever before. Such advances are, however, highly dependent on the skills and knowledge of clinicians, access to health-care services, and the availability and affordability of diagnostic technologies. Most health-care providers follow a conventional model in which a patient presents with a set of symptoms and signs, which the provider uses to make a "most likely" diagnosis. The provider then prescribes a treatment that he or she thinks will be most effective. If this treatment fails, the process is repeated until a correct diagnosis or more effective treatment is found. In such a model, **preventive health maintenance** is encouraged. Compliance, however, is challenging because information about risk factors, as well as the patient's perception of risk, is at best approximate.

Personalized medicine is a model of practice in which each person's personal risk for rare and common conditions and the effectiveness of various treatments are estimated directly from his or her unique combination of genetic and environmental risk factors. Accordingly, a health-care provider can predict a person's risk for common diseases, select diagnostic tests to confirm the presence of disease, and prescribe the best therapeutic regimen to treat it. Ideally, knowledge of disease risk promotes interventions (e.g., modification of diet, choice of drug therapy) that not only can treat disease early in its course but also can delay its onset or prevent it altogether.

The effectiveness of personalized medicine depends on a number of factors. These include identifying genetic and environmental risk factors (and their interactions) that enable accurate prediction of clinically significant risk; demonstrating that individual risk assessment improves diagnostic accuracy and treatment outcome; developing technologies for cost-efficient assessment of a person's genome; building an infrastructure for clinicians to access risk data, interpret risk information, and explain risk estimates to patients; and developing guidelines and policies for how risk assessment information should be used in clinical and research applications. Not all of these aims will be achieved for every common disease. Indeed, for many complex diseases, it is likely that there will be no alternative to the conventional model of practice in the near future because so little is known about their etiology and pathophysiology. Nevertheless, for some common diseases and drug responses, genetic testing and, in several cases personalized medicine, are already being adapted to the clinical setting.

In this chapter, we discuss how new technologies are making the assessment of individual human genomes widely accessible, how such genome-wide information is being used currently to make personal decisions about health, and the implications of personalized care.

 Personalized medicine is the use of each person's unique combination of genetic and environmental risk factors to make predictions about his or her disease risk and response to various treatments.

A TECHNOLOGY-DRIVEN TRANSFORMATION

Traditionally, the search for genetic variants that influence risk for mendelian conditions and common complex diseases has been a daunting task and has been one of the major obstacles to developing personalized medicine. The most common approach to finding such variants involved testing whether polymorphisms in candidate genes were associated with disease risk in a small group of unrelated patients with the same phenotype (e.g., diabetes, obesity). This was problematic, in part because choosing the most appropriate candidate genes was difficult, small cohorts provided limited statistical power, and the process of genotyping or sequencing was labor intensive and expensive. This situation has changed dramatically with the development of technologies to interrogate millions of polymorphisms per person cheaply and efficiently (Box 11-1) and more recently the development of exome and genome sequencing. These technologies, coupled with advances in statistics and computing, enabled the application of new approaches such as genome-wide association studies, as well as the study of much larger cohorts of tens or hundreds of thousands of persons. In addition, these new technologies for genotyping and DNA sequencing have made it possible to develop cost-effective clinical tests that take advantage of newly discovered risk variants. The major challenge nowadays to implementing personalized medicine is translating discoveries of risk variants into clinical practice.

THE IMPACT OF GENOMICS

Pharmacogenetics

Many of the drinks (e.g., coffee, tea) and foods that we ingest each day contain thousands of complex compounds that each of us must process. Some of these compounds never leave the gastrointestinal tract, but most are absorbed, distributed, metabolized, and eliminated (i.e., biotransformed) to a variety of products that are used immediately, stored, or excreted. Exogenously synthesized compounds that are administered to achieve a specific effect on the human body (e.g., pharmaceuticals) also undergo **biotransformation**, and humans vary in the efficiency and speed with which they do this. Moreover, the response of a drug's target (e.g., enzymes, receptors) can also vary among individuals. The study of the individual genetic variants that modify human responses to pharmacological agents is called **pharmacogenetics**; the assessment of the action of many genes simultaneously is called **pharmacogenomics**.

Genetic Prediction of Serious Adverse Drug Responses

Over the last decade, ambitious efforts have been undertaken to advance the knowledge of pharmacogenetics. This has been driven, in part, by the expec-

BOX 11-1 Assessing Your Genome

Knowledge of a person's genetic makeup will clearly be an important tool for making better decisions about health, medical care, and perhaps lifestyle as well. Until recently, assessing the genome as a whole was fairly expensive and done only in research laboratories. However, new technologies have dramatically lowered the cost of whole-genome analysis and have spurred the development of consumer services that offer whole-genome studies directly to the public (see Chapter 10). These services have rapidly made headlines, as much for their novelty as for their potential to inform persons about their genetic composition.

Most whole-genome consumer services offer to genotype millions of common single nucleotide polymorphisms (SNPs). The SNPs typed for consumers are the same ones commonly being used by researchers to identify disease-gene associations for common multifactorial disorders such as hypertension, diabetes, and obesity. As gene-disease associations are reported, consumers who have

access to their genetic information can evaluate their risk for genetic diseases. Also, because each person's genetic data are permanent, evaluation of risk can be reassessed with each new discovery However, many of the SNP-disease associations reported to consumers are relatively weak and may be misunderstood or misinterpreted by the lay consumer (see Chapter 10).

More recently, exome sequencing and whole-genome sequencing have been made available to the public. This service is still expensive and therefore very limited in application. It remains unclear whether a person's understanding of health-related risks will be increased by knowing about some or all of the genetic risk variants that they carry. Most of the caveats raised in the previous paragraph for whole-genome SNP typing apply equally to **whole-genome sequencing**. However, since risk variants for mendelian conditions are frequently detected by sequencing, some variants of potential clinical utility are virtually always found.

tation that through the use of pharmacogenetics, we will be able to profile DNA differences among individuals and thereby predict responses to different medicines. For example, a **genetic profile** (i.e., a summary of a person's risk alleles) might predict who is more or less likely to respond to a drug or to suffer a **serious adverse drug reaction (SADR)**.

Many drugs have a response rate between 25% and 75%. For example, ACE inhibitors and beta blockers have been found to be ineffective or only partially effective in up to 70% of hypertensive patients. The use of such drugs in persons who are unlikely to respond increases the incidence of SADRs and adds to the burden of health-care costs. Yet, for most drugs, no tests are available to determine who will or will not respond, so these drugs are administered largely on a trial-and-error basis.

Many drugs have adverse effects that are of clinical importance, and of the approximately 1200 drugs approved for use in the United States, about 15% are associated with a significant incidence of SADRs. A widely cited analysis conducted in the mid-1990s suggested that nearly 2 million people are hospitalized each year as a result of adverse drug effects, and approximately 100,000 people die from them, even when the drugs are appropriately prescribed and administered. Studies in Europe and Australia have yielded similar results. Thus, identification of genetic profiles that predict a person's response to drugs is likely to increase the overall efficacy and safety of pharmaceuticals.

Testing is currently available for a handful of alleles that predict SADRs. For example, thiopurine methyl transferase (TPMT) is an enzyme that inactivates thiopurine drugs (e.g., 6-mercaptopurine, azathioprine), which are frequently used to treat acute lymphatic leukemia and to prevent rejection of organ transplants. A mutation of the ***TPMT* gene** reduces enzyme activity. About one in 300 persons of European ancestry is homozygous for this mutation, and these patients can experience life-threatening bone marrow suppression upon exposure to thiopurine drugs. The presence of such variants can be assessed by genotyping or by enzyme assays, which are now

commonly done before administering thiopurines. Large-scale **exome sequencing** studies have demonstrated that each person carries at least several alleles that alter drug metabolism compared to the general population.

 Each person's response to natural and synthetic chemicals is determined in part by polymorphisms in genes that control pathways of biotransformation and the chemical's target.

Individualized Drug Therapy

One of the major challenges of pharmacogenetics is the selection of appropriate targets (e.g., a specific enzyme, cytokine, or cell-surface receptor) that might be amenable to manipulation by a drug. The results of genetic studies are used to identify polymorphisms associated with varying susceptibility to disease (i.e., a potential target for a drug) or polymorphisms that modify the human response to a drug. For example, long QT syndrome (LQT syndrome; see Chapter 5) can be caused by mutations in one of at least a dozen different genes whose protein products affect ion channel function in heart cells (e.g., sodium and calcium channels). Because sodium channels and calcium channels are blocked by different drugs, a person's genetic profile can be used to choose the best drug for treatment of LQT syndrome. In this case, the relationship between disease and target is well characterized.

Polymorphisms in genes that encode angiotensinogen, angiotensin-converting enzyme (ACE), and the angiotensin II type 1 receptor have been associated with differential responses to antihypertensive agents. For example, the *ACE* gene contains a 190-bp sequence that can be either present (the *I* allele) or deleted (the *D* allele). Persons who are homozygous for the *D* allele are more responsive to ACE inhibitors. Response to antihypertensive beta blockers has been associated with polymorphisms in genes that encode subunits of the β-adrenergic receptor (Table 11-1). None of these variants are commonly tested prior to initiating antihypertensive therapy, but studies are under way to determine when such information, in conjunction with environmental risk factors such as smoking and diet, might facilitate the development of individualized treatment.

Many of the physiological effects of variation in drug response have been known for decades. A deficiency of glucose-6-phosphate dehydrogenase (G6PD), which is estimated to affect more than 200 million people worldwide, causes increased sensitivity to the antimalarial drug, primaquine, producing an acute hemolytic anemia. The metabolism of isoniazid (a drug commonly used to treat tuberculosis) is strongly influenced by an allele of the gene that encodes N-acetyltransacetylase 2 (*NAT2*), the enzyme that is used to acetylate, and thereby inactivate, isoniazid. Persons who are homozygous for this allele are known as slow inactivators and are at higher risk for developing side effects than persons who metabolize isoniazid more quickly. About half of persons of European or African ancestry are slow inactivators, but this figure is lower among East Asians. Succinylcholine is a drug widely used in anesthesia to induce short-term muscle paralysis. Typically, the effects

of succinylcholine last only a few minutes before it is rapidly degraded in the plasma by circulating butyrylcholinesterase. Several alleles of the gene that encodes butyrylcholinesterase cause reduced enzyme activity. Persons who are homozygotes or compound heterozygotes for such alleles have a diminished ability to inactivate succinylcholine. This can result in prolonged paralysis and respiratory failure that requires mechanical ventilation for up to several hours.

In each of these examples, a person who has a relatively common allele might, upon exposure to a specific chemical, experience an unanticipated pharmacological effect. Variants have been discovered in enzymes that produce a much broader effect on the body's response to multiple drugs. An example is debrisoquine hydroxylase, an enzyme encoded by the gene *CYP2D6*. This gene is a member of the cytochrome P450 superfamily, which encodes many different enzymes responsible for the biotransformation of compounds with widely divergent chemical structures. Polymorphisms of *CYP2D6* affect the metabolism of more than 25% of all pharmaceuticals, includ-

TABLE 11-1	**Examples of Effects of Gene Polymorphisms on Drug Response**		
GENE	ENZYME/TARGET	DRUG	CLINICAL RESPONSE
CYP2D6	Cytochrome P4502D6	Codeine	Persons homozygous for an inactivating mutation do not metabolize codeine to morphine and thus experience no analgesic effect
CYP2C9	Cytochrome P4502C9	Warfarin	Persons heterozygous for a polymorphism need a lower dose of warfarin to maintain anticoagulation
VKORC1	Vitamin K epoxide reductase	Warfarin	Persons heterozygous for a polymorphism need a lower dose of warfarin complex, subunit 1, to maintain anticoagulation
NAT2	N-Acetyl transferase 2	Isoniazid	Persons homozygous for slow-acetylation polymorphisms are more susceptible to isoniazid toxicity
TPMT	Thiopurine S-methyltransferase	Azathioprine	Persons homozygous for an inactivating mutation develop severe toxicity if treated with standard doses of azathioprine
ADRB2	β-Adrenergic receptor	Albuterol	Persons homozygous for a polymorphism get worse with regular use of albuterol
KCNE2	Potassium channel, voltage-gated	Clarithromycin	Persons heterozygous for a polymorphism are more susceptible to life-threatening arrhythmias
SUR1	Sulfonylurea receptor 1	Sulfonylureas	Persons heterozygous for polymorphisms exhibit diminished sensitivity to sulfonylurea-stimulated insulin secretion
F5	Coagulation factor V (Leiden)	Oral contraceptives	Persons heterozygous for a polymorphism are at increased risk for venous thrombosis

ing β-adrenergic receptor antagonists, neuroleptics, and tricyclic antidepressants (Fig. 11-1). Another example is variants in *CYP2C19* that diminish the rate at which the pro-drug clopidogrel, an antiplatelet drug, is metabolized to its active form. Clopidogrel is commonly used in the more than 2 million persons who undergo stenting of their coronary arteries, and persons with a variant in *CYP2C19* that reduces function are at substantially higher risk of stent thrombosis-which can precipitate a heart attack and death. All of these are examples of relatively simply genetic profiles (i.e., single polymorphisms) that affect drug response. Many drug responses are likely to be determined by much more complex profiles that are composed of multiple polymorphisms at multiple loci.

Two common variants of *CYP2C9* (*CYP2C9*2* and *CYP2C9*3*), another cytochrome P450 gene, influence the metabolism of warfarin, an anticoagulant drug. The frequencies of these alleles vary between 6% and 12% in populations of European origin, but each is found at a substantially lower frequency in sub-Saharan Africans and East Asians. Warfarin is widely used to prevent thrombosis, but because of variation in dose requirements, hemorrhagic complications from warfarin therapy are common. Therefore, a person's level of anticoagulation needs to be checked regularly so that warfarin is given at a dose that prevents thrombosis but avoids excessive bleeding. Persons with at least one copy of either *CYP2C9*2* or *CYP2C9*3* require less warfarin for effective anticoagulation than the general popula-

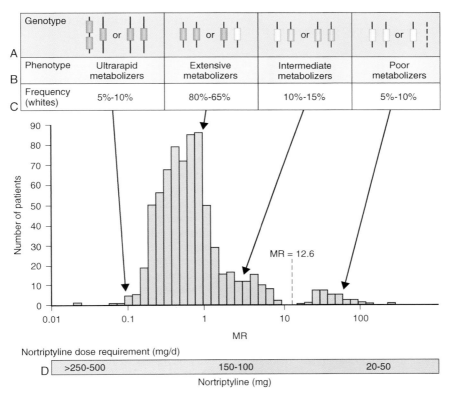

FIG 11-1 Genotype-phenotype relationships between *CYP2D6* polymorphisms and drug metabolism. **A**, Possible genotypes at the *CYP2D6* locus. Fully functional alleles of the *CYP2D6* gene are indicated by *dark purple* boxes, alleles with reduced function in *pink*, and null (i.e., inactive) *CYP2D6* alleles in *light purple*. **B**, The ability to metabolize many drugs varies depending on an individual's *CYP2D6* genotype. **C**, Distribution of phenotype frequencies assessed in a population of European Americans as determined by the urinary metabolic ratio (MR) of debrisoquine to 4-hydroxy-debrisoquine. **D**, Poor metabolizers require a smaller dose of the antidepressant drug nortriptyline, and ultrarapid metabolizers require a higher dose to achieve the same plasma concentration. (Adapted from Meyers U. Pharmacogenetics—five decades of therapeutic lessons from genetic diversity. *Nat Rev Genet.* 2004; 5: 669-676.)

tion. Consistent with this observation, hemorrhagic complications are, on standard dosing, more common in persons who carry the *CYP2C9*2* or the *CYP2C9*3* alleles. Thus, *CYP2C9* variants influence both warfarin metabolism and adverse outcomes associated with warfarin. Genetic variation in one of warfarin's pharmacologic targets, vitamin K epoxide reductase (VKORC1; see Table 11-1), also helps to predict a person's response to this drug. Genetic testing can be done on both *CYP2C9* and *VKORC1* to help to calibrate warfarin dosage.

Pharmacogenetics and pharmacogenomics are slowly beginning to change the way that medicine is practiced, although the pace of change is likely to accelerate over the next few decades (Box 11-2). A primary issue for all alleles that are associated with drug response is whether testing these alleles will affect the clinical management of patients and, if so, to what extent. The genetic profile of a drug response may be important if the drug is widely used in clinical practice and the response to the drug is medically important, if the drug's therapeutic and toxic effects are difficult to assess and titrate clinically, if adverse effects are difficult to predict with existing information, and if a profile provides easily interpretable results with high sensitivity and specificity. It is unclear how many drug-and-genetic profile combinations are likely to meet these criteria, although to date more than a hundred drugs now carry a label indicating that genetic testing should be performed prior to use.

 Genetic testing for polymorphisms associated with variation in drug metabolism or effectiveness can lead to better predictions of a person's response to drugs and can reduce the incidence of drug-related side effects.

BOX 11-2   Personal Genomics

It is 2025. Jonathan is a 1 hour-old baby sleeping comfortably in his mother's arms in the room in which he was just born. Jonathan's parents are comforted by the knowledge that Jonathan does not have a serious childhood-onset genetic condition such as cystic fibrosis, sickle cell disease or one of several hundred inborn errors of metabolism (e.g., galactosemia, PKU). Testing for these conditions used to be part of newborn screening programs, but nowadays testing for these conditions occur prenatally. In most cases, this screening is done via whole genome sequencing of the fetal genome from fetal free-DNA found in a pregnant mother's blood. Jonathan's parents did learn that he is a carrier for sickle cell disease. An electronic summary of Jonathan's complete genome sequence is deposited in a national health information database prior to his birth. A subset of genotypes that represent a unique genetic profile are put into a national forensics database.

Jonathan's parents can access his genome sequence information, specifically information about risk variants that he has, at any time. They also control who has access to these risk data, and they elect to provide Jonathan's pediatric care providers with risk variants for conditions that commonly manifest in childhood. On Jonathan's well-child visit at 1 month of age, a genetic counselor explains that Jonathan has a higher-than-average genetic risk for autism, peanut allergy, chronic otitis media, and adverse responses to penicillin. It is recommended to his parents that he avoid both penicillin and products containing peanuts until he can undergo direct testing. Jonathan is

also found to have a lower-than-average genetic risk for asthma.

At 1 year of age, it is apparent that Jonathan's speech and language development is delayed. His genetic profile confirms that he has no risk variants known to be associated with hearing loss, suggesting that his delay might be an early indication of autism. An optimal therapy for autism is selected based on his genetic profile. Jonathan responds well to this intervention and, in conjunction with speech training, his development by the age of 5 years is appropriate.

Jonathan remains healthy throughout childhood, and, when he turns 18 years old, control over his genetic risk data is switched from his parents to him. At the same time, Jonathan's medical care is transferred to a family physician. At his first appointment, Jonathan's physician explains his risk for heart disease, hypertension, obesity, type 2 diabetes, and colon cancer. Jonathan is alerted to his high risk of developing both diabetes and obesity, and a program of exercise and diet that has been shown to delay disease onset is recommended to him.

Ten years later, Jonathan informs his physician that he and his wife are planning to start a family. His wife is also a carrier for sickle cell disease and has several risk variants for asthma, so they are referred for further counseling about prenatal genetic testing options. When Jonathan is 45, he develops hypertension, and, based on his profile of drug response variants, therapy is initiated with a specific antihypertensive agent to which he is likely to respond.

Diagnosing and Monitoring Common Disease

In the previous sections, we have explained how genomic information can be used to personalize risk assessments for rare and common diseases as well as drug responses. Genomic information can also be used to facilitate disease diagnosis and to monitor therapeutic responses. For example, a microarray or RNA sequencing (see Chapter 3) can be used to estimate the expression level of each gene (i.e., the amount of mRNA that is transcribed) in a specific tissue. These gene-expression profiles can be used to identify patterns of gene expression that are associated with specific conditions (e.g., increased transcription of an oncogene or reduced transcription of a tumor suppressor gene in tumor tissue). Such information can help to distinguish different types of cancers, different types of infections, or other phenotypes associated with disease. It should be appreciated that genomic information is just one of many types of data about a person and their environment that can be assessed to make predictions about disease states. This includes information about protein expression (i.e., **proteome**), metabolic functions (i.e., **metabolome**), normal body flora (i.e., microbiome), and environmental exposures (i.e., exposome).

Cancer Genomics

Every cancer cell harbors numerous alterations in DNA sequence and copy number that affect genes or regulatory sequences, often accompanied by reversible, epigenetic modifications. These changes perturb the expression and/or function of hundreds to thousands of gene. Collectively, these changes result in the activation or inhibition of various cellular pathways that control the characteristics of cancers such as growth or metastasis, and they determine, in part, prognosis and response to treatment. Cancer genomics is the study of the DNA-associated changes that accompany cancer with the overall goal of better preventing, detecting, diagnosing, and treating common cancers.

A particularly powerful application of genomics to cancer has been the use of genome-wide gene expression analyses to provide a snapshot of gene activity within a tumor at a given point in time. This has facilitated the development of classification schemes based on expression profiles for many types of cancer, including leukemia, lymphoma, and cancers of the breast, lung, colon, and brain. This information can be used, for example, in refining prognosis, directing the application of conventional and targeted biological therapies, and identifying targets for new drug development (Fig. 11-2).

Currently, it is often difficult to predict the prognosis of cancer patients based on traditional phenotypic information such as the type of tumor (T), whether the cancer is found in nearby lymph nodes (N), and evidence of metastasis (M). Staging using this TNM system is currently the standard for most solid tumors, yet these stages are often not predictive of prognosis or treatment response. **Gene-expression profiling** can help to distinguish between cancers that are easily confused (e.g., Burkitt lymphoma vs. diffuse large B-cell lymphoma). It can also facilitate the identification of subsets of tumors of the same TNM stage that might have quite different outcomes. Several gene-expression profiles are currently available for assessing breast cancer prognosis, and gene-expression profiles that predict recurrence of several other types of cancer have been established. Prospective trials will determine the extent to which the use of expression profiling is of clinical benefit, but it is anticipated that its use will lead to a substantial improvement in cancer management.

The conventional approach to cancer therapy has been to provide treatment based on the tissue or organ in which the cancer originated. However, persons with the same type of cancer often have different genetic abnormalities in their tumors, resulting in differential responses to treatment. For example, among young women whose breast cancer has not spread to their lymph nodes and who are treated by resection of the tumor and local radiation, only 20% to 30% will experience a recurrence. This subgroup of women might benefit the most from receiving adjuvant chemotherapy, and those at lower risk of recurrence (the majority) might benefit less from

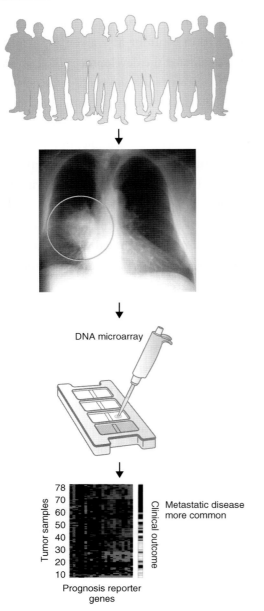

FIG 11-2 Prediction of disease outcome by gene-expression profiling. The clinical outcome of individuals with lung cancer (*circled tumor on radiograph*) is predicted by testing the expression of a set of genes known to be abnormally regulated in lung cancer cells. For each individual tumor, RNA is extracted and placed onto a microarray, and the expression of each gene is measured. *Bottom*, Each column represents the expression profile of a different tumor. Diminished expression of a gene in one lung tumor compared to other lung tumors is indicated by *green*, and increased expression is indicated by *red*. The outcome of the disease is shown at the *right*, where white indicates persons with metastatic disease (poor outcome) and *black* indicates no metastasis (good outcome).

chemotherapy. Yet, because the high- and low-risk groups can not be distinguished reliably, 85% to 95% of all women with this type of breast cancer receive adjuvant chemotherapy. This means that many women might undergo such treatment unnecessarily, putting them at risk for drug-related complications and increasing the overall cost of health care. Expression profiling has the potential to help delineate subsets of cancers that are likely to be more responsive to various therapeutic regimens and to guide the optimal selection of agents for each individual.

Gene-expression profiling of cancers is helping to improve the classification of different types of tumors and may help to guide therapy

Common Disease

Gene-expression profiling is being used to study the pathogenesis of common diseases and to monitor tissue-specific gene activity in order to facilitate diagnosis and monitor disease progression and treatment. For example, expression profiling of circulating white blood cells in patients with type 1 diabetes has revealed increased expression of a large number of proinflammatory genes. The expression of some of these genes is also increased in persons with rheumatoid arthritis, suggesting that some autoimmune disorders might share expression profiles. A screening test based on these profiles might enable earlier diagnosis and/ or identify high-risk persons who could benefit from preventive care. Gene profiling has also been used effectively to monitor immunosuppression in individuals who have undergone organ transplantation. Studies are also under way to identify whether gene-expression profiles can predict outcome in persons infected with pathogens such as malaria, HIV-1, and tuberculosis.

Race and Genetic Assessment of Individual Ancestry

An important and controversial issue in personalized medicine is whether a person's **race**—using its historical meaning as a descriptor of Africans, Asians, Europeans, Native Americans, and Pacific Islanders—and/ or **genetic ancestry** is useful for making predictions about health-related risks. Traditionally, it has been commonplace to use race to predict the likelihood that a person carries a particular genetic variant that influences susceptibility to disease or drug response. This practice was based partly on the observation that disparities in health are common among racial groups. For example, the incidence of prostate cancer is twofold higher in African American men than in European American men. Other disorders that vary in prevalence or outcome among racial groups include hypertension, end-stage renal disease, preterm birth, and type 2 diabetes. It remains unclear, however, whether genetic risk factors explain, even partly, these disparities. Many health-related disparities probably are influenced more strongly instead by environmental factors such as dietary differences and inequities in the provision of health-care services. Accordingly, the use of race to make predictions about whether a person has such risk factors is still the subject of considerable debate.

It is important to distinguish between race and genetic ancestry. Race has traditionally been used to categorize large groups of persons and can reflect geographic origin, language, and various cultural attributes that describe a group (e.g., Native Americans or Asians). Ancestry refers to the geographic, historical, or biological origins of one's ancestors and, for any person, can be complex. For example, a person might have ancestors from Africa, Europe, and North America (i.e., a complex ancestry), but he or she might still self-identify as an African American. Therefore, race captures some biological information about ancestry, but the two concepts are not equivalent. Knowledge of a person's ancestry can provide information about his or her genetic makeup and thus can be useful for identifying genetic and environmental factors that underlie common diseases. Accordingly, over the past several years, it has become increasingly common to use genetic markers such as single nucleotide polymorphisms (SNPs) to directly estimate the genetic ancestry of a person (Fig. 11-3). The extent to which race helps us to pre-

dict genetic differences that influence health depends partly on how well traditional classifications of race correspond with such genetic inferences of individual ancestry.

On average, persons chosen at random from different populations, such as sub-Saharan Africans, Europeans, and East Asians, will be only slightly more different from one another than persons from the same population, reflecting the fact that all humans are quite similar in their DNA sequence

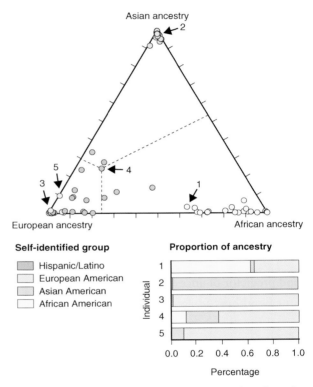

FIG 11-3 Genetically inferred ancestry fractions for persons (*colored circles*) sampled from the United States and geno-typed for 6000 single nucleotide polymorphisms (SNPs). Each circle represents one person, color-coded to correspond to one of four self-identified groups. The distance of a circle to the edge of the triangle is proportional to the amount of the person's ancestry contributed by each of the three ancestral populations in the corners of the triangle (African, Asian, and European). For example, the Hispanic/Latino American labeled number 4 received about 60% of his genetic ancestry from Europe, 30% from Asia (due to Native American ancestry), and 10% from Africa. The circles representing Hispanic/Latino and African Americans are less tightly clustered because the proportion of ancestry among persons is more varied than in Asian Americans and Americans of European descent. A bar graph indicates the estimated ancestry proportions for each of the subjects labeled 1-5.

(see Chapter 3). Common disease-associated polymorphisms, such as those associated with response to antihypertensive agents (see earlier), often differ in these populations only in their frequency. Few, if any, genetic variants are found in all members of one major population and in no members of another major population. For this reason, population affiliation or race is not a reliable predictor of individual genotypes.

It is possible, however, to allocate individuals to groups that correspond to different geographic regions by simultaneously analyzing several hundred or more variants, such as SNPs (see Fig. 11-3). These variants differ in frequency among geographic regions because our ancestors were more likely to mate with close neighbors than with distant ones. Thus, proxies for geographic ancestry such as race can sometimes be used to make reasonably accurate predictions of a person's genetic ancestry. Indeed, several studies done in the United States have reported that classification of persons by self-identified population group is highly correlated with inferences based on genetic data.

In many circumstances, however, race is not a good predictor of ancestry. For example, populations from neighboring geographical regions typically share more recent common ancestors, and therefore their allele frequencies can be very similar. Consequently, persons sampled at regular intervals across some intercontinental regions (e.g., the Middle East or Central Asia) are more difficult to allocate into genetic groups that are concordant with common notions of race. Correspondence with geography is also less apparent for populations (e.g., Latin Americans, South Asians) that have been influenced by recent historical mixtures of multiple ancestral populations.

In the United States, race is only a crude predictor of a person's genetic ancestry. For example, the average portion of African ancestry among self-identified African Americans is about 80%, but it ranges from 100% to 20% or even less in some persons. The genetic composition of self-identified European Americans also varies, with about 30% of European

Americans estimated to have less than 90% European ancestry. Similarly, Hispanics from different regions of the United States have highly variable ancestries (e.g., more African ancestry in Hispanics living in the Southeast and more Native American ancestry in the Southwest). Accordingly, membership in a group does not mean that all members of the group necessarily have similar genetic ancestries.

Although it is clear that explicit genetic information, rather than race, can be used to make more accurate inferences of ancestry, it is not yet known to what extent personal ancestry information can make useful predictions about one's risk of common disease. The consequences of using detailed ancestry information in a clinical setting are also largely unknown. It is possible that personal ancestry information could have adverse effects on a person's perception of risk and cultural identity. Similarly, such information could reinforce unfair stereotypes about specific populations. Further research is needed to examine the potential benefits and risks of using ancestry information in clinical practice.

The relationship between ancestry and traditional concepts of race is complex. Genetic information, rather than race, is a better predictor of ancestry.

THE FUTURE OF PERSONALIZED MEDICINE

Genetic variants that influence the risk of common disease or response to treatment are now being found with increasing speed and efficiency (see Chapter 5), but only a small fraction of the genetic basis of disease risk and treatment response has thus far been defined. In addition, the interactions of multiple disease-predisposing gene products, and their interactions with nongenetic factors, remain almost completely unknown. Thus, the promise of predictive medicine, in which a detailed genetic profile can provide clinically useful risk information for common diseases such as diabetes, cancer, or heart disease, remains largely unfulfilled. It is hoped that with increasing knowledge of alleles that predispose persons to disease, genetic testing will begin to contribute more substantially to the diagnosis and treatment of disease. It must also be borne in mind that nongenetic factors, such as diet and exercise, are also part of each person's risk profile. These factors can and should be assessed and modified to maximize each person's potential for a long and healthy life.

SUMMARY

When the reference sequence of the human genome was initially introduced, widespread genomic variations were unknown. As the science has advanced, appreciation and understanding of the genomic variations among individuals has grown. Personalized medicine is becoming established as a new and exciting field. This emerging medical model uses the unique combination of genetic and environmental factors to predict an individual's disease risk as well as response to various treatments. This chapter provides an overview of personalized medicine as it pertains to new genomic technologies, and the role of an individual's genomic information in medical practice and health care.

This chapter also provides an introduction to pharmacogenetics, which aims to identify individual genetic variations associated with drug response features, treatment efficacy, and safety. Via illustrative examples in which genetic polymorphisms can be associated with drug reactions, we may be able to predict an individual's response to drug metabolism in a more efficient manner. Therefore, we may be able to reduce the incidences of drug-related side effects and serious adverse drug reactions. This will facilitate the development of individualized treatments for patients. Personalized medicine can also be used for individualized risk assessments for common and rare diseases. Cancer genomics and gene-expression profiling will improve the classification of different types of tumors and will lead to better diagnostics and treatments for common cancers. As the chapter to follow illustrates, gene-expression profiling of individuals with lung cancer may iden-

tify persons with metastatic disease, or the lack of it, and this can be used to refine prognoses and provide direction with respect to the application of conventional and targeted biologic therapies. This chapter also discusses the use of genetic markers to estimate individual race and genetic ancestry; genetic information rather than race can be used to make more accurate inferences regarding ancestry, and this has provided insight into the genetic diversity of the human population.

Personalized medicine has emerged over the past decade and is a rapidly growing field in health care. It will drive profound change in clinical medicine. However, the identification and management of personal genome sequences for clinical applications are challenging, and the numbers of useful pharmacogenetic biomarkers are still relatively few. Nonetheless, the goal of personalized medicine is to optimize preventive health care strategies and drug therapies in the early stages of disease, which will be beneficial to both patients and health care providers and drive significant change in clinical medicine.

IMPORTANT TERMINOLOGY

preventive health maintenance　预防保健
personalized medicine　个性化医学
biotransformation　生物转化
pharmacogenetics　药物遗传学
pharmacogenomics　药物基因组学
whole-genome sequencing　全基因组测序
genetic profile　遗传档案
serious adverse drug reaction (SADR)　严重药物不良反应
TPMT gene　巯嘌呤甲基转移酶基因
exome sequencing　外显子组测序
proteome　蛋白质组
metabolome　代谢组
cancer genomics　肿瘤基因组学
gene-expression profiling　基因表达谱
race　种族
genetic ancestry　遗传学祖先

REVIEW QUESTIONS

1. Explain how genetic information can be used to enhance the practice of predictive medicine compared to a conventional model of medical service. Give at least one example.
2. Different individuals with the same type of cancer often respond differently to therapy. Provide at least two possible explanations of this observation.
3. Define race and ancestry; explain the differences between them.
4. Consider how explicit genetic information about your ancestry might change your perception of your biological and cultural identities.
5. Give an example of a polymorphism that affects drug metabolism and/or the response to a drug.
6. Explain some of the possible obstacles to the use of genetic information in practicing precision medicine.
7. Distinguish between genetic medicine and genomic medicine.
8. Give examples of how the availability of whole-genome data from individuals might change the ways medicine is currently practiced.

SUGGESTED READINGS AND WEBSITES

1. Bamshad MJ. Genetic influences on health: does race matter? *JAMA*. 2006; 294: 937-946.
2. Harper AR, Topol EJ. Pharmacogenomics in clinical practice and drug development. *Nat Biotechnol*. 2012; 30: 1117-1124.
3. McDermott U, Downing JR, Stratton MR. Genomics and the continuum of cancer care. *N Engl J Med*. 2011; 364: 340-350.
4. Pirmohamed M. Personalized pharmacogenomics: predicting efficacy and adverse drug reactions. *Annu Rev Genomics Hum Genet*. 2014; 15: 1-22.
5. Rotimi CN, Jorde LB. Ancestry and disease in the age of genomic medicine. *N Engl J Med*. 2010; 363: 1551-1558.
6. Royal CD, Novembre J, Fullerton SM, et al. Inferring genetic ancestry: opportunities, challenges and implications. *Am J Hum Genet*. 2010; 86: 661-673.
7. Topol EJ. Individualized medicine from prewomb to tomb. *Cell*. 2014; 157: 241-253.
8. Weitzel JN, Blazer KR, MacDonald DJ, et al. Genetics, genomics and cancer risk assessment: state of the art and future directions in the era of personalized medicine. *CA Cancer J Clin*. 2011; 61: 327-359.
9. National Institutes of Health-sponsored pharmacogenetics research network: http://www.nigms.nih.gov/Initiatives/PGRN
10. National Cancer Institute-sponsored tutorial on cancer genomics: http://www.cancer.gov/cancertopics/understandingcancer/cancergenomics

(Yongshu He)

Chapter 12

Clinical Genetics and Genetic Counseling

In the last 2 decades medical genetics has clearly emerged as a recognized specialty in mainstream medicine. In the 1960s, the fields of biochemical genetics, clinical cytogenetics, and **dysmorphology** (the study of abnormal physical development) arose as disciplines primarily within pediatrics. The 1970s witnessed the establishment of the techniques necessary for the prenatal diagnosis of genetic disorders. By the end of the 1970s, discussions about forming the American Board of Medical Genetics had occurred, and in 1981 the first certification examination was administered. The American Board of Genetic Counseling was established in the early 1990s, and now various types of geneticists, including genetic counselors, medical geneticists, and basic human geneticists, can be certified as specialists within the discipline. In 1991 the American Board of Medical Specialties recognized this new field, and medical genetics has now become an integral part of medicine.

Whereas medical genetics involves the study of the genetics of human disease, **clinical genetics** deals with the direct clinical care of persons with genetic diseases. The diagnostic, counseling, and management issues surrounding genetic disease are the principal foci of clinical genetics.

In this chapter, we summarize the principles of clinical genetics and the process of genetic counseling. In addition, we provide an overview of the field of dysmorphology, because the growth of this area has influenced and paralleled the emergence of clinical genetics.

THE PRINCIPLES AND PRACTICE OF CLINICAL GENETICS

As mentioned in Chapter 1, genetic conditions as a group are common and are a significant cause of human mortality and morbidity. Typically, genetic disorders are complex, multiorgan, systemic conditions, and the care of persons with these disorders can also involve multiple medical specialties. Thus, genetic disorders are among the differential diagnosis of most symptoms and clinical presentations. For example, when evaluating an infant with a blistering skin disease, the ability to distinguish between one of the many forms of epidermolysis bullosa (an inherited disorder of keratinocytes in which skin blisters develop after mild trauma) and staphylococcal skin disease must be part of the clinician's repertoire.

Because of the complexity and number of human genetic diseases, their clinical diagnosis and treatment can seem overwhelming. To help manage this information, we provide an overview of the most important concepts, including the importance of accurate diagnosis, the application of the tenets of medical genetics to medical practice, and the role of genetic counseling in the care of persons with genetic disease.

Accurate Diagnosis

The significance of the basic medical principle of accurate diagnosis cannot be overemphasized. The process of genetic counseling, one of the principal components of the service of medical genetics, begins with correct diagnosis. All discussions of natural history, prognosis, management, risk determination, options for prenatal diagnosis and referral to genetic support groups (also termed *genetic advocacy groups*) depend on an accurate diagnosis of the patient's condition. For example, genetic counseling for a family who has a son with an intellectual disability usually involves questions of risk for this condition in future offspring. An accurate answer requires the clinician to identify a condition of known etiology. Once a specific diagnosis (e.g., fragile X syndrome) is made, then the genetic counseling process begins: Current information can be shared and management can be initiated (Clinical Commentary 12-1).

 In clinical genetics, as in all of medicine, accurate diagnosis is the most important first step in patient care.

The process of diagnosing a genetic disorder is a complex sequence of events. It depends upon diagnostic decision making, recognition of important phenotypic signs, application of principles of dysmorphology and medical genetics and laboratory diagnosis. For diseases in which the diagnostic criteria are well established, the practitioner has guidelines for making a diagnosis. An example of such criteria is the criteria recommended by the National Institutes of Health Consensus Development Conference for the diagnosis of neurofibromatosis type 1

CLINICAL COMMENTARY 12-1
Reasons for Making a Diagnosis of a Syndrome

The long list of syndromes associated with congenital malformations can be overwhelming to the clinician. More than 400 conditions are listed in *Smith's Recognizable Patterns of Human Malformations*, and more than 1000 are accessible through the POSSUM or London Dysmorphology computerized databases (see Suggested Readings and Websites at the end of this chapter). This number imparts a sense that the diagnosis of a malformation syndrome lies in the arena of academic trivia. However, this is not the case.

Consider, for example, the child who is large for gestational age and has a number of physical abnormalities: omphalocele (intestinal protrusion at the umbilicus), large tongue, facial hemangioma, flank mass, and asymmetrical limb length (Fig. 12-1). His family has questions such as, "What does he have?" "How will he do?" "Will he look different?" "Will he have developmental delays?" "What is the chance of his condition occurring again in another child?"

FIG 12-1 A child with Beckwith-Wiedemann syndrome. Note the prominent eyes and large, protruding tongue.

By putting these features together and making the pattern recognition diagnosis of the Beckwith-Wiedemann syndrome, the clinician is able to answer all of the parents' questions fairly precisely. Most cases of Beckwith-Wiedemann syndrome occur sporadically, but some are inherited. In addition, the genes that are involved in causing the condition exhibit imprinting effects (see Chapter 4). If the child has the typical methylation alteration that causes the majority of cases, the sibling recurrence risk is low and likely less than 1%. If the results of the methylation analysis are normal, the recurrence risk is higher, and linkage or mutation analysis can provide a more precise risk estimate. In future pregnancies, prenatal diagnosis using ultrasound can test for an omphalocele in the second trimester and for large size for gestational age, excessive amniotic fluid (polyhydramnios) and large tongue. If a fetus is thought to have Beckwith-Wiedemann syndrome, then the delivery plan would change and the baby should be born in a tertiary care center.

Children with the Beckwith-Wiedemann syndrome do not usually have cognitive disabilities. Although the large tongue can cause orthodontic problems, speech difficulties, and occasionally upper airway problems, these conditions usually improve as the child gets older. The facial appearance is not strikingly abnormal in later childhood.

Chromosome analysis should be considered, although most Beckwith-Wiedemann patients do not have the chromosome 11 duplication that has been reported in a small number of cases. Otherwise, the main emphases of the medical care plan include regular abdominal sonogram until age 7 years to look for intra-abdominal malignancies, especially Wilms tumor and hepatoblastoma. Children with Beckwith-Wiedemann syndrome have a 5% to 10% risk of developing these tumors, and both types are treatable if detected early.

In this example, it was important to diagnose the Beckwith-Wiedemann syndrome. The correct label led to precise information for genetic counseling, prediction of natural history (including reassurance), organization of appropriate laboratory studies, a health supervision plan, and referral to a lay advocacy group. Diagnosis was helpful to the parents, the family physician and the child.

(NF1; see Chapter 4). For conditions that are defined by a specific laboratory marker, such as an abnormal karyotype or biochemical assay, the diagnostic procedure is generally straightforward. For many genetic diseases, however, there are no well-established criteria, the definition and delineation of the disorder are not clear-cut, and diagnosis can be challenging.

Dysmorphic syndromes require knowledge and skills in the recognition of mild malformations, minor anomalies, and phenotypic variations. The diagnosis of other genetic diseases, including cancer syndromes and inborn errors of metabolism, can require expertise from a variety of disciplines. For instance, the diagnosis of any of the forms of retinitis pigmentosa (see Chapter 8) necessitates input from an ophthalmologist who is familiar with this group of retinal degenerative conditions. The diagnostic process is further complicated by the variable expres-sion, incomplete penetrance and heterogeneity of many genetic diseases. These concepts are discussed in Chapter 4.

Application of the Principles of Medical Genetics

Developing a genetic approach to human disease in the clinical setting requires the application of all of the basic principles of medical genetics discussed in this book. This is often called "thinking genetically." For example, making or excluding the diagnosis of NF1 requires knowledge of the clinical variability and age of onset of certain features of the condition (Clinical Commentary 12-2). Recognition of the various forms of neurofibromatosis (i.e., heterogeneity) is also important in developing a management plan.

Knowledge of the other formal principles of medical genetics is also necessary in the care of persons

---

CLINICAL COMMENTARY 12-2
The Negative Family History

One of the common discussions on ward rounds is the notation that a person's family history is negative or "non-contributory." This is often thought to rule out a genetic disorder. However, the majority of persons who have a genetic disease do not have a positive family history. A quick review of the mechanisms of mendelian, chromo-somal, and multifactorial disease inheritance shows that a lack of other affected persons in the family is common and does not by any means exclude the presence of a genetic disease. For example, the sibling recurrence risk is 25% for diseases with autosomal recessive inheritance. Thus, a significant number of families with multiple offspring have only one affected child and no family history. Even some well-established autosomal dominant disorders often present a negative family history because of high proportions of new mutations (examples include Marfan syndrome, neurofibromatosis type 1 [NF1], and achon-droplasia, in which the percentages of cases caused by new mutations are 30%, 50% and 80%, respectively). Chromosomal syndromes usually have a low recurrence risk. Even when a parent carries a balanced chromosome rearrangement, the recurrence risk among the offspring is usually less than 15%. The sibling recurrence risks for multifactorial conditions are usually 5% or less.

Case

A family comes in with a 6-year-old boy who has 10 café-au-lait spots exceeding 0.5 cm in diameter widely distrib-uted on the trunk and arms and an optic glioma detected on a brain MRI (Fig. 12-2). The family has questions about the diagnosis and the recurrence risk in future pregnan-cies. On initial telephone contact it is learned that there is no history of a family member with similar features.

FIG 12-2   A 6-year-old boy with multiple *café-au-lait* spots. (From Burger P, Scheithauer B, Vogel FS: *Surgical Pathology of the Nervous System and Its Coverings*, 4th ed. Philadelphia: Churchill Livingstone; 2002.)

There are several possible explanations for this finding. Exploring them underscores the implications of a negative family history:

CLINICAL COMMENTARY 12-2
The Negative Family History (Continued)

- *New mutation of the NF1 gene.* Because of the relatively high percentage of new mutations for this disorder, this is the most likely explanation.
- *Variable expression.* It is also possible that one of the parents carries the gene but has mild expression of the phenotype. Occasionally a parent has multiple *café-au-lait* spots and a few unrecognized neurofibromas, but a diagnosis of NF1 has never been made. Thus, it is important to evaluate the parents for mild expression of NF1.
- *Incomplete penetrance.* This is a possibility; however, it is unlikely for NF1, in which penetrance is close to 100%. If a family has two children with NF1 and neither parent has the gene, germline mosaicism would be the more likely explanation.

- *Incorrect diagnosis.* One of the assumptions and basic principles of medical genetics is accurate diagnosis. This patient meets the National Institutes of Health established criteria for NF1 (see Chapter 4). However, if this patient had only *café-au-lait* spots, then the diagnosis would have been an issue. One would need to know the differential diagnosis of multiple *café-au-lait* spots.
- *False paternity.* Although it is relatively unlikely, this possibility must be kept in mind.

We began with an individual who had a classic autosomal dominant disorder with no family history. This can be explained in a number of ways. The statement that there is "a negative family history" should not be considered conclusive evidence against the presence of a heritable condition.

---

with genetic conditions. The accumulation of family history data and the interpretation of pedigree information are important in answering a family's questions regarding risk of recurrence. An understanding of the various modes of inheritance is required in any explanation of recurrence risk. Discussion of the concepts of new mutation and pleiotropy are commonplace in reviewing the cause and pathogenesis of a genetic disease with a family. Even an understanding of meiosis is a requirement for discussions of etiology with the family of a newborn with Down syndrome (Clinical Commentary 12-3).

Genetic Counseling: Definition and Principles

Genetic counseling represents one of the central foci of medical genetics and with accurate diagnosis comprises the cornerstones of the field. At first glance, use of the term "counseling" implies that this service lies in the domain of mental health, social work, or psychotherapy. In fact, genetic counseling is centered in the conventional medical model because it depends significantly on accurate diagnosis and knowledge of medical genetics. As a tradition, genetic counseling grew out of the field of human genetics rather than from behavioral science, unlike other counseling disciplines.

In 1975 the American Society of Human Genetics adopted a definition of genetic counseling. Newer language has been proposed recently to modernize

and clarify this definition, but the original language stands the test of time:

Genetic counseling is a communication process that deals with the human problems associated with the occurrence or risk of occurrence of a genetic disorder in a family. This process involves an attempt by one or more appropriately trained persons to help the individual or family to (1) comprehend the medical facts, including the diagnosis, probable course of the disorder, and the available management; (2) appreciate the way heredity contributes to the disorder and the risk of recurrence in specified relatives; (3) understand the alternatives for dealing with the risk of recurrence; (4) choose a course of action that seems to them appropriate in their view of their risk, their family goals, and their ethical and religious standards, and act in accordance with that decision; and (5) make the best possible adjustment to the disorder in an affected family member and/or to the risk of recurrence of that disorder.

This definition illustrates the complex tasks that face the practitioner. The first task involves establishing the diagnosis and discussing the natural history and management of the condition. In this regard, the medical care of a patient with a genetic disease does not differ from that of a patient with any other type of human disease.

The second task requires an understanding of

CLINICAL COMMENTARY 12-3

Talking to the Parents of a Newborn with Down Syndrome

The birth of a newborn with Down syndrome presents many challenges. Typically, the infant is not acutely ill and the parents are not aware of the diagnosis before the birth. Thus, the practitioner must approach the parents, often strangers, with unexpected and sometimes disappointing news. The family can experience a series of emotions that are somewhat similar to the reactions after a loss: anger, denial, sadness, and then usually reorganization and adaptation. Families face these situations with markedly different backgrounds: varying attitudes toward crisis, different demographic and socioeconomic circumstances, and even a wide range of differences in the cultural meaning of a disability or defect. All of these variables, plus the fact that physicians are often not trained in being the bearers of difficult news, can make this a challenging situation. Parents remember in detail the way the news is presented. The practitioner has both the opportunity and the challenge to help the family through these events.

A number of practical suggestions have come from studies investigating the recommendations of parents who have experienced this event:

- *Prepare yourself.* Set up the interview scenario, and think about how you will begin the discussion.
- *Talk to both parents together whenever possible.* This is sometimes not practical, but when it can be accomplished, it is critical.
- *Communicate the diagnosis as soon as possible.* All studies of parental interviews show that they prefer early communication of the diagnosis.
- *Choose a place that is private and quiet where both the parents and the professionals can sit down.* Avoid standing up with the parents seated. Always be sure to introduce yourself. Structure the interview from the beginning.
- *Humanize the situation as much as possible.* Learn the baby's first name if it has been decided on, and always know the baby's gender. Refer to the infant by name or as a son or daughter, and be aware of the use of all language. Phrases. such as "mental retardation" have

great Impact, and currently that term is not considered the appropriate designation by professionals in pediatrics, psychology, and medical genetics (it has been replaced by intellectual disability or cognitive disability). Terms such as "mongolism" are not appropriate because they are stigmatizing, pejorative, and incorrect.

- *Develop a sense of realistic positivism.* It is important to discuss the developmental limitations in a patient with Down syndrome, but it is also important to have an optimistic and positive attitude. This suggestion comes from the advocacy and parents' organizations that have developed in the last four decades.
- *Answer the parents' questions, but avoid technical overload.* It is important to be accurate and current on the biological and medical aspects of the condition under discussion. When an answer is not known, mention that the question can be reviewed or referred to a consultant.
- *Listen actively.* Assume that almost all feelings are natural and that parents will be wrestling with their own guilt and shame. Validate all feelings that arise. Most parents can meet this challenge quite effectively and do not require psychiatric consultation.
- *Refer the family to the appropriate resources early.* This would include parent advocacy groups or even individual parents who have a child with Down syndrome. Share available written material and web pages, but make certain that it is accurate and current.

Above all, be aware of the unique plight of families in such a situation, and make an effort to spend time with them. Although it is difficult to present in written form how one can develop attributes such as kindness and empathy, it is important for physicians in training to learn from their mentors and use their own individual communication style as a strength. Clearly, the recommendations provided here apply not only to genetic counseling but also to any situation in which difficult information is presented to patients or families. (See Suggested Readings at the end of the chapter.)

---

the basic tenets of medical genetics, especially the principles of human genetics and risk determination discussed throughout the text. For chromosomal and multifactorial disorders, empirical figures are used to estimate recurrence risk. Knowledge of inheritance patterns is applied to predict the recurrence risk of mendelian disorders. However, the clinical issues are often complicated by incomplete penetrance, variable expression, delayed age of onset, and allelic and locus heterogeneity. In some cases, incorporation of additional information using the Bayesian probability approach can significantly assist in providing estimates (Box 12-1).

The third and fourth objectives of the genetic counseling process underlie the primary differences between the genetic model and the traditional biomedical approach. These tasks involve discussing reproductive options and facilitating decision making. Implicit in the fourth part of the definition is the notion of respect for the family's autonomy and their perceptions of risk and of the disorder itself. This approach has been called **nondirectiveness:** the counselor leaves all decisions about future reproduction up to the family. This differs somewhat from the more traditional medical approach, in which *recommendations* for treatment or intervention are often made in a more directed fashion. This is an important issue, because nondirectiveness sometimes conflicts with the broader view of preventive medicine, which might suggest that the principal goal of genetic counseling should be the reduction of the incidence of genetic diseases.

BOX 12-1 Recurrence Risks and Bayes Theorem

The estimation of recurrence risks was treated at some length in Chapter 4. A typical example of recurrence risk estimation is a case in which a man with hemophilia A, an X-linked recessive disorder, produces a daughter (individual II-1 in the following diagram). Because the man can transmit only the X chromosome carrying the hemophilia A mutation to his daughter, she must be a carrier. The carrier's daughter, individual III-6, has a 50% chance of receiving the X chromosome carrying the mutation and being herself a carrier. Even though the daughter in generation III has five normal brothers, her risk remains 50% because we know that the mother in generation II is a carrier.

Suppose now that the woman in generation III produces three sons (generation IV), none of whom has hemophilia A. Intuitively, we might begin to suspect that she is not a carrier after all. How can we incorporate this new information into our recurrence risk estimate?

A statistical principle that allows us to make use of such information is called **Bayes theorem** (the application of Bayes theorem is often termed Bayesian analysis or Bayesian inference). The table below summarizes the basic steps involved in Bayesian analysis. We begin with the **prior probability** that the woman in generation III is a carrier. As its name suggests, the prior probability denotes the probability that she is a carrier before we account for the fact that she has produced three normal sons. Because we know her mother is a carrier, this woman's prior probability must be 1/2. Then the prior probability that she is not a carrier is 1 − 1/2, or 1/2.

	SHE IS A CARRIER	SHE IS NOT A CARRIER
Prior probability	1/2	1/2
Conditional probability	1/8	1
Joint probability	1/16	1/2
Posterior probability	1/9	8/9

Next we take into account the woman's three normal sons by estimating the probability that all three of them would be normal given that she is a carrier. Because this probability is *conditioned* on her carrier status, it is termed a **conditional probability.** If she is a carrier, the conditional probability that all three of her sons are normal would be $(1/2)^3$, or 1/8. We also estimate the probability that all of her sons would be normal given that she is *not* a carrier. This conditional probability is, of course, very close to 1.

Next we want to find the probability that the woman is a carrier *and* that she is a carrier with three normal sons. To obtain the probability of the co-occurrence of these two events, we multiply the prior probability times the conditional probability to derive a **joint probability** (i.e., the probability of both events occurring together, a concept discussed in Chapter 4). The joint probability that she is a carrier is then $1/2 \times 1/8 = 1/16$. Similarly, the joint probability that she is not a carrier is $1/2 \times 1 = 1/2$. These joint probabilities indicate the woman is 8 times more likely not to be a carrier than to be a carrier.

The final step is to standardize the joint probabilities so that the two probabilities under consideration (i.e., being a carrier versus not being a carrier) sum to 1. To do this, we simply divide the joint probability that the woman is a carrier (1/16) by the sum of the two joint probabilities (1/16 + 1/2). This yields a **posterior probability** of 1/9 that she is a carrier and 8/9 that she is not a carrier. Notice that this standardization process allows us to provide a risk estimate (1/9, or 11%), while preserving the odds of non-carrier versus carrier status indicated by the joint probabilities.

Having worked through the Bayesian analysis, we see that our intuition was confirmed: The fact that the woman in question produced three normal sons reduced her risk of being a carrier substantially, from an initial estimate of 50% to a final probability of only 11%.

Another common application of Bayesian analysis is illustrated in part A of the diagram that follows. The male in generation II is affected with Duchenne muscular dystrophy (DMD), a lethal X-linked recessive disease (see Chapter 4). Either his unaffected mother is a carrier of the mutation, or he received a new mutation on the X chromosome transmitted by his mother. It is important to determine whether the mother is a carrier or not, because this fact will influence recurrence risks for DMD in her subsequent offspring. If the mother has only one affected offspring, the probability that she is a carrier can be evaluated directly, because one third of all cases of X-linked lethal recessive disorders arise as a result of new mutations. (To understand this, consider the fact that because females have two X chromosomes and males have only one, 2/3 of all X-linked disease-causing mutations in a population must be found in females. For a lethal X-linked recessive, all of the male X chromosomes are eliminated from the population in each generation. Yet the frequency of the

BOX 12-1   Recurrence Risks and Bayes Theorem (Continued)

mutation remains the same, generation after generation. This is because new disease-causing mutations arise at the same rate as the loss of mutation-containing X chromosomes. Because one third of the mutation-containing X chromosomes are lost in each generation, it follows that one third of the mutations in the population must occur as the result of new mutation.) If the probability that the affected son received a new mutation is 1/3, then the probability that the mother is a carrier—the alternative possibility—must be 1–1/3, or 2/3.

In the table below, we use Bayesian analysis to evaluate the probability that the mother is a carrier. As in the previous example, we derive a prior probability that she is a carrier, assuming no knowledge that she has produced an affected son. This probability is given by 4μ, where μ is the mutation rate for the *DMD* locus (i.e., the probability, per generation, that a disease-causing mutation arises at this locus in an individual). The derivation of the probability, 4μ, is beyond the scope of this text, but it can be found elsewhere (see Suggested Readings, Hodge, 1998). Because the prior probability that the mother is a carrier is 4μ, the prior probability that she is not a carrier is $1 - 4\mu$, which is approximately equal to 1 because μ is very small. The conditional probability that the woman transmits the mutation given that she is a carrier is 1/2 (there is also a very small probability that she transmits her normal allele, which is then mutated, but this can be ignored). The conditional probability that she transmits a mutation given that she is not a carrier (i.e., the probability that a new mutation arises in the gamete she transmits) is μ. We then multiply the prior probability that she is a carrier, 4μ, by the corresponding conditional probability, 1/2, to obtain a joint probability of 2μ. The same procedure produces a joint probability of μ that she is not a carrier. Finally, we standardize the joint probabilities to get the posterior probabilities. The posterior probability that she is a carrier is $2\mu \div (2\mu + \mu) = 2/3$, and the posterior probability that she is not a carrier is $\mu \div (2\mu + \mu) = 1/3$. As expected, these probabilities correspond to the ones we obtained by simple direct observation.

	SHE IS A CARRIER	SHE IS NOT A CARRIER
Prior probability	4μ	$1-4\mu \approx 1$
Conditional probability	1/2	μ
Joint probability	2μ	μ
Posterior probability	2/3	1/3

Suppose, however, that the woman has had an affected son and an unaffected son (see part B of the figure below). This gives us additional information, and intuitively it increases the possibility that she is not a carrier (i.e., that the one affected offspring is the result of a new mutation). In the table below, we incorporate this new information. The prior probabilities remain the same as before (i.e., we assume no knowledge of either of her offspring). But the conditional probability of transmission, given that she is a carrier, changes to account for the fact that she now has two offspring: $1/2 \times 1/2 = 1/4$ (i.e., the probability that she did not transmit the mutation to one off- spring times the probability that she did transmit the mutation to the other

offspring). The conditional probability that she transmitted a new mutation to the affected offspring is μ, and the probability that she did not transmit a mutation to the unaffected offspring is $1 - \mu$. Thus, the probability of both events, given that she is not a carrier, is $\mu \times (1 - \mu) \approx \mu$. The joint and posterior probabilities are obtained as before, and we see that the woman's chance of being a carrier is now reduced from 2/3 to 1/2. Again, this confirms (and quantifies) our expectation.

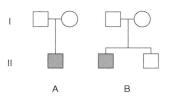

	SHE IS A CARRIER	SHE IS NOT A CARRIER
Prior probability	4μ	$1-4\mu \approx 1$
Conditional probability	1/4	$\mu \times (1-\mu) \approx 1$
Joint probability	μ	μ
Posterior probability	1/2	1/2

Before the advent of disease diagnosis through linked markers or mutation detection, Bayesian analysis was often the only way to derive a risk estimate in situations such as these. Now, of course, an attempt would be made to identify the factor VIII or *DMD* mutation that causes hemophilia A or DMD in these families directly, or, failing that, linked markers would be used. This is a much more direct and accurate approach for determining carrier status. However, as discussed in Chapter 10, it is not always possible to identify the responsible mutation, particularly when a large number of mutations can cause the disorder (as is the case for hemophilia A, DMD, or cystic fibrosis). Bayesian inference can be used in such cases to incorporate the sensitivity of the genetic test (e.g., if a standard mutation analysis of the *CFTR* gene reveals 85% of the mutations [see Chapter 10], there is a 15% probability that the person in question has the mutation even though the test did not reveal it). In addition, linkage analysis is not always informative. Thus, Bayesian analysis is still sometimes a useful tool for refining risk estimates.

The additional information incorporated in Bayesian analysis is not confined to the assessment of health status in relatives, as was shown in these examples. Another type of information is a biochemical assay, such as factor VIII activity level, that could help to indicate carrier status. Because there is usually overlap between carriers and normal homozygotes for such tests, the assay cannot determine carrier status with certainty, but it does provide a *probability* estimate for incorporation into Bayesian analysis. In diseases with delayed age of onset, such as adult polycystic kidney disease, the probability of being affected at a certain age can be used in a Bayesian analysis. Here, one considers the fact that the at-risk person is less and less likely to possess the disease gene if he or she remains unaffected beyond a certain age.

Historically, the principle of nondirectiveness developed in the arena of reproductive counseling and in the context of decisions surrounding prenatal diagnosis. If prevention or reduction of disease is the primary goal, then one's approach would logically be more directive. However, the main goal of genetic counseling is to help an individual family understand and cope with genetic disease, not to reduce the incidence of genetic disease.

Although most geneticists subscribe to the principles of autonomy and nondirectiveness, it may be challenging to the clinician to be entirely nondirective, simply because of the limitations of a time-restricted session. Additionally it is challenging as a clinician to avoid reflecting one's own biases. For example, an explanation of nutritional management of an infant with a disease detected by newborn screening (see Chapter 10) would require a more directive approach than the discussion of disease risks in future pregnancies. Nondirectiveness may be challenging when the consequences of disease are serious, as in high-risk cancer counseling (see the discussion of the newly proposed definition later). In addition, information may be presented quite differently in different contexts. Information about Down syndrome, for example, may be communicated differently depending on whether the diagnosis was made prenatally or after the birth of an affected newborn (see Clinical Commentary 12-3) (although we would suggest that the information needs to be presented in a balanced manner in either situation).

In 2006, leaders in the field of genetic counseling and the National Society of Genetic Counselors reached a consensus on an updated and revised definition of genetic counseling:

Genetic counseling is the process of helping people understand and adapt to the medical, psychological, and familial implications of genetic contributions of disease. The process integrates the following: (1) interpretation of family and medical histories to assess the chance of disease occurrence or recurrence; (2) education about inheritance, testing, management, prevention, resources, and research; and (3) counseling to promote informed choices and adaptation to the risk of the condition.

The revised definition emphasizes the dual and integrated roles of education and counseling.

The majority of geneticists subscribe to the principle of nondirectiveness in reproductive counseling: Information about risks, natural history, treatment, and outcome is presented in a balanced and neutral manner, and decisions about reproduction are left to the family.

The facilitation of discussion about reproductive decision making is central to the task of genetic counseling. Several factors are involved in a family's decision about future pregnancies when there is an increased risk. The obvious ones are the magnitude of the risk figure and the burden or impact of the disorder. However, these are not the only significant issues. The individual family's perception of the impact of the condition is probably more important in their decision making than the professional's perception of the burden. The meaning of children to the individual family, according to their own cultural, religious, or personal preferences, is weighed heavily in the reproductive decision-making process. In addition, families frequently play out the scenario of coping with a recurrence of the condition in another child. Identification of these issues for a family often helps to stimulate their own discussions. Some families perceive a recurrence risk qualitatively rather than quantitatively: They consider themselves to be either "at risk" or not, with the actual risk estimate being a secondary consideration. The fact that there is so much variation in the importance people assign to each of these factors (perception of risk, perception of impact, meaning of children, and possibility of recurrence) underscores the point that the professional should be a facilitator and not the decision maker. Awareness of the family's views and values is needed to help in this complex undertaking.

A central task of genetic counseling is to help the family cope with the presence of the disorder or its recurrence risk, or both. This task is similar to the physician's support of a family dealing with any chronic disease or disability. What is unique, perhaps, is the family's perception of the meaning of a genetic disorder (Boxes 12-2 and 12-3). In many acquired conditions, such as infections or accidents, the ultimate meaning of the condition is externalized. In genetic disorders, the condition is more intrinsic to the individual and the family; it thus often presents a complex personal dilemma. Validation of the plight of families is vital and is probably more effective than simplistic attempts to remove guilt. Feelings of guilt and shame are natural to the situation and also need acknowledgment.

The primary care practitioner plays a vital role in the ongoing support of families in which a member has a genetic disease. Additional support strategies include referral of the family to a genetic support and advocacy group, distribution of current printed and Internet information on the disorder, referral to mental health professionals for ongoing counseling, and frequent follow-up visits that include time for discussions of feelings and thoughts.

 Genetic counseling includes many themes: medical diagnosis and management, determining risk of recurrence, options for addressing the risk, reproductive decision making, and support services.

Numerous studies in the past four decades have attempted to evaluate the effectiveness of genetic

---

BOX 12-2 Birth of a Child with Trisomy 18

Our daughter Juliett arrived on a beautiful summer afternoon in 1984. Late in my pregnancy, an ultrasound had showed an enlarged heart, dilated left kidney, and possible malformation of the cerebellum. During labor, our daughter's heart rate decelerated significantly, and we were given the option of an emergency C-section. Without hesitation, we opted for the C-section. A drape was hung so that I could not see, and I only knew that the baby was born when the pediatrician ran out of the room with something in his arms. My husband quickly followed, and then I waited for what seemed an eternity.

Juliett weighed 4 pounds, 6 ounces and was 18 inches long. I had graduated as an RN just before Juliett was conceived and had worked in a pediatric ICU. I had just enough experience to pick up a few of her obvious problems, but many escaped me. She was clearly much too thin, and her rib cage looked too short and prominent. But compared to the mental images I had formed after the ultrasound, I was relieved to see how beautiful she was. Her most striking feature was her incredible blue eyes, which were wide open and very alert. Her nose and mouth were beautifully formed and very petite. As my husband and I sat in awe over her, a neonatologist entered the room. He pointed out several characteristics, the only one of which I clearly remember was the clenched fist with the index finger lying over the middle finger. He concluded that she probably had trisomy 18. Of the grim things he rattled off, the only thing I remembered was that he said she would be a vegetable and that she would most likely die within the next couple of days. He then walked away, and we sat there, stunned. In this state of grief and turmoil I tried to understand how this clenched fist could lead to death, and how these bright, alert eyes could belong to a vegetable.

In the days that followed, I often opened up her fist and laid her fingers straight, hoping that the blood tests would not confirm the doctor's suspicions. Our bonding with Juli-

ett had been instant, and our great desire was to be able to take her home before she died. As she began to tolerate feedings and was weaned away from oxygen, our pleas to take her home were granted.

We left with no follow-up or care plan. Each time she went to sleep, we prayed she would wake up again and that we could complete another feeding. At 3 months of age, she started to smile at us, and our hopes brightened. We have been fortunate to see her outlive the grim statistics, and we have learned that there is no clear explanation why some children with this condition live longer than others. Juliett's heart was enlarged because of a defect similar to a tetralogy of Fallot. Mild scoliosis at birth has now progressed to a 100-degree lumbar curve and a 90-degree thoracic curve. Despite her many physical challenges, Juliett has continued at her slower pace to learn and develop new skills. Her personality is delightful, and people are often surprised to see how responsive and interactive she is.

We have often been asked if we were afraid to have more children. Perhaps we were crazy, but we felt that another like Juliett would be great. We have had four more girls. To everyone's surprise, our fifth child, Camille, was born with Down syndrome. With Juliett, the grieving process had been covered up with the gratitude we felt that she was even alive. With Camille, we experienced the more typical grieving process.

On the day of Juliett's birth, a pediatrician came forward, put his arms around us, and told us he thought she was beautiful and to love her for as long as she could be with us. He turned her into a human being with a life to be highly valued. In the 13 years that have followed, Juliett has seen many doctors. Most of them, although they could not cure her problems, gave us the most important thing we needed: to know that our daughter's life was of great worth and that, if they could, they would do anything to help her.

BOX 12-3 Raising a Child with Bloom Syndrome

Tommy was born via an emergency cesarean section, because 1 week before his delivery date his fetal movements markedly decreased. At birth, he weighed only 4 pounds, and the first time that I saw him, he was in an incubator connected to all sorts of tubes. He spent his first month of life in the neonatal intensive care unit so that his weight gain could be closely monitored. Because he was so small, he was fed through a feeding tube for many months, and as a consequence, he refused to drink from a bottle. Eventually, he overcame his aversion to using his mouth to eat but only after substantial training. Nevertheless, despite our care, Tommy remained small for his age.

The following summer, Tommy developed dark red marks on his cheeks and under his eyes. Our pediatrician referred us to a dermatologist, who suspected that the marks on Tommy's face were related to his growth failure. We were very surprised. How could these two findings be related? That is when we were told that Tommy might have a genetic disorder called Bloom syndrome. We hoped that the doctor was wrong, but soon thereafter Tommy had a genetic test that measured the number of sister chromatid exchanges per cell (see Chapter 2). This test confirmed that Tommy had Bloom syndrome. Although I insisted that it was a false-positive result, I learned to accept that our son had a very rare cancer syndrome.

We were barraged by questions from family, friends, and doctors. As a result, we became very protective of our son and his privacy. Nevertheless, there was only so much we could do to protect him because he is such a social little boy, loving to play with family and friends. This also made choosing an appropriate elementary school a very difficult decision for us. We expected that children would pick on him because of his small size. However, to our surprise, he easily developed friendships and adjusted well to his classmates. In fact, the problems that he did develop were largely because of his misbehavior. Thus, we struggled to find a balance between protecting Tommy while not permitting him special privileges because of his small stature.

In our home, we try to treat Tommy like any of our other children. One challenge for us is that because of Tommy's small size, people wrongly perceive that he is much younger than his chronological age. This is very frustrating for Tommy, yet we occasionally reinforce this image because of our concern for his safety. For example, although Tommy is 6 years old, he weighs only 21 pounds. Thus, he must sit in an infant seat when he travels in a car and we explain to Tommy's friends that it helps him see through the windows. Another safety problem is that many of the sensors for the automatic doors at supermarkets cannot detect his presence and easily slam into him.

Overall, Tommy has adapted well. He climbs or jumps in order to reach things. To keep up with his peers, he often runs, hops, or jumps instead of walking. We constantly worry about his safety, but we cannot control all that happens to him. To date, he has been healthy, and although it seems like we have been riding an emotional roller-coaster, we wouldn't trade our experiences for anything.

---

counseling. The methodology of these studies is complicated, and the evaluation of the results depends on one's interpretation of the goal of genetic counseling. A few general points, however, can be made. Families tend to recall recurrence risks relatively well. A letter sent to them after the visit improves this recall. Families who perceive their offspring's condition as being serious and one of impact recall risk figures better. Most studies suggest that genetic counseling is relatively effective in providing information about the medical aspects and genetic risks of the condition. Effectiveness regarding issues surrounding decision making and psychosocial support is more complex to define and assess and requires additional investigation.

Genetic Counselors and the Delivery of Genetic Counseling

As the discipline of medical genetics including genetic counseling evolved in the 1970s, it became clear that the delivery of this service is multifaceted and time-consuming. Not only did the geneticist need to have skills in most specialties of medicine, but facilitation of decision making and provision of psychological support were also necessary. As a need for genetics professionals other than physicians became apparent, a number of genetic counseling training programs emerged in the United States and Canada. Currently, 34 accredited programs in North America provide master's level training in genetic counseling. Genetic counselors have become integral partners with physicians and other professionals in the delivery of medical genetic services. From this growth evolved a professional society, The National Society of Genetic Counselors, and the certifying body, the American Board of Genetic Counseling, and the accrediting body, the Accreditation Council of Genetic Counseling. Although the range of skills is wide and job descriptions vary in different medical centers, genetic counselors have established themselves as experts in the determination of recurrence risk, reproductive decision making, and psychosocial support (Box 12-4). In the prenatal and cancer genetics settings, genetic counselors function relatively independently as practitioners and can often bill for their services. More recently, genetic counselors have become important professionals on research teams and in genetics laboratory services.

Genetic Advocacy Groups

These support groups can provide critical assistance to families who have a member with a genetic disorder (see, for example, Genetic Alliance under Suggested Readings and Websites at the end of this chapter). These organizations give the family the sense of a fellow traveler in a way that the professional is not able to do. The feeling of isolation that often accompanies genetic disorders (and rare conditions in general) is potentially alleviated by meeting someone else in the same situation. Immediate bonds are formed that can assist in the coping process. In the last few decades, a clear partnership of professionals and persons with genetic disorders and disabilities has developed. Not only have these groups provided a needed service, but they also have promoted the establishment of databases and research studies. Referral to a genetic support group and distribution of their written information are now a routine part of the care and management of all genetic disorders.

 The delivery of genetic services including genetic counseling involves a partnership of physicians, genetic counselors, and genetic advocacy groups.

Clinical Genetics Evaluation and Services

With the development of medical genetics as a medical specialty, clinical genetics services have become part of the health-care delivery system. Most university medical centers in North America include a genetics clinic whose major objective is to provide genetic diagnosis, management, and counseling services. In recent years adult genetics services and hereditary cancer clinics have developed as part of this growth.

As in all medical visits, evaluation of a person or family for a potential genetic condition requires a thorough history and physical examination. The history includes information about the family's concerns, the prenatal period, labor, delivery (in the assessment of a child), and documentation of family relationships (the pedigree). The physical examination should focus on the physical variations or minor anomalies that provide clues to a diagnosis. Additional family members might need evaluation for the presence or absence of a genetic disorder. Photographs and recording of certain physical measurements are a standard component of the genetic evaluation of a person for the consideration of a syndrome. Ancillary tests may be required to document specific physical features (e.g., an echocardiogram or MRI for aortic dilatation in Marfan syndrome or radiographs to diagnose achondroplasia).

One important component of clinical data gathered in this process is the family history (Box 12-5). The data obtained in a family history are often useful in obtaining an accurate diagnosis of a condition. For example, a strong family history of early-onset coronary disease might indicate the presence of a low-density lipoprotein-receptor defect causing familial hypercholesterolemia. A family history of early-onset colon cancer could indicate that a gene for familial adenomatous polyposis or hereditary nonpolyposis colorectal cancer is present in the family. An affected sibling with congenital sensorineural hearing loss suggests the presence of autosomal recessive deafness. Family history information can also guide the estimation of recurrence risks by helping to determine whether a genetic disease has been transmitted by one's parents or has occurred as a new mutation (this is especially important for diseases with reduced penetrance). The knowledge and skills required to take an accurate and thorough family history are important for all clinicians, not only clinical geneticists.

Routinely, the clinician sends the family a letter summarizing the diagnosis, natural history, and risk information regarding the condition. This letter is a valuable resource for the family, because it helps to document the risk information for later review. Information regarding lay advocacy groups, including the group's webpage, social network contact information, pamphlets, and booklets, is often provided. Follow-up visits are recommended depending on the individual situation. Box 12-6 provides a list of clinical genetics services.

BOX 12-4 An Insider's View of Genetic Counseling

What Is a Genetic Counselor?

In its most general usage, the term *genetic counselor* refers to any medical professional who is professionally qualified to provide genetic counseling. Typically, a genetic counselor is a genetic professional with a master's degree, with some genetic counselors having advanced degrees, generally in related fields. Degree programs in genetic counseling provide education and clinical training in medical genetics and counseling. A certified genetic counselor has also passed a certification examination administered by the American Board of Genetic Counseling or the American Board of Medical Genetics.

What Do Genetic Counselors Do?

The majority of genetic counselors practice in a clinical setting, often working as part of a team that may include medical geneticists, other physicians (e.g., obstetricians, oncologists, neurologists, social workers, psychologists, nutritionists, nurses). Genetic counselors collect and assess medical information leading to a diagnosis; provide patient education; provide psychosocial support and counseling; provide genetic counseling and risk assessment for genetic/genomic testing; help physicians with the management of genetic/genomic conditions; and provide patient follow-up. They often triage inquiries and referrals to the service in which they practice. They might manage or coordinate clinics and personnel. They are active in genetic education programs for medical professionals and the lay public.

In What Settings Do Genetic Counselors Work?

Genetic counselors work in obstetrics settings, providing counseling for prenatal diagnosis and screening, genetic testing for couples with multiple pregnancy loss, diagnosis and management of pregnancies affected with abnormalities detected by radiological imaging, and alternative reproductive technologies. They work in cancer genetics clinics, providing genetic counseling services for families with suspected or known cancer genetic syndromes. Genetic counselors also work in general genetics/genomics settings in pediatrics and adult medicine, as well as multidisciplinary specialty clinics for groups of diseases (e.g., metabolic, craniofacial, bone dysplasia, neurogenetic, cardiovascular) or for single diseases (e.g., Down syndrome, neurofibromatosis, hemophilia).

Many counselors participate in research related to clinical genetics/genomics and genetic counseling. For example, predictive testing for disorders such as Huntington disease and hereditary cancers was initiated mainly in research studies aimed at assessing the medical, ethical, legal, and social consequences. More recently, genetic counselors have participated in clinical trials evaluating the transmission of information from tests such as whole exome sequencing, which provides information not just about the condition tested for, but information about many other "actionable" genetic traits. These studies are examining patient preferences and the consequences of providing this ancillary information in a clinical setting. Within a research setting, genetic counselors provide counseling and help to design, implement, evaluate, and publish research.

Many genetic counselors are employed by laboratories to provide an interface between the laboratory and its clients (health-care practitioners, patients, or both), as part of the sales force, and to help develop laboratory protocols, policies, and educational materials. A small percentage of genetic counselors are in private practice, and some work in administrative positions for the state or federal government or other agencies. Many genetic counselors are active at regional and national levels in professional organizations, and some counselors help to start, maintain, or advise lay advocacy groups for genetic disorders.

What Skills and Personal Qualities Make a Good Genetic Counselor?

A good genetic counselor needs both a strong background in the biological sciences and genetics and training in the theory and practice of psychosocial techniques (e.g., family systems, crisis counseling, interviewing skills, aid with decision making, health promotion). Because most genetic counselors provide direct patient service, it is essential to work well with people. Genetic counselors must work well both independently and on a team. There is a high level of responsibility involved in direct and indirect patient care aspects and participation in policy decisions, and counselors must successfully learn to handle the stress of the difficult situations of the families and agencies with whom they work.

What Is the Future of Genetic Counseling?

In the last 10 years, clinical genetics/genomics has moved solidly into mainstream medicine. Genetic counselors continue to increase in number, but the rapid increase of genetic/genomic tests into all aspects of medicine also requires genetic counselors and other geneticists to participate in education and support for other health-care providers. As genomic testing becomes the norm, genetic counselors will help develop and carry out the techniques for clinical interpretation of the vast amount of personal data generated. The National Society of Genetic Counselors is currently examining workforce issues and the Association of Genetic Counseling Program Directors is examining advanced training options for certified genetic counselors. What is undisputed is the striking emergence of medical genetics from an obscure medical subspecialty to an area of knowledge that is fast becoming integrated into every field of medicine.

(Courtesy Bonnie J. Baty, M.S.)

BOX 12-5 The Family History

A thorough, accurate family history is an indispensable part of a medical evaluation, and a pedigree should be part of the patient's chart. At a minimum, the following items should be included.

- The sex of each individual and his or her relationship to other family members. This information should be indicated using standard pedigree symbols (see Chapter 4).
- A three-generation family history should be obtained. For example, male relatives on the mother's side of the family will be especially important when considering an X-linked recessive disorder.
- The age of each individual. A record must be kept of whether each individual is affected with the disease in question, and inquiries should be made about diseases that may be related to the disease in question (e.g., ovarian cancer in a family being seen for familial breast cancer).
- All known miscarriages and stillbirths.
- The ethnic origin of the family. This is important because many diseases vary considerably in prevalence among different ethnic groups.
- Information about consanguinity. Although it is relatively rare in most Western populations, consanguinity is common in many of the world's populations, and immigrant populations often maintain relatively high rates of consanguinity (see Chapter 4).
- Changes in family histories. Family members develop newly diagnosed diseases, and additional children are born. These changes can affect diagnosis and risk estimation, so the family history and pedigree should be updated periodically.

(see Guidelines in Suggested Readings and Websites, Benentt et al.)

BOX 12-6 Types of Clinical Genetic Services and Programs

Center-based genetics clinics
Outreach clinics
Inpatient consultations
Specialty clinics
- Metabolic clinics
- Cancer genetics clinics
- Spina bifida clinics
- Hemophilia clinics
- Craniofacial clinics
- Other single-disorder clinics (e.g., NF1 clinics)
Prenatal diagnosis programs: Perinatal and reproductive genetics clinics
- Amniocentesis and chorionic villus sampling clinics
- Ultrasound programs
- Maternal serum screening programs (see Chapter 10)
- Preimplantation diagnosis programs
- Presymptomatic diagnosis in families (e.g., familial breast cancer diagnosis)
Genetic screening
- Newborn screening program/follow-up clinics
- Other population screening programs (e.g., Tay-Sachs disease)
Education and training
- Health-care professionals, including clinical geneticists and genetic counselors
- General public
- School system
- Teratology information services

> Clinical genetic evaluations include physical examination, detailed family history, ancillary tests as needed, and communication of information to the family through letters and the distribution of published literature.

The care of persons with genetic disease includes the development of guidelines for follow-up and routine care. Knowledge of the natural history of a condition, coupled with a critical review of screening tests and interventions, can provide a framework for health supervision and anticipatory guidance. The management plan can subsequently be used by the primary care provider. It is primarily for this purpose that many of the specialized clinics, such as those for NF1 or hemophilia, have been established. An example of this approach is the management checklist for the health maintenance of infants and children with Down syndrome (see Chapter 6). Gene Reviews, a highly important resource for practitioners in any setting, provides these guidelines for all of the genetic conditions included in their database (see Suggested Readings and Websites below).

As treatment options for mendelian disorders become more numerous (e.g., the treatment of aortic dilatation in Marfan syndrome; see Chapter 4), the role of clinical geneticists will likely change. Since the turn of the 21st century, geneticists have become increasingly involved in the design and implementation of clinical trials, and this trend will certainly continue and change the nature of the practice.

BOX 12-7 Common Indications for Genetics Referral

Evaluation of a person with cognitive disability or developmental delay

Evaluation of a person with single or multiple malformations; question of a dysmorphic syndrome

Evaluation of a person with a possible inherited metabolic disease

Presence of a possible single-gene disorder

Presence of a chromosomal disorder, including balanced rearrangements

Person at risk for a genetic condition, including questions of presymptomatic diagnosis or cancer risk

Person or family with questions about the genetic aspects of any medical condition

Couples with a history of recurrent miscarriages

Consanguinity in a couple, usually first cousin or closer relationship

Teratogen counseling

Preconceptional counseling and risk-factor counseling, including advanced maternal age and other potential indications for prenatal diagnosis

---

Traditionally, genetic counseling involves the family who comes in with questions about the diagnosis, management, and recurrence risk of the condition in question. Thus, in the majority of situations, genetic counseling is carried out retrospectively. With the increased availability of prenatal, carrier, and presymptomatic testing, and the expected rise in the personalized health-care model, prospective genetic counseling will become more common. Box 12-7 lists common reasons for referral for genetic evaluation.

DYSMORPHOLOGY AND CLINICAL TERATOLOGY

Dysmorphology was defined at the beginning of this chapter as the study of abnormal physical development (**morphogenesis**). Congenital defects are caused by altered morphogenesis. Although the term *dysmorphology* may seem synonymous with **teratology,** the latter term usually implies the study of the environmental causes of congenital anomalies, even though its literal meaning does not refer to etiology. (The term *teratology* is derived from *teras*, the Greek word for "monster." The term dysmorphology was proposed by Dr. David Smith as a reaction to the pejorative connotation of teratology.)

Congenital defects represent an important cause of infant mortality and morbidity. Current studies indicate that the frequency of medically significant malformations diagnosed in the newborn period is about 2%. Investigations that have observed children for a longer period demonstrate that this frequency increases to about 3% by the age of 1 year. In the United States, congenital malformations represent the most common cause of mortality during the first year of life. Table 12-1 lists some of the most common and important malformation syndromes.

There are several ways to classify congenital abnormalities. The most common classification approach is by organ system or body region (e.g., craniofacial,

TABLE 12-1 Examples of Common Multiple Congenital Anomaly and Dysplasia Syndromes Referred to a General Medical Genetics Clinic

SYNDROMES	ETIOLOGY
Down syndrome	Chromosomal
Neurofibromatosis type 1	Single gene (AD)
Angelman syndrome	Microdeletion of chromosome 15q; uniparental disomy
Amnion disruption sequence	Unknown
Osteogenesis imperfecta	Single gene; heterogeneous, AD, AR; type I collagen, and related genes
Trisomy 18	Chromosomal
VATER association	Unknown
Marfan syndrome	Single gene (AD)
Prader-Willi syndrome	Microdeletion of chromosome 15q; uniparental disomy
Noonan syndrome	Single gene (AD)
Williams syndrome	Microdeletion of chromosome 7
Achondroplasia	Single gene (AD)
Trisomy 13	Chromosomal
Turner syndrome	Chromosomal (45,X)
Rett syndrome	X-linked gene
Rubinstein-Taybi syndrome	Single gene (AD)
Klippel-Trenaunay	Heterogeneous; one susceptibility syndrome gene identified
Fetal alcohol syndrome	Excessive alcohol
Cornelia de Lange syndrome	Single gene (AD)

AD, Autosomal dominant, *AR*, autosomal recessive; *VATER*, vertebral anomalies, anal atresia, tracheoesophageal fistula, esophageal atresia, renal anomalies.

limb, heart). More clinically useful classification schemes include (1) single defect versus multiple congenital anomalies, including a recognizable syndrome, (2) major (medically or surgically significant defects) versus minor anomalies, (3) categorization by pathogenic process, and (4) etiological classification.

Regarding etiologic classification, there has been only one investigation in North America that examined the causes of the malformations in a cohort of infants with congenital defects (see Nelson and Holmes on the Readings list). These authors list the causes of the various defects in their study conducted in Boston. Three key messages emerged from these data: the cause of two thirds of the congenital defects is either unknown or falls into the multifactorial category (see Chapter 5); well-established environmental causes of congenital malformations are infrequent (less than 4%); and a known genetic component is identified in approximately 30% of cases.

Principles of Dysmorphology

In discussing the basic principles of dysmorphology, it is important to define certain key terms. The following definitions, based on pathogenic processes, are used in clinical practice:

- **Malformation** is a congenital morphologic anomaly of a single organ or body part due to an alteration of a primary developmental program (e.g., cleft lip, polydactyly).
- **Dysplasia** is a morphologic anomaly involving a dynamic or ongoing alteration of cellular constitution or tissue organization within a specific organ or tissue type (e.g., ectodermal dysplasia).
- **Sequence** is one or more secondary morphologic anomalies known or presumed to cascade from a single malformation or dysplasia (e.g., Pierre Robin sequence, a disorder in which a primary defect in mandibular development produces secondarily a small jaw, glossoptosis, and a cleft palate).
- **Syndrome** is a pattern of multiple primary malformations known or thought to be causally related (e.g., trisomy 13 syndrome).
- **Deformation** is alteration of the shape or position of a normally formed body part due to aberrant mechanical forces. It usually occurs in the fetal period, not in embryogenesis. A deformation is a secondary alteration and can be extrinsic, as in oligohydramnios (reduced amniotic fluid), or intrinsic, as in congenital myotonic dystrophy.
- **Disruption** is a congenital morphological defect of an organ, part of an organ, or a larger region of the body resulting from the breakdown of a body structure that had a normal developmental potential. It is by definition a secondary malformation (e.g., secondary limb defect resulting from a vascular event).

Note that malformations and dysplasias are morphologic anomalies whose primary events occur in embryogenesis and histogenesis, whereas disruptions and deformations are by definition secondary. All of these terms were recently updated and clarified by an international working group called the Elements of Morphology; see Suggested Readings at the end of the chapter.

When evaluating a child with a congenital malformation, the most important question is whether the abnormality represents a single, isolated anomaly or is instead one component of a broader, organized pattern of malformation (i.e., a syndrome). This concept is exemplified by the evaluation of a baby with a cleft lip. If a baby has an isolated, nonsyndromic cleft lip with no other malformations, the discussion of natural history, genetics, prognosis, and management is markedly different than if the baby's cleft lip is one feature of the trisomy 13 syndrome (see Chapter 6). The former condition can be repaired surgically and has a relatively low recurrence risk (see Chapter 5) and few associated medical problems. Trisomy 13 is a serious chromosomal disorder. In addition to orofacial clefts, these infants usually have a congenital heart defect and central nervous system malformations. More importantly, 50% of children with trisomy 13 die in the newborn period, and 90% die before 1 year of age. Thus, prediction of the natural history and medical management in these two examples are quite different.

Another example is a child with cleft lip who also has pits or fistulas of the lower lip. The combination of orofacial clefts and lip pits signifies an autosomal dominant condition called the van der Woude syndrome. Although the natural history of this condition differs little from that of nonsyndromic cleft lip, the discussion of genetic recurrence risks is much different. In the evaluation of a child with van der Woude syndrome, it is very important to determine whether one of the parents carries the gene. If so, the sibling recurrence risk is 50%. This is much greater than the 4% sibling recurrence risk usually given for nonsyndromic cleft lip (see Chapter 5). Because van der Woude syndrome has variable expression and often is manifested only by lip fistulas, it is quite commonly overlooked. Thus, a careful physical examination, combined with a knowledge of the genetics of isolated malformations and syndromes, is necessary to determine accurate recurrence risks.

▶ The most important question to ask when evaluating a child with a congenital malformation is whether the defect is isolated or part of a syndrome pattern.

Increasing knowledge of the pathogenesis of human congenital defects has led to a better understanding of the developmental relationship of the defects in multiple congenital anomaly patterns. Some well-established conditions that appear to be true syndromes at first glance are really a constellation of defects consisting of a primary malformation with its secondary, localized effects (i.e., a sequence). In a sequence, the pattern is a developmental unit in which the cascade of secondary pathogenic events is well understood. In contrast, the pathogenic relationship of the primary malformations in a syndrome is not as well understood, although pathogenesis may be clarified when the syndrome is the result of the pleiotropic effects of a single gene (e.g., Marfan syndrome; see Chapter 4).

One of the best examples of a sequence is the Potter phenotype or oligohydramnios sequence. It is currently believed that any significant and persistent condition leading to oligohydramnios can produce this sequence, whether it be intrauterine renal failure due to kidney malformations (such as missing kidneys, renal agenesis) or chronic leakage of amniotic fluid. The fetus will develop a pattern of secondary growth deficiency, joint contractures (deformations), characteristic facial features, and pulmonary hypoplasia (Fig. 12-3). Before the cause of these features was understood, the phenotype was termed the *Potter syndrome*. Now, with the understanding that all of the features are secondary to oligohydramnios, the disorder is more properly called the *oligohydramnios sequence*. As with any malformation, the renal defect can occur by itself, or it can be a part of any number of syndromes in which renal malformations are component features (such as autosomal recessive Meckel-Gruber syndrome or the more common nonsyndromic multifactorially caused disorder, bilateral renal agenesis). Distinguishing between syndromes and sequences can often improve understanding of the underlying cause of a disorder and aid in prediction of prognosis.

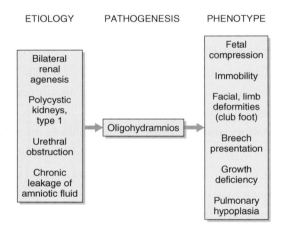

FIG 12-3 The oligohydramnios sequence. Oligohydramnios can arise from a number of distinct causes. It produces a constellation of secondary phenotypic features.

▶ It is important to distinguish between a sequence, which is a primary defect with secondary structural changes, and a syndrome, which is a collection of malformations whose relationship to one another tends to be less well understood.

Clinical Teratology

A **teratogen** is an agent external to the fetus's genome that induces structural malformations, growth deficiency, and/or functional alterations during prenatal development. Although teratogens cause only a small percentage of all congenital defects, the preventive potential alone makes them worthy of study. Table 12-2 lists the well established human teratogens due to medications or drugs. Other categories of agents include infectious diseases during pregnancy (e.g., cytomegalic virus), maternal disease states (e.g., maternal diabetes mellitus), and ionizing radiation.

It is important to understand the reasoning process that leads to the designation of a substance or exposure as a teratogen. This process is based on an evaluation of epidemiological, clinical, biochemical, and physiological evidence. Animal studies can also help to establish whether an agent is teratogenic and provide insight into pathogenesis.

The key issues involved in determining whether an agent is teratogenic are summarized in Clinical Commentary 12-4. A key clinical point is that it is common for families to ask their health-care professionals questions about the risks of certain exposures during pregnancy. When faced with such a question, the clinician has a number of options. One is to review the literature on particular exposures in humans, make a judgment regarding the degree of risk, and then provide counseling. Various online and printed sources available to the clinician are listed at the end of the chapter. An alternative is to refer the patient to a teratology information service or to a clinical genetics unit. Because of the complexity of these issues, teratology information services have sprung up throughout the United States,

---

CLINICAL COMMENTARY 12-4

The Bendectin Saga

Bendectin, or doxyclamine, was an agent introduced in the 1960s for "morning sickness" (nausea and vomiting during pregnancy). The agent was particularly efficacious, and during the 1970s about one third of American women took Bendectin at some time during their first trimester of pregnancy.

Bendectin has probably been studied more than any other individual pregnancy medication. Several epidemiological studies have found no conclusive evidence of an increased risk of congenital malformations with use of Bendectin during pregnancy. The few studies that have demonstrated weak associations between Bendectin and birth defects did not reveal any consistent patterns. Animal studies also indicate no association. Despite these data, a number of lawsuits were filed in the 1980s against the company that marketed Bendectin. As a result, the company removed the drug from the market.

The reasoning process used to determine causation in such cases is complex. Before judgments about etiology are made, a critical review of the literature is required. The available epidemiological studies must be evaluated in terms of their methodology, design, and biases. Up-to-date knowledge of the etiology and pathogenesis of congenital malformations must be included in the design of the study. The basic principles of teratology must be applied. This includes an evaluation of the critical period (i.e., did exposure occur during the period of pregnancy in which the malformed fetal structures were developing?). Clinical evidence includes the search for a pattern of defects (i.e., a specific syndrome), because all well-established teratogens produce consistent patterns. Animal models never prove causation in humans but can provide supportive evidence and information about pathogenesis. In addition, the proposed effect of the agent should be biologically plausible.

A review of the evidence regarding Bendectin shows that it meets none of these criteria. Indeed, because of its extensive testing, Bendectin satisfies standard criteria for safety as well as any known medication. What, then, could have produced this litigation? An important part of the answer to this question involves the coincidental occurrence of congenital malformations and Bendectin exposure. Considering that a major congenital malformation will be diagnosed in 3% of infants by 1 year of age and that about one third of women were taking Bendectin in the first trimester of pregnancy, then about 1% ($1/3 \times 3\%$) of all pregnancies in the 1970s would have experienced the co-occurrence of these two events by chance alone. Because about two thirds of congenital malformations have no known cause, it is not surprising that many families of children with these disorders (and their lawyers) would attribute them to Bendectin use.

Bendectin was removed from the market in 1983. Since then, the percentage of babies born with congenital malformations has remained the same, and the number of women admitted to hospitals for complaints of morning sickness has doubled.

It is very difficult to prove epidemiologically that any exposure is "safe." The statistical power of such studies does not permit an absolute statement that there is no effect. All that can be demonstrated is that there is no definitive evidence that a particular agent (in this case, Bendectin) causes an adverse outcome. Blanket reassurance or absolute statements of complete safety are not appropriate. On the other hand, when the evidence is relatively conclusive, as in the case of Bendectin, it is clinically appropriate to have a reassuring tone in discussing exposure in the pregnancy setting. Notably the generic form of Bendectin has recently been rereleased onto the Canadian markets.

TABLE 12-2 Well-Established Human Teratogens[*]

DRUG	POTENTIAL DEFECT	CRITICAL EXPOSURE PERIOD	PERCENTAGE OF THOSE EXPOSED WHO ARE AFFECTED
Angiotensin-converting enzyme (ACE) inhibitors	Renal dysgenesis; oligohydramnios; skull ossification defects	Second to third trimester	NE
Alcohol, chronic	Craniofacial and central nervous system anomalies; heart defects	<12 wk	10-15
	Low birth weight; developmental delay	>24 wk	NE
Aminopterin	Spontaneous abortion	<14 wk	NE
	Craniofacial anomalies; limb defects; craniosynostosis; neural tube defects	First trimester	NE
	Low birth weight	>20 wk	NE
High-dose androgens or norprogesterones	Masculinization of external female genitalia	>10 wk	0.3
Carbamazepine	Spina bifida	<30 days after conception	≈1
Carbimazole/ methimazole	Hypothyroidism; goiter, Choanal atresia, scalp defects, other anomalies?	NE	NE
Cocaine	Abruptio placentae	Second to third trimester	NE
	Intracranial hemorrhage; premature labor and delivery	Third trimester	NE
Diethylstilbestrol	Uterine abnormalities; vaginal adenosis; vaginal adenocarcinoma; cervical ridges; male infertility	<12 wk	NE
Fluconazole (high-dose)	Limb and craniofacial defects	First trimester	NE
Isotretinoin	Fetal death; hydrocephalus; central nervous system defects; microtia or anotia; small or missing thymus; conotruncal heart defects; micrognathia	>15 days after conception	45-50
Methotrexate	Craniosynostosis; underossified skull; craniofacial dysmorphology; limb defects	6-9 wk after conception	NE
Mycophenolate mofetil	Ear malformation, orofacial clefts, and heart defects	First trimester	NE
Penicillamine	Cutis laxa, joint contractures	NE	NE
Phenytoin	Craniofacial anomalies; hypoplastic phalanges and nails	First trimester	10-30
Solvents, abuse (entire pregnancy)	Small size for gestational age; developmental delay		NE
Streptomycin	Hearing loss	Third trimester	NE
Tetracycline	Stained teeth and bone	>20 wk	NE
Thalidomide	Limb deficiencies; ear anomalies	38-50 days post-LMP	15-25
Thiouracil	Spontaneous abortion	First trimester	NE
	Stillbirth	>20 wk	NE
	Goiter		NE
Trimethadione	Developmental delay; V-shaped eyebrows; low-set ears; irregular teeth	First trimester	NE
Valproic acid	Spina bifida	<30 days after conception	≈1-2
	Craniofacial anomalies; preaxial defects	First trimester	NE
Warfarin	Nasal hypoplasia; stippled epiphyses	6-9 wk	NE
	Central nervous system defects secondary to cerebral hemorrhage	>12 wk	NE

Data from Martinez LP, Robertson J, Leen-Mitchell M: Environmental causes of birth defects. In: Rudolph CD, Rudolph AM, Hostetter MK, et al: *Rudolph's Pediatrics*. 21st ed. New York: McGraw-Hill; 2002:9.

NE, Not established; *post-LMP*, after last menstrual period.

[*]Other established teratogens include maternal infections (rubella, cytomegalovirus, toxoplasmosis, varicella, Venezuela equine encephalitis, syphilis, parvovirus), maternal disease states (diabetes mellitus, phenylketonuria, systemic lupus erythematosus, Graves' disease), and ionizing radiation.

Canada, and Europe. The Organization of Teratology Information Services (OTIS) provides current and comprehensive information on exposures in pregnancy, lists the available teratology information services in North America, and provides connections to a regional resource.

 Teratogens are external agents that cause a small but important percentage of congenital malformations. It is often difficult to prove conclusively that a substance is teratogenic.

Prevention of Congenital Malformations

Because the majority of structural defects have no obvious cause, their prevention presents a challenge. An example is fetal alcohol syndrome (FAS), one of the more common preventable causes of human malformation (Clinical Commentary 12-5). The institution of rubella immunization programs and the preconceptional administration of folic acid exemplify successful prevention (Clinical Commentary 12-6).

Preconceptional counseling is a model for primary prevention. Women who have diabetes mellitus, phenylketonuria, or systemic lupus erythematosus (an autoimmune disorder involving production of autoantibodies that affect multiple organs) can decrease their risk of producing an infant with a structural defect through appropriate preconceptional management, a primary prevention strategy. Examples of secondary and tertiary levels of prevention, respectively, include newborn screening for hearing loss and the provision of high-quality medical care for infants and children with congenital malformations. Instituting appropriate guidelines for health supervision and anticipatory guidance can decrease some of the complications of these disorders. Also important is public education regarding the limitations of scientific knowledge and the emotional difficulties of families in which a child has a congenital defect. Such information has the potential to diminish anxiety, improve the family's coping process, and reduce the stigma that surrounds congenital malformations and genetic disorders.

CLINICAL COMMENTARY 12-5
Fetal Alcohol Syndrome

Among the human teratogens, one of the most common and potentially preventable exposures is excessive alcohol consumption. Women who are chronic alcoholics are at significant risk of bearing a child with the fetal alcohol syndrome (FAS). This condition consists of prenatal and postnatal growth deficiency, microcephaly (small head), a wide range of develop- mental disabilities, and a constellation of facial alterations (Fig. 12-4).The more distinctive and consistent facial features include short palpebral fissures, underdeveloped philtral folds, and a thin upper lip vermilion. (See the Elements of Morphology reference at the end of the chapter for the precise definition of these terms.) Although most of these signs are not specific for FAS, their mutual occurrence in the context of maternal alcohol abuse allows the clinician to make the diagnosis.

In addition to these findings, infants and children with FAS are at risk for a number of structural defects, including congenital heart malformations, neural tube defects, and renal anomalies. Most children with FAS have a mild degree of developmental delay, ranging from mild cognitive disability to learning difficulties. Additionally many children with FAS have significant behavioral problems.

There are still many unanswered questions regarding alcohol use in pregnancy. These include the extent of genetic predisposition to FAS, the risk of binge drinking, the role of moderate and social drinking, and the safe level of alcohol in pregnancy. Although there is no conclusive evidence that light drinking in early pregnancy is harmful, avoidance of alcohol during pregnancy is the most prudent approach.

FIG 12-4 A 2-year-old child with fetal alcohol syndrome. Note the depressed nasal root, short palpebral fissures, smooth philtrum, and thin upper lip vermilion.

CLINICAL COMMENTARY 12-6
Folate and the Prevention of Neural Tube Defects

The primary prevention of congenital malformations is an important goal of clinical genetics. Because the ultimate cause of most congenital malformations is currently unknown, there are relatively few opportunities for primary prevention. A recent approach to the prevention of congenital malformations is the periconceptional use of folate and multivitamin regimens to prevent the occurrence and recurrence of neural tube defects (NTDs).

NTDs consist of malformations of the developing neural tube and express themselves as anencephaly, encephalocele, and spina bifida (see Chapter 5). Their impact is serious: Anencephaly is invariably fatal, and the medical complications of spina bifida (lower limb paralysis, hydrocephalus, urinary obstruction) are significant. Because of the potential influence of nutritional elements on embryogenesis, a series of epidemiological studies were performed in the 1970s and 1980s. With one exception, they demonstrated that the use of vitamins and folate in the periconception period reduced the recurrence risk of spina bifida and anencephaly in families that had previously had a child with one of these conditions. In 1991 the Medical Research Council of the United Kingdom published a double-blind study* in which 4 mg of folate with or without vitamins was administered to women who had had a child with an NTD. The group receiving folate alone experienced a 70% reduction in the recurrence of these malformations in their offspring. In 1992, a Hungarian group demonstrated the usefulness of vitamins and folic acid in preventing the initial occurrence of NTDs. In this study, two groups of women, one receiving vitamins and folic acid and the other not, were followed for the duration of their pregnancies. The vitamin-and-folic acid regimen significantly decreased the occurrence of NTDs. Numerous additional studies have confirmed these results.

Although it is still not clear whether the purported protective effect is due to folic acid or a combination of folic acid and other vitamins, these data indicate that periconceptional vitamin use is an effective prevention strategy. The mechanism for the apparent effect remains unknown. Nonetheless, the encouraging results of these studies have prompted the Centers for Disease Control and Prevention to publish two recommendations regarding the use of folate. The first is that all women who have previously had a child with an NTD should take 4 mg/d of folic acid if they are planning to become pregnant. The second recommendation is that all women of reproductive age should take 0.4 mg/d of folic acid (the amount available in a typical multivitamin tablet) throughout their reproductive years. The latter recommendation is prudent in light of the fact that approximately half of pregnancies in the United States are unplanned. These recommendations have led to the folic acid fortification of wheat and other grain products in the United States and other nations. In the past decade, studies in a variety of countries throughout the world have demonstrated a decrease in the occurrence of NTDs after the initiation of a food fortification program.

*A double-blind study is one in which, during the treatment phase of the study, neither the subjects nor the investigator knows which subjects are receiving an active ingredient and which are receiving placebo.

BIOETHICS AND MEDICAL GENETICS

With new discoveries and advances in medical technology come new choices for patients, families, and society. As medical genetics came to be defined as a medical specialty during the past several decades, a number of new issues in bioethics also emerged. Because of the significance and complexity of these issues, a significant portion of the budget of the Human Genome Project was devoted to the ethical, legal, and social implications of human genetics. Some of these implications have been touched upon previously in this textbook (e.g., genetic testing, gene therapy, embryonic stem cell research). Our goal here is to provide a sampling of the major ethical questions currently confronting the medical and genetics communities.

The combination of advances in prenatal diagnosis (e.g., ultrasound, amniocentesis), the ability to determine the human karyotype, and the option of pregnancy termination set the stage for the rise of prenatal diagnosis as a clinical service in the 1970s. By that time, most tertiary medical centers in developed nations offered amniocentesis for various indications, most commonly advanced maternal age (see Chapter 10). In the early discussions of the ethics of prenatal diagnosis, the central controversy involved a woman's (or couple's) right to terminate a pregnancy. In the 1990s, the issue took on a new dimension with the concern that persons with disabilities may be devalued by society when prenatal diagnosis can lead to the selective termination of fetuses with a disability. Similar concerns revolve around the issue of withdrawal of support for newborns with serious birth defects (e.g., trisomy 13, some neural tube defects). The main principles guiding decisions about these issues are to consider the best interests of the child and to provide genetic counseling so that the parents can make an informed decisio.

Ethical concerns have arisen about other types of genetic testing, including carrier testing and pre-symptomatic testing (see Chapter 10). Genetic tests differ from other types of medical testing because genes (including mutations that predispose to disease) can be shared in families. Thus, a genetic test performed in one person might reveal risk information about a relative who might not wish to know about his or her risk (e.g., testing of a young adult for an autosomal dominant disease might indicate that one of the parents must have transmitted the disease-causing mutation). In addition, many people perceive that their genetic inheritance is very much an intrinsic part of themselves (and their families). Genetic risk is often misperceived as "unchangeable." All of these factors can lead to unfair stigmatization of individuals, families, and even whole populations. To help counter this, care providers must be sensitive to the needs and concerns of individuals and their families. They should avoid making value judgments that could lead to or reinforce stigmatization. They should dispel notions of genetic determinism, making it clear to families that genes are but one part of the cause of a disease. Nongenetic factors, which often can be altered, can also play an important role. As with all medical information, privacy and confidentiality must be respected.

Genetic testing also raises the specter of discrimination by insurance companies or employers. Insurance companies have long collected information about family history as a means of assessing risk. In some cases (e.g., an individual at risk for inheriting a *BRCA1* mutation), a genetic test can provide a much more accurate measure of disease risk. At-risk persons are understandably concerned about the possibility of losing their insurance benefits or their employment because of the outcome of a genetic test. A paradoxical result is that some choose not to be tested, even when it could lead to a potentially life-saving intervention. Insurance providers and employers reason that denying coverage (or increas-

ing premiums) to at-risk individuals serves the general interest by minimizing costs. Others respond that, unlike lifestyle choices such as cigarette smoking or exercise, one does not choose one's genes, so it is unfair to discriminate on the basis of genetic tests.

Because of concerns in the United States regarding discrimination in employment and health insurance, the genetics community and supportive legislators worked together during the early 2000s to enact legislation to ensure the confidentiality of genetic test results. The Genetic Information Nondiscrimination Act (GINA) was formulated to prevent the discriminatory use of genetic test results by employers or health insurers. GINA became a federal law in 2008 and took effect in 2009.

Preimplantation genetic testing (see Chapter 10) has also been the focus of ethical debates. For example, this form of testing can be used to determine the sex of an embryo. Indeed, an early application was to avoid implanting male embryos that had an increased risk of carrying an X-linked recessive mutation. Many scientists and ethicists believe that pre-implantation diagnosis solely for sex selection is inappropriate, and the practice is currently banned in the United Kingdom. Preimplantation diagnosis could also be used to select preferentially for embryos that *do* carry disease-causing mutations. For example, an embryo that is homozygous for mutations causing autosomal recessive deafness could be selected to match the phenotypes of deaf parents (a case was reported in which deaf parents deliberately conceived a deaf child by artificial insemination). Such applications might put the interests of the parents and the interests of the child in conflict. Another controversial application of pre-implantation diagnosis was in the selection of a human leukocyte antigen (HLA)-matched embryo that could later provide bone marrow cells for an older sibling who had Fanconi anemia. It is argued that such persons could feel that their life was devalued because they had been selected partly on the basis of their suitability as a bone marrow donor.

Questions have arisen about the genetic testing of children. When such testing can lead to useful diagnostic measures or interventions, it may be warranted. An example would be the genetic testing of children at risk for inheriting a mutation in the adenomatous polyposis coli (*APC*) gene. As discussed in Chapter 8, colonoscopy should begin in gene carriers by age 12 years and is potentially life-saving. In contrast, childhood diagnosis of Huntington disease currently provides no preventive or therapeutic benefits and increases the potential for anxiety and stigmatization. A consensus has emerged that childhood genetic testing should not be pursued unless it provides an avenue to clinically beneficial intervention.

With the advent of whole exome and genome sequencing in the clinical arena (see Chapter 10), significant controversy arose in the field surrounding the reporting of **incidental** (or secondary) **findings** that were commonly detected in the testing process. These findings represent variations unrelated to the original indication for ordering the study but of potential medical value in patient care. Some geneticists felt that all variations should be reported to the patient (or family) while others argued that only "medically actionable" findings should be shared. A Working Group of the ACMG was convened in 2012, and after a year-long process of consensus provided a set of recommendations now widely adopted in the field (see Suggested Readings and Websites, Green et al). The panel recommended that laboratories performing these new tests analyze and report variants of genes for a specified group of 56 conditions; they encouraged the development of an ongoing process for updating the guidelines.

Intense controversy has surrounded the issues of cloning and embryonic stem cell research (see Chapter 10). It is important to repeat the distinction between *reproductive* cloning and *therapeutic* cloning. Because of the high failure rate of reproductive cloning in other mammals, and because the benefits of reproductive cloning are unclear, the scientific community is nearly unanimous in its opposition to the creation of human beings through reproductive cloning. The use of cloning to create embryonic stem cells for therapeutic purposes (e.g., pancreatic islet cells for patients with diabetes or neurons for those

with Alzheimer disease) is more controversial and, like pregnancy termination, involves highly charged questions about the definition of human life and the limits of medical intervention. As noted in Chapter 10, these issues require informed and thoughtful input from the scientific community and from patient advocacy groups, ethicists, philosophers, legal scholars, the clergy, and others.

The science of genetics is no stranger to controversy and even to abuse. The **eugenics** movement (Greek, "good birth"), popular in the United States and some European countries in the early part of the 20th century, advocated both "positive eugenics" (preferential reproduction of those deemed to be genetically more fit) and "negative eugenics" (the prevention of reproduction of those thought to be genetically less fit). Eugenics, in concert with the political thinking of the times, led to a series of abuses that culminated in the atrocities of Nazi Germany. These events are a sobering reminder of the potential for misuse of genetic information. Geneticists must help to ensure that their science is used for maximum benefit while adhering to the time-honored maxim *primum non nocere* ("first, do no harm").

SUMMARY

Clinical genetics and genetic counseling are two main approaches to the early detection and prevention of disease. The field of dysmorphology has influenced and paralleled the emergence of clinical genetics. In clinical genetics, accurate diagnosis is the most important first step in patient care. The process of diagnosing a genetic disorder involves a complex sequence of events and depends on diagnostic decision making, recognition of important phenotypic signs, and application of principles of dysmorphology and medical genetics as well as laboratory diagnosis. Genetic counseling is a central focus of medical genetics and with accurate diagnosis comprises the cornerstone of the field. In fact, genetic counseling is centered in the conventional medical model because it depends on accurate diagnosis and knowledge of medical genetics. Genetic counseling includes many aspects: medical diagnosis and management, determining risk of occurrence, options for addressing risk, reproductive decision making, and support services. A central task of genetic counseling is to help families cope with the presence of a disorder or its risk of occurrence, or both. With the development of medical genetics as a medical specialty, clinical genetics services have become part of the health care delivery system. As in all medical visits, evaluation of an individual or family for a potential genetic condition requires a thorough history and physical examination. Clinical genetic evaluations include physical examination, detailed family history, ancillary tests as needed, and communication of information to the family via letters and the distribution of published literature. Congenital defects are caused by altered morphogenesis. Congenital defects represent an important cause of infant mortality and morbidity. When evaluating a child with a congenital malformation, the most important determination is whether the abnormality represents a single, isolated anomaly or is instead one component of a broader, organized pattern of malformation (ie, a syndrome).

IMPORTANT TERMINOLOGY

desmorphology　畸形学
clinical genetics　临床遗传学
nondirectiveness　非指导性原则
Bayes theorem　拟概率定律
prior probability　前概率
conditional probability　条件概率
joint probability　联合概率
posterior probability　后概率
morphogenesis　形态发生
teratology　畸胎学
dysplasia　发育不良
deformation　变形过程
teratogen　致畸剂
eugenics　优生学

■ REVIEW QUESTIONS

1. Allen, a 40-year-old man, comes to your office because he is concerned about his family history of heart disease. His father had a fatal myocardial infarction (MI) at 45 years of age, and his paternal grandfather had a fatal MI at age 47 years. Allen's father had two brothers and two sisters. One of the brothers had an MI at age 44 years, and one of the sisters had an MI at age 49 years. Allen's mother had a brother and sister, both of whom are still alive. Allen's mother's parents both survived into their 80s and died of "natural causes." Draw a pedigree summarizing the information you have taken about Allen's family, and make a recommendation for further study and/or treatment.

2. Mary's two brothers and her mother's brother all had Duchenne muscular dystrophy (DMD) and are now dead. Based on only this information, what is the probability that Mary is a heterozygous carrier for this disorder? What is the probability that she will produce affected offspring? Suppose Mary has a serum creatine kinase (CK) test and is told that her level is above the 95th percentile for homozygous normal individuals. Approximately two thirds of DMD carriers have CK levels above the 95th percentile. Given this information, use Bayes theorem to calculate the probability that Mary is a carrier and the probability that she will produce affected offspring.

3. Bob's father had Huntington disease and is now deceased. Bob is now 51 years old and has no symptoms of Huntington disease. Age-of-onset curves show that approximately 85% of individuals with an affected father show symptoms by this age (the percentage is slightly lower, about 80%, if the mother is affected). Based on this information, use Bayes theorem to estimate the probability that Bob inherited the Huntington disease mutation from his father.

SUGGESTED READINGS AND WEBSITES

1. Aase J. Dysmorphologic diagnosis for the pediatric practitioner. *Pediatr Clin North Am.* 1992; 39: 135-156.

2. Allanson JE, Biesecker LG, Carey JC, Hennekam RC. Elements of morphology: introduction. *Am J of Med Genet A.* 2009; 149A: 2-5. (Introduction to issue that includes 6 articles on standardized definitions of morphologic terms).

3. Baty B, Biesecker B. Evidence-based genetic counseling. (Special issue on genetic counseling). *Am J Med Genet C Semin Med Genet.* 2007; 142C: 220.

4. Bennett RL, French KS, Resta RG, et al. Standardization of human pedigree nomenclature. *J Genet Couns.* 2008; 17: 424-433.

5. Boulet SL, Yang Q, Mai CL, et al. Trends in the postfortification prevalence of spina bifida and anencephaly in the United States. *Birth Defects Res A Clin Mol Teratol.* 2008; 82: 527-532.

6. Brent RL. The Bendectin saga: an American tragedy. *Teratology.* 1983; 27: 283-286.

7. Cassidy SB, Allanson JE. *Management of Genetic Syndromes.* 3rd ed. Hoboken, NJ: John Wiley; 2010.

8. Clarke A. Ethical and social issues in clinical genetics. In: Rimoin DL, Connor JM, Pyeritz RE, Korf BR, eds. *Emery and Rimoin's Principles and Practice of Medical Genetics*, Vol. 1. 4th ed. Philadelphia: Churchill Livingstone; 2002: 897-928.

9. Dent K, Carey JC. Breaking difficult news in the newborn setting: Down syndrome as a paradigm. *Am J Med Genet C Semin Med Genet.* 2006; 142C: 173-179.

10. Green RC, Berg JS, Grody WW, et al. ACMG Recommendations for reporting of incidental findings in clinical exome and genome sequencing. *Gen Med.* 2013; 15: 565-572.

11. Hennekam RCM, Allanson J, Krantz I. *Gorlin's Syndromes of the Head and Neck.* 5th ed. New York: Oxford University Press; 2009.

12. Hodge SE. A simple, unified approach to Bayesian risk calculations. *J Genet Couns.* 1998; 7: 235-261.

13. Hunter AG. Medical genetics: 2. The diagnostic approach to the child with dysmorphic signs. *CMAJ.* 2002; 167: 367-372.

14. Jones KL. *Smith's Recognizable Patterns of Human Malformation.* 7th ed. Philadelphia: WB Saunders; 2014.

15. Koren G. *Medication Safety in Pregnancy and Breast Feeding.* New York: McGraw-Hill; 2007.

16. Rudolph C, Rudolph A, Lister G, eds. *Rudolph's Pediatrics.* 22nd ed. New York: McGraw-Hill; 2009:774-779.

17. Nelson K, Holmes LB. Malformations due to presumed spontaneous mutations in newborn infants. *N Engl J Med.* 1989; 320: 19-23.

18. Rasmussen SJ, Friedman JM. Issues in teratology. *Am J Med Genet Part C Semin Med Genet.* 2011; 157: 147-152. (Entire issue or review articles on teratology.)

19. Walker AP. Genetic counseling. In: Rimoin DL, Connor JM, Pyeritz RE, Korf BR, eds. *Emery and Rimoin's Principles and Practice of Medical Genetics*, Vol. 1. 4th ed. New York: Churchill Livingstone; 2002: 842-874.

20. Elements of Morphology (definitions and exemplary figures of over 400 phenotypic variations): http://elementsofmorphology.nih.gov

21. Gene Reviews (current and comprehensive review of many genetic condition): http://www.genetests.org/resources/genereviews.php

22. Gene Tests (directory of genetic tests and laboratories performing them): http://www.genetests.org

23. Genetic Alliance (descriptions of genetic conditions, information on health insurance, and links to advocacy groups): http://www.geneticalliance.org/

24. Genetic and Rare Conditions Site (links to lay advocacy groups for a large number of genetic disorders): http://www.kumc.edu/gec/support/

25. Genetic Interest Group (alliance of organizations, with a membership of more than 120 charities that support children, families, and individuals affected by genetic disorders): http://www.gig.org.uk/

26. London Dysmorphology Database (computer-aided diagnosis of genetic disorders and other syndromes; paid subscription required): http://www.lmdatabases.com

27. National Institutes of Health Office of Rare Diseases (information on more than 6000 rare diseases): http://rarediseases.info.nih.gov/

28. Organization of Teratology Information Specialists (reviews of various exposures in pregnancy): http://www.otispregnancy.org

29. POSSUM (computer-aided diagnosis of genetic disorders and other syndromes; paid subscription required): http://www.possum.net.au/

(Jinbo Zhang, Sha Sha)